Lecture Notes in Computer Science   9184

Commenced Publication in 1973
Founding and Former Series Editors:
Gerhard Goos, Juris Hartmanis, and Jan van Leeuwen

More information about this series at http://www.springer.com/series/7409

Vincent G. Duffy (Ed.)

Digital Human Modeling

Applications in Health, Safety, Ergonomics and Risk Management: Human Modeling

6th International Conference, DHM 2015
Held as Part of HCI International 2015
Los Angeles, CA, USA, August 2–7, 2015
Proceedings, Part I

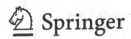 Springer

Editor
Vincent G. Duffy
Purdue University
School of Industrial Engineering
West Lafayette, IN
USA

ISSN 0302-9743   ISSN 1611-3349   (electronic)
Lecture Notes in Computer Science
ISBN 978-3-319-21072-8   ISBN 978-3-319-21073-5   (eBook)
DOI 10.1007/978-3-319-21073-5

Library of Congress Control Number: 2015942490

LNCS Sublibrary: SL3 – Information Systems and Applications, incl. Internet/Web, and HCI

Springer Cham Heidelberg New York Dordrecht London
© Springer International Publishing Switzerland 2015

Printed on acid-free paper

Springer International Publishing AG Switzerland is part of Springer Science+Business Media
(www.springer.com)

Foreword

The 17th International Conference on Human-Computer Interaction, HCI International 2015, was held in Los Angeles, CA, USA, during 2–7 August 2015. The event incorporated the 15 conferences/thematic areas listed on the following page.

A total of 4843 individuals from academia, research institutes, industry, and governmental agencies from 73 countries submitted contributions, and 1462 papers and 246 posters have been included in the proceedings. These papers address the latest research and development efforts and highlight the human aspects of design and use of computing systems. The papers thoroughly cover the entire field of Human-Computer Interaction, addressing major advances in knowledge and effective use of computers in a variety of application areas. The volumes constituting the full 28-volume set of the conference proceedings are listed on pages VII and VIII.

I would like to thank the Program Board Chairs and the members of the Program Boards of all thematic areas and affiliated conferences for their contribution to the highest scientific quality and the overall success of the HCI International 2015 conference.

This conference could not have been possible without the continuous and unwavering support and advice of the founder, Conference General Chair Emeritus and Conference Scientific Advisor, Prof. Gavriel Salvendy. For their outstanding efforts, I would like to express my appreciation to the Communications Chair and Editor of HCI International News, Dr. Abbas Moallem, and the Student Volunteer Chair, Prof. Kim-Phuong L. Vu. Finally, for their dedicated contribution towards the smooth organization of HCI International 2015, I would like to express my gratitude to Maria Pitsoulaki and George Paparoulis, General Chair Assistants.

May 2015

Constantine Stephanidis
General Chair, HCI International 2015

Foreword

HCI International 2015 Thematic Areas
and Affiliated Conferences

Thematic areas:

- Human-Computer Interaction (HCI 2015)
- Human Interface and the Management of Information (HIMI 2015)

Affiliated conferences:

- 12th International Conference on Engineering Psychology and Cognitive Ergonomics (EPCE 2015)
- 9th International Conference on Universal Access in Human-Computer Interaction (UAHCI 2015)
- 7th International Conference on Virtual, Augmented and Mixed Reality (VAMR 2015)
- 7th International Conference on Cross-Cultural Design (CCD 2015)
- 7th International Conference on Social Computing and Social Media (SCSM 2015)
- 9th International Conference on Augmented Cognition (AC 2015)
- 6th International Conference on Digital Human Modeling and Applications in Health, Safety, Ergonomics and Risk Management (DHM 2015)
- 4th International Conference on Design, User Experience and Usability (DUXU 2015)
- 3rd International Conference on Distributed, Ambient and Pervasive Interactions (DAPI 2015)
- 3rd International Conference on Human Aspects of Information Security, Privacy and Trust (HAS 2015)
- 2nd International Conference on HCI in Business (HCIB 2015)
- 2nd International Conference on Learning and Collaboration Technologies (LCT 2015)
- 1st International Conference on Human Aspects of IT for the Aged Population (ITAP 2015)

Conference Proceedings Volumes Full List

Digital Human Modeling and Applications in Health, Safety, Ergonomics and Risk Management

Program Board Chair: Vincent G. Duffy, USA

The full list with the Program Board Chairs and the members of the Program Boards of all thematic areas and affiliated conferences is available online at:

http://www.hci.international/2015/

HCI International 2016

The 18th International Conference on Human-Computer Interaction, HCI International 2016, will be held jointly with the affiliated conferences in Toronto, Canada, at the Westin Harbour Castle Hotel, 17–22 July 2016. It will cover a broad spectrum of themes related to Human-Computer Interaction, including theoretical issues, methods, tools, processes, and case studies in HCI design, as well as novel interaction techniques, interfaces, and applications. The proceedings will be published by Springer. More information will be available on the conference website: http://2016.hci.international/.

General Chair
Prof. Constantine Stephanidis
University of Crete and ICS-FORTH
Heraklion, Crete, Greece
Email: general_chair@hcii2016.org

http://2016.hci.international/

Contents – Part I

Modeling Human Work and Activities

Contents – Part II

Human Modeling in Medicine and Surgery

Quality in Healthcare

Modeling Human Skills
and Expertise

Comparison Knitting Skills Between Experts and Non-experts by Measurement of the Arm Movement

Kontawat Chottikampon[✉], Shunyu Tang, Suchalinee Mathurosemontri,
Porakoch Sirisuwan, Miyako Inoda, Hiroyuki Nishimoto, and Hiroyuki Hamada

Kyoto Institute of Technology, Matsugasaki, Sakyo-Ku, Kyoto, 606-8585, Japan
ruklongtime@hotmail.com

Abstract. This research focused on the developing the capacity of knitting skill. The comparison of skill between the experts with non-expert was study. The movement of arms was measure to investigate the effect of arm movement on quality of knitting fabric. The experiment was carried out on a video camera to record and analyze the differences of the knitting speed and manner in knitting. The quality of the fabric is measured by a loop of fabric to see the consistency of the loop fabric is important and beautiful fabrics. The result is a procedure used to crochet knitting machines are very different in appearance, knitting and speed. The quality of the fabric is beautiful, similar to the use of a knitting machine knitting. The main difference between them is only part of the seams.

Keywords: Knitting · Arm movement measurement · Knitting skill · Plain pattern

1 Introduction

The knitting is a process of manufacturing a fabric by inters looping of yarns. Knitting is the second most important method of fabric formation. It can be defined as a needle technique of fabric formation, in which, with the help of knitting needles, loops are formed to make a fabric or garment. Fabric can be formed by hand or machine knitting, but the basic principle remains.

A knitting machine is a device used to create knitted fabrics in a semi or fully automated fashion. There are numerous types of knitting machines, ranging from simple spool or board templates with no moving parts to highly complex mechanisms controlled by electronics. All, however, produce various types of knitted fabrics, usually either flat or tubular, and of varying degrees of complexity. Pattern stitches can be selected by hand manipulation of the needles, or with push-buttons and dials, mechanical punch cards, or electronic pattern reading devices and computers.

Manual knitting machines require the knitter to move the specific needles, based on a chart, into pattern position. In this research I study the knitting structure is plain and rib. Plain knit, the basic form of knitting can be produced in flat knit or in tubular (or circular) form. It is also called jersey stitch or balbriggan stitch. A row of latch or beard needles is arranged in a linear position on a needle plate or in a circular position on a cylinder. Rib stitch produces alternate lengthwise rows of plain and purl stitches and as

© Springer International Publishing Switzerland 2015
V.G. Duffy (Ed.): DHM 2015, Part I, LNCS 9184, pp. 3–13, 2015.
DOI: 10.1007/978-3-319-21073-5_1

such the face and back of the fabrics are a lookalike. Rib stitch can be produced on a flat rib machine as well as circular rib machine.

2 Experiment

In this research, the expert and non-expert were observed their arm moment during knitting process. Both of them fabricated the knitted products through the same knitting machine. Two types of yarns as cotton yarn and glass fiber yarn were selected to compare a knitted skill between the expert and non-expert. The knitted fabric was prepared, knitted and steaminess process following as show in Figs. 1, 2 and 3.

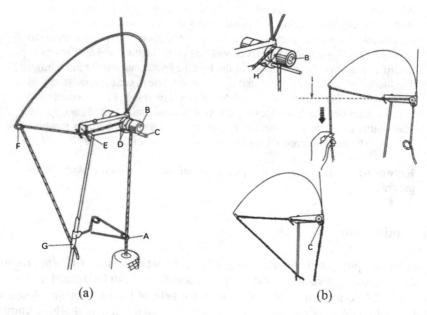

(a)   (b)

Fig. 1. The preparation of knitting process

2.1 Knitting Preparation

1. Through right tension guide eyelet "A".
2. Between tension dial "B" and guide bar "C".
3. Between two tension discs "D".
4. Through right yarn guide eyelet "E".
5. Through right tension spring eyelet "F".
6. Put the yarn end under tarn clip "G".

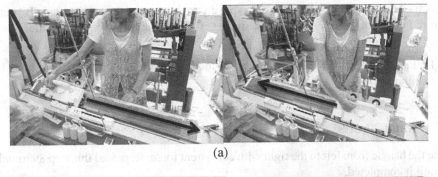

(a)

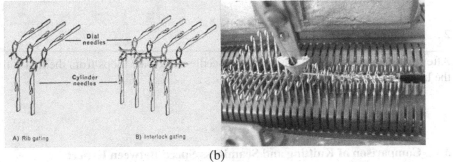

(b)

Fig. 2. Knitting process

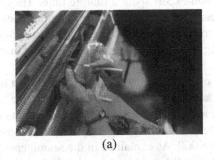

(a)

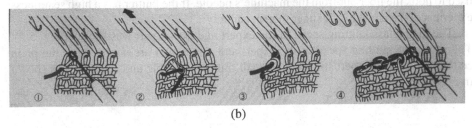

(b)

Fig. 3. Seaminess process

Adjust the tension dial according to type of yarn by turning the tension dial "B" until required number corresponds to the < shape "H" using the following as a guide

1. Yarn comes out freely from the yarn bell.
2. Distance between the tension spring and the horizontal line "I" 10~20 cm must be maintained.

2.2 Knitting Process

Slide the handle from left to the right with consistent force. Repeated this step 89 rounds or until it completed.

2.3 Seaminess Process

After that seam the fabric by inserting the needle and create loops from the first roll to the last.

3 Results and Discussion

3.1 Comparison of Knitting and Seaminess Speed Between Expert and Non-expert (Plain Cotton and Plain Glass)

Figure 4 indicate the plain cotton knitting speed of the expert and non-expert. For the knitting speed, the non-expert spent a longer time per one cycle when compared the expert's speed as shown in Fig. 4(a). There is show the unstable speed of non-expert. Some knitting cycle the non-expert spent a double time. Thus, the video was used to investigate this strangeness. It was pound that the main problem is the entanglement of fiber during process. Whereas the speed of the non-expert are quite constant. The expert shows the average knitting speed of 0.61 s/cycle that is faster than non-expert obviously as shown in Fig. 4(b).

The seaminess speed of expert and non-expert were shown in Fig. 4(c). The results of both knitters indicate an extremely deviation especially the result of non-expert. In Fig. 4(d) the average seaminess speed of the expert is clearly faster than the non-expert. In this process the seaminess skill of knitter is required. The cause of the lateness in this process is the needle usage skill. As explained in the seaminess method, the needle was used to hook the fiber out from the machine's needle. If the knitter has a high seaminess experience, she can hook the fiber loop accurately.

The plain glass knitting speed of the expert and non-expert was show in Fig. 5(a). The results of knitting speed of the expert and non-expert are similar with the plain cotton results. The expert still spent a small time for knitting and seaminess as shown in Fig. 5(b).

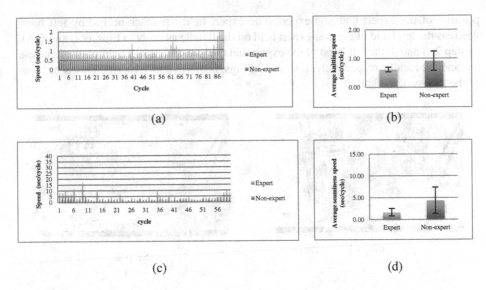

Fig. 4. Knitting and seaminess speed of plain cotton of the expert and non-expert

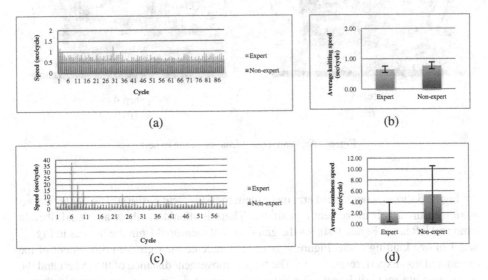

Fig. 5. Knitting and seaminess speed of plain glass fiber of the expert and non-expert

3.2   The Arm Movement Measurement of the Expert and Non-expert

The arm movement of the knitters was analyzed from four movement steps in one knitting cycle. The first different point before the knitters move the handle is the left hand position of the expert and non-expert. The expert held the machine bar by left hand whereas the left hand of the non-expert held on the handle as show in Figs. 6(a) and 7(a). In step 2, 3 and 4, the left hand of the expert and the non-expert still held on the machine bar and the handle, respectively as shown in Figs. 6(b)–(d) and 7(b)–(d). This is because of the fitness of the knitter.

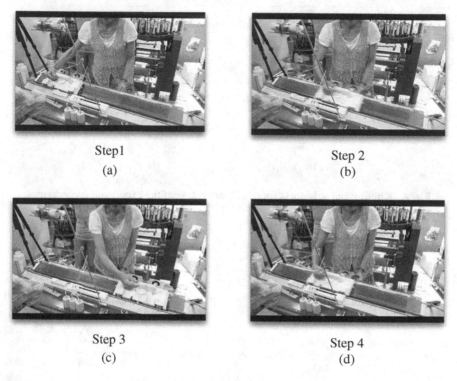

Step 1

(a)

Step 2

(b)

Step 3

(c)

Step 4

(d)

Fig. 6. Arm movement images of the expert

Figure 8 shows schematic of arm movement measurement position. The knitter's arms were measured their movement 6 positions. There is shoulder, elbow and hand of right hand and left hand. Figure 9 shows the gait data that measured from the images in Figs. 6 and 7 in one knitting cycle. Figure 9(a) and (c) indicate the right arm movement of the expert and non-expert, respectively. The handle movement distance of the expert and the non-expert are quite different. The handle movement distance of the expert is shorter than the non-expert. These results were supported by the image as shown in Figs. 6(c) and 7(c). The handle position of the non-expert in step 3 was held over the knitting bed groove whereas the expert stopped the handle at the knitting bed groove edge. It can say that the long handle movement distance impact on the knitting speed of the expert and non-expert. Figure 9(b) and (c) show the left arm movement of the expert and non-expert, respectively. As mentioned before, the left hand of the expert held on the machine bar. Therefore, there are no movement of the expert's hand and elbow. However, the shoulder

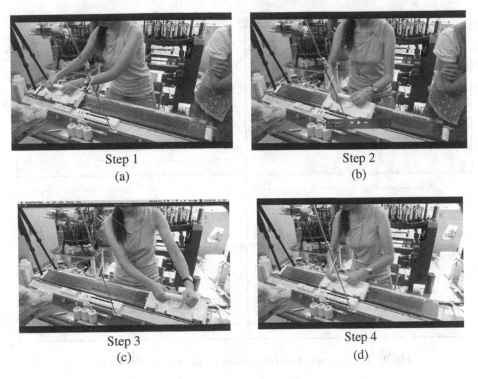

Step 1
(a)

Step 2
(b)

Step 3
(c)

Step 4
(d)

Fig. 7. Arm movement images of the non-expert

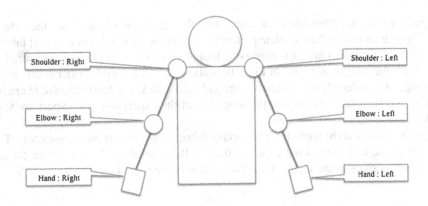

Shoulder : Right

Shoulder : Left

Elbow : Right

Elbow : Left

Hand : Right

Hand : Left

Fig. 8. Schematic of arm movement measurement position

of the expert shows a small movement. The non-expert arm movement shows the similar movement direction with the right arm.

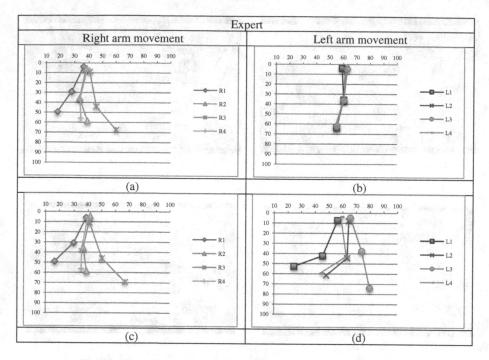

Fig. 9. The gait data of arm movement of the expert and non-expert

3.3 The Quality of Knitting Fabric

The pattern of plain cotton fabric was control by the knitting machine. Thus, the defects do not appear and show the complete pattern in both of the expert and non-expert fabrics as shown in Fig. 10(a) and (b). However, loop size of plain fabric was measured to investigate the quality of them. In Fig. 10(c) show the loop length distribution curve. The range of loop length of the expert is around 0.24 to 0.33 cm and 0.25 to 0.33 cm for the non-expert. It can be seen that the loop size of the expert and non-expert are very similar.

Figure 11(a) and (b) show the plain glass fabric of the expert and non-expert. The majority of the loop size of the expert is 0.24 to 0.28 cm and 0.23 to 0.29 cm for the non-expert as show in the loop length distribution curve (Fig. 11(c))

3.4 The Quality of Knitting Seam

Figure 12 shows the quality of the cotton seams of the expert and non-expert. Which can be seen that the seams of the expert do not reveal the defects. All of loop seams are beautiful and regular. The seaminess of the non-expert indicates the defects as a wide gap of loop. This is because of the accuracy of the non-expert skill. The seam

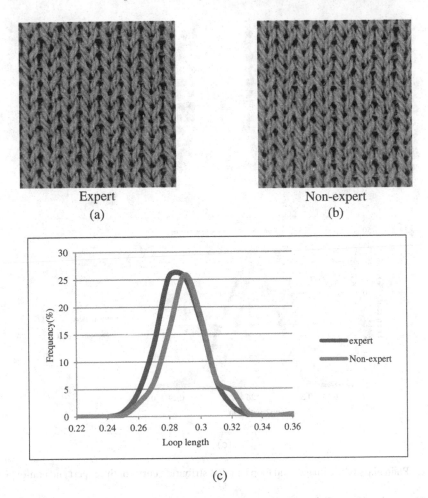

Expert   Non-expert
(a)   (b)

(c)

Fig. 10. Plain cotton fabric images and loop length distribution curve of the expert and non-expert.

photograph of the glass seam of the expert and non-expert are show in Fig. 13. The seaminess of both knitters do not show the desirable products. However, the non-expert seam appears many defects. Besides the human error that effected on the quality of seam, a sliding of glass fiber impacted on the difficulty of hooking by needle and tension of seam.

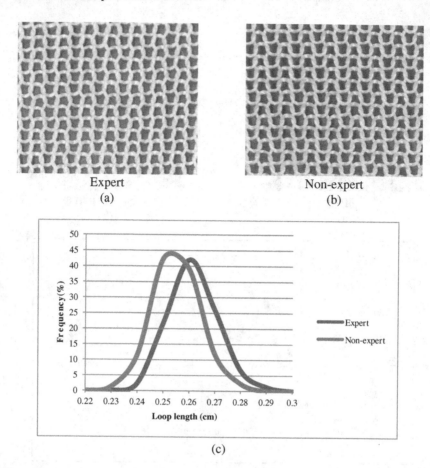

Expert
(a)

Non-expert
(b)

(c)

Fig. 11. Plain glass fabric images and loop length distribution curve of the expert and non-expert.

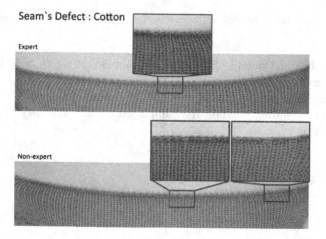

Fig. 12. The plain cotton seaminess images of the expert and non-expert

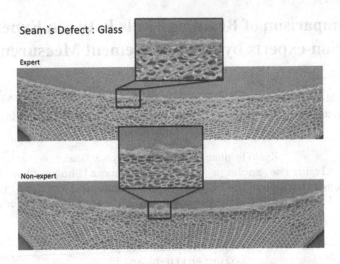

Fig. 13. The plain glass fiber seaminess images of the expert and non-expert

4 Conclusion

The plain knitting of cotton and glass fiber were studied in this research. The skill of knitters do not affect on the a quality of knitting fabric significantly. However, the seaminess process is required the skill of knitting. The expert show the high knitting and seaminess speed and a good fabric quality when compared with the non-expert.

References

1. Munden, D.L.: 26—The geometry and dimensional properties of plain-knit fabrics. J. Text. Inst. Trans. **50**(7), T448–T471 (1959)
2. Knapton, J.J.F., Munden, D.L.: A study of the mechanism of loop formation on weft-knitting machinery Part II: The effect of yarn friction on yam tensions in knitting and loop formation. Text. Res. J. **36**(12), 1081–1091 (1966)
3. Spencer, D.J.: Knitting technology: a comprehensive handbook and practical guide, vol. 16. CRC Press, Leicester (2001)
4. Lee, J.R., Ruppenicker, G.: Effects of processing variables on the properties of cotton knitting yarns. Text. Res. J. **48**(1), 27–31 (1978)

Comparison of Braiding Skills Between Expert and Non-experts by Eye's Movement Measurement

Kontawat Chottikampon[1(✉)], Suchalinee Mathurosemontri[1], Hitoshi Marui[1], Porakoch Sirisuwan[1], Akihiko Goto[2], Tadashi Uozumi[3], Miyako Inoda[1], Makiko Tada[1], Hiroyuki Nishimoto[1], and Hiroyuki Hamada[1]

[1] Kyoto Institute of Technology, Kyoto, Japan
{ruklongtime,zucha_k_t_89,p-sirisuwan}@hotmail.com
rugger.hitoshi@gmail.com, {Inoda,hhamada}@kit.ac.jp
makiko@texte.co.jp, hiroyuki.nishimoto@outlook.com
[2] Osaka Sangyo University, Daito, Japan
gotoh@ise.osaka-sandai.ac.jp
[3] Gifu University, Gifu, Japan
uozumi@gifu-u.ac.jp

Abstract. A braiding rope is the Japanese traditional rope that a quality and beauty of them have depended on the skill and experience of a braider. In this research, the skill of a expert and two non-experts who practice the braiding everyday and every week, respectively were measured and compared through the eye's movement measurement and observed the braiding rope quality. The measurement was carried out every month for three times. It was found that the expert show the constant of eye's focus at the center of marudai plate and reveled a complete pattern of braiding rope. For two non-experts, their eye's movement wobbled around marudai plate for all trials. However, the braiding speed and quality were developed by the regular training. There are no the defects in the ropes in the trial 2 and 3.

Keywords: Braiding · Kumihimo · Eye's movement measurement · Braiding skill

1 Introduction

Kumihimo is a traditional Japanese braiding technique that is used for making of long decorative rope. In that past, kimihimo is the important accessories for Japanese kimono and samurai armor. The styles and uses for the braids have changed over time. Nowadays, these braiding ropes are used in a variety of decorative ways. Some people wear them as bracelets or necklaces. In general silk was used as a braiding material due to its beauty and strength. However, many types of fiber can be used to braid kumihimo such as cotton floss or pearl cotton even metallic thread is used also. Because the beauty of the braid is accomplished by the color of threads. For the processing, the Japanese braiding technique is braided by specialized stands. The most common pattern of kumihimo is carried out on the

© Springer International Publishing Switzerland 2015
V.G. Duffy (Ed.): DHM 2015, Part I, LNCS 9184, pp. 14–23, 2015.
DOI: 10.1007/978-3-319-21073-5_2

marudai, which means round stand. The braiding is done on top of the marudai plate and the finished braid goes down the center of the plate. The sequence of moving the treads creates the shape. The initial placement of the colors will create a repeating pattern. The shape is usually round. However, there are many shapes that can created from the different specialized stand such as square shape, which is braided from kakudai or square stand.

In this research, the comparison of braiding skill between the expert and non-experts were carried out by using the common method as a marudai. In order to study the basic braiding skill, The braiding speed is the first parameter that was investigated in this experiment. The eye's movement measurement was selected to study and explain the concentration position of braider's eyes during the process. The braiding ropes were observed and measured the diameter to evaluate the quality of ropes.

2   Braiding Method

The cotton strands and marudai stand were prepared for braiding experiment. The first braiding step start by gathering all eight strands and tie a knot at one end (Fig. 1(a)). And then drop the knotted end into the center hole on the marudai (Fig. 1(b)). Next separate the strands out into four groups with two strands each and lay them over the marudai (Fig. 1(c)). After that reel strands around the bobbins tightly as shown in Fig. 1(d).

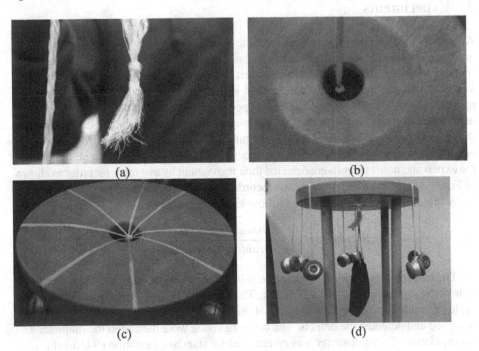

(a)　　　　(b)

(c)　　　　(d)

Fig. 1. Strand and marudai stand preparation

The braiding method is shown in Fig. 2. First step, start by moving the strand A across strand B and strand E across strand F. After that move strand C across strand D and strand G across strand H. Next the strands are braided anticlockwise. Start by moving the strand F across strand C and strand B across strand G. Finally move strand D across strand A and strand H across strand E. Continue the braiding from first step until finish.

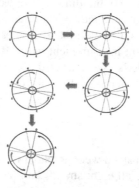

Fig. 2. Braiding method

3   Experiments

An expert and two non-experts were measured theirs braiding skill by eye's movement analysis. Before started the experiment, two non-experts studied a braided method from the expert. After braiding class, non-expert 1 practiced his braided skill everyday. Whereas non-expert 2 practice his braided skill only once time per week. For eye's movement analysis, the expert and non-experts were measured their eye's movement once time per month for 3 times. The first measurement was conducted on the first day that non-experts studied the braiding technique. The second and third times were conducted after 1 month and 2 month, respectively. During the experiment, the eyes of the expert and non-experts were detected their movement by eye mark recorder as shown in Fig. 3 and the braiding process was recorded by video camera.

A braiding speed was calculated follow Eq. (1) as show below.

$$Braiding\ speed = \frac{Braid\ length\ (cm)}{Braiding\ time\ (min)} \tag{1}$$

The braided rope position in the marudai hole during braiding process was measured to investigate the tension of each thread. Those positions were determined from each cycle of braiding process. Finally the final products of the expert and non-experts were observed and detected the defects. The braiding ropes were measured the diameter and the regularity of rope diameter was determined by standard deviation (S.D.) values.

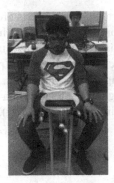

Fig. 3. Eye's movement experiment

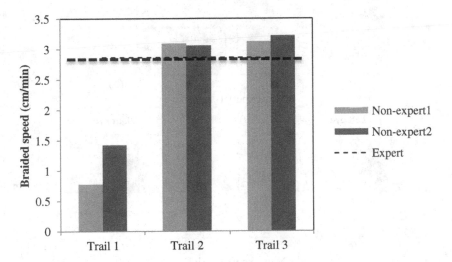

Fig. 4. Comparison of braiding speed between expert and non-experts

4   Results and Discussion

4.1   Comparison of Braiding Speed between the Expert and Non-experts

The braiding speed of expert and non-expert are compared as shown in Fig. 4. For the first braiding trial, the braiding speed of the expert show significantly higher speed than both non-expert samples. This is due to the difference of the experience and skill between expert and non-experts. However after non-expert samples have already understood the braiding process, the braiding speed in the second and third trials of non-expert samples obviously increase when compared with the first trial.

4.2   Eye's Movement Analysis of the Expert and Non-experts

The details of the different braiding skill between expert and non-expert are evaluated by the determination of eye`s movement during braiding. The comparison of the movement of eyes between expert and non-experts are shown in Figs. 5, 6 and 7. The origin point of the plot is based on the center of the hole of the marudai. The movement of eyes of expert mainly changes in the horizontal direction. In addition, during the braiding process an expert focused on the center position of the marudai plate as the eyes movement data clustering in the center area. In the case of non-expert, both non-expert samples show the higher scattering data and the vertical movement of eyes during the first trail of braiding process (Fig. 5).

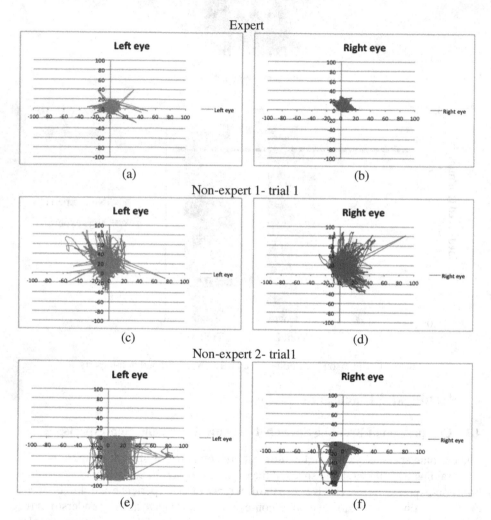

Fig. 5. Eye's movement direction of trial 1 (a) Expert – left eye, (b) Expert – right eye, (c) Non-expert 1 – left eye, (d) Non-expert 1 – right eye, (e) Non-expert 2 – left eye and (f) Non-expert 2 – right eye.

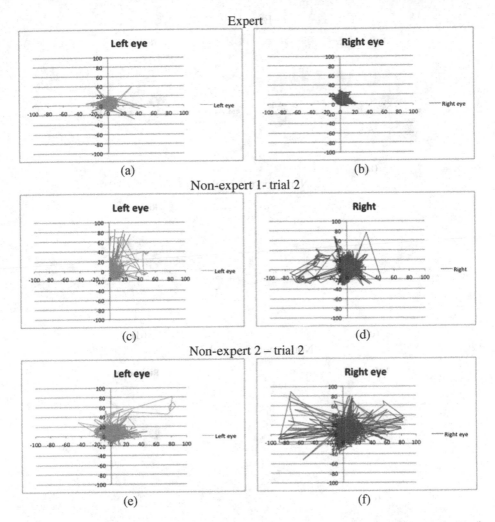

Fig. 6. Eye's movement direction of trial 2 (a) Expert – left eye, (b) Expert – right eye, (c) Non-expert 1 – left eye, (d) Non-expert 1 – right eye, (e) Non-expert 2 – left eye and (f) Non-expert 2 – right eye

After non-expert samples experienced the braiding technique, the eyes's movement in the second and third braiding trials changes from vertical movement to more horizontal direction as shown in Figs. 6 and 7. This is due to the non-expert samples' eyes are focused on the movement of the thread during braiding.

4.3 Braiding Rope Position

Figure 8(a)–(b) shows the position of the braided rope during braiding process. The position of the rope is directly influenced by the tension of each thread. The braided rope positions of an expert scatter around the center of the marudai while the non-experts

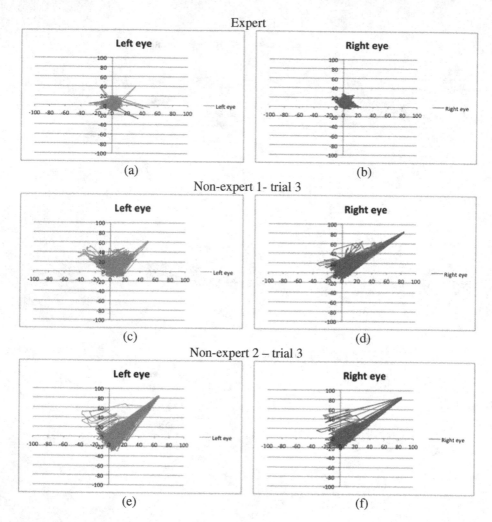

Fig. 7. Eye's movement direction of trial 3 (a) Expert – left eye, (b) Expert – right eye, (c) Non-expert 1 – left eye, (d) Non-expert 1 – right eye, (e) Non-expert 2 – left eye and (f) Non-expert 2 – right eye

show the unsymmetrical scattering of the rope positions. The unsymmetrical distribution of the rope position is caused by the instability of the tension of the thread during braiding process.

4.4 Comparison of Braiding Rope Quality

A quality and beauty of braiding rope of the expert and non-experts were observed. The photographs of braiding ropes were shown in Fig. 9. A braiding rope of the expert shows the complete braiding pattern along a rope. The quality of braiding ropes that were fabricated by non-expert at the first trial shows the defects due to the incorrect pattern.

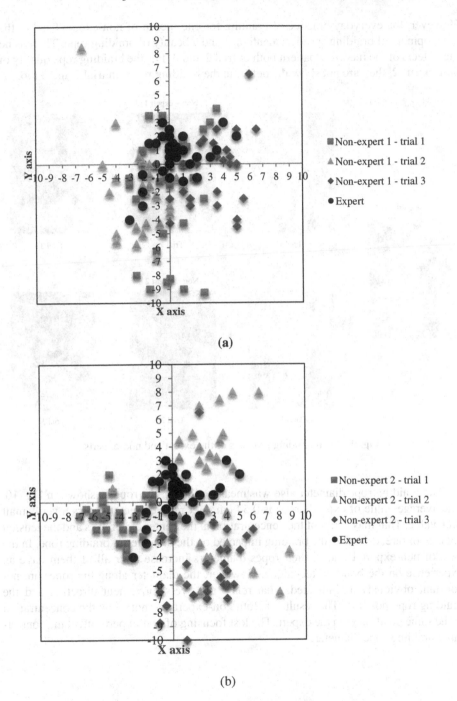

(a)

(b)

Fig. 8. Braiding rope position (a) Non-expert 1 and (b) Non-expert 2

However, the everyday practice of braiding for one month of non-expert 1 led to the development of braiding speed as mentioned and a beauty of braiding rope. There is no the defects of the incorrect pattern both of trial 2 and 3. For the braiding rope quality of non-expert 2, they are not show the defect in the braiding ropes in trial 2 and 3 too.

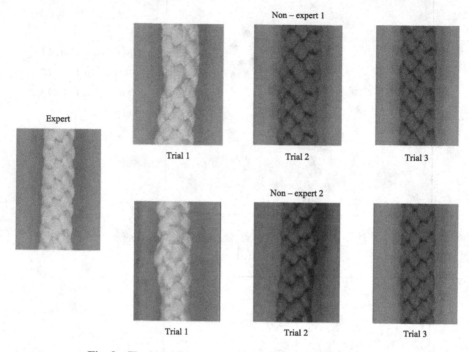

Fig. 9. Final braiding products of the expert and non-experts

The braiding rope diameter also was measured along the rope as shown in Fig. 10. The average value of expert's rope is 0.54 cm. Her rope diameter shows a very small S.D. value. That may cause of the concentration at the center of her eyes and the tension balance of threads during the braiding impacted on the diameter of braiding rope. In the case of non-expert 1 and 2, their ropes diameters increase after all of them have an experience on the braiding technique. However, the diameter along the ropes are not constant obviously as indicated. That relate the eye's movement direction and the braiding rope position. The results of Both non-experts do not show the concentration at the same position with the expert. The lost focusing of non-experts affect the controllable braiding rope diameter.

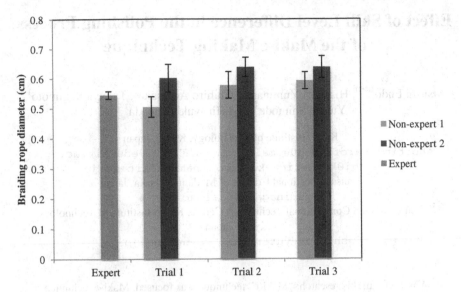

Fig. 10. Braiding rope diameter of the expert and non-experts

5 Conclusion

The expert shows the high performance and constant of braiding skill. Her eye's movement focused at the center of marudai plate that accorded with the braiding rope position. The expert can balance the rope tension during the braiding process well. Whereas the eye's movement of non-experts did not relate with the braiding rope position. However, the braiding experience of non-experts led to the increasing on their braiding speed and a quality of braiding ropes.

References

1. Catherine, M.: Kumihimo: Japanese silk braiding techniques. Old Hall, UK (1986)
2. Keijo, S.: Exquisite: the world of Japanese kumihimo braiding. Kodansha Amer Inc, New York (1988)
3. Dixon, A.: Introduction to Kumihimo (1995)

Effect of Skill Level Difference in the Polishing Process of the Maki-e Making Technique

Atsushi Endo[1(✉)], Hisanori Yuminaga[2], Chihiro Akatsuka[1], Takuya Sugimoto[1], Yutaro Shimode[3], and Hiroyuki Hamada[1]

[1] Kyoto Institute of Technology, Kyoto, Japan
shootingstarofhope30@gmail.com, d2851502@edu.kit.ac.jp,
t-sugi@koyo-kinzoku.com, hhamada@kit.ac.jp
[2] Kansai Vocational College of Medicine, Osaka, Japan
yuminaga@kansai.ac.jp
[3] Future-Applied Conventional Technology Centre, Kyoto Institute of Technology,
Kyoto, Japan
shimode-yutaro@xa2.so-net.ne.jp

Abstract. In this research, "Maki-e" technique was focused. Maki-e technique is a decoration technique of Urushi crafts technique. There is a polishing process in the Maki-e making process. Maki-e surface is polished by a charcoal and whetstone in the polishing process. Time-served technique is needed for this process. Because this process affects a finish of Urushi crafts work, this research aimed to clarify a relationship between a skill level difference of craftspeople and a finish of Urushi crafts work in the polishing process by using charcoal. Characteristics of the finish Urushi crafts work and how to use a body of craftspeople was analyzed. As the results of this research, it was confirmed that; 1. The expert's Maki-e specimen was more brightness and yellow than the non-expert. 2. There was not much difference about the gloss and surface roughness between the expert and the non-expert. 3. The expert took the rhythmic activity in each muscle. Therefore it seemed that the finish of the work became more beautiful. These results suggest that how to use the body affects the finish of the Urushi crafts work in the polishing process. The non-expert can improve the finish of the work and the level of polishing skill by training the body position and motion like the expert.

Keywords: Urushi crafts · Maki-e · Polishing · Color · Gloss · Surface roughness · Electromyogram

1 Introduction

There are many traditional crafts in Japan. Urushi crafts is one of the Japanese traditional crafts. In the past, it was very famous in the world, Urushi resin and Urushi crafts work was called "japan". It was exported to the European countries by the East India Company et al. in the Age of Discovery about 400 years ago. As a result, Urushi crafts work collection was made by the royalty and the aristocracy. After Age of Discovery, Japan closed the country to foreign commerce, but Urushi crafts work continued to be exported to foreign countries

© Springer International Publishing Switzerland 2015
V.G. Duffy (Ed.): DHM 2015, Part I, LNCS 9184, pp. 24–34, 2015.
DOI: 10.1007/978-3-319-21073-5_3

through Netherlands, England, China et al. In the modern age, Urushi crafts work was focused once again because of the Japonisme and exhibition of the World Exposition. However Urushi crafts work is not used now because a synthetic resin and substitute material was developed. In this current situation, Urushi crafts work was collected and exhibited as an art or cultural property by the domestic and overseas museum and art museum.

To this day, Urushi crafts technique is needed to make a new work and repair or restore the old work now. This technique was kept by craftspeople. Craftspeople technique has much wisdom and knowledge called a knack and hunch. They are called the "implicit knowledge", and it takes a long time to understand and master them. Therefore, year of ascetic training for craftspeople is too long. And then researchers have turned implicit knowledge into explicit knowledge, they invent a new method of manufacturing base on it, and apply it to short-time ascetic training [1–4].

In this research, "Maki-e" technique was focused. Maki-e technique is a decoration technique of Urushi crafts technique. After painting an Urushi resin on the surface of base body, rough design is drawn by the mixture of raw Urushi and Bengal red powder. After that a metallic powder is sprinkled on the rough design. There is a polishing process in the Maki-e making process. Maki-e surface is polished by a charcoal and whetstone in the polishing process. Time-served technique is needed for this process. Because this process affects a finish of Urushi crafts work, this research aimed to clarify a relationship between a skill level difference of craftspeople and a finish of Urushi crafts work in the polishing process by using charcoal. Characteristics of the finish Urushi crafts work and how to use a body of craftspeople was analyzed. In the previous researches, physical property and polishing performance of the charcoal for polishing was analyzed [5], the body movement of polishing process was not analyzed yet. On the other hand, the difference of muscle activity of expert and non-expert's finger was pointed out in the sprinkling metallic powder process [6]. The relationship between a grip force of expert craftspeople and a surface roughness of industrial component was analyzed in the polishing process of the manufacturing industry [7]. As these results, this research is effective to making a high quality Urushi crafts work and training non-expert Urushi craftspeople.

2   Measurement

2.1   Subject

There were two subjects in this research. One was an expert Urushi craftspeople, the other was a non-expert Urushi craftspeople. They had engaged in the making Maki-e especially. Expert was a right-handed male, his age was 59 years old, and his year of experience was 41 years and 8 months. Non-expert was a right-handed female, her age was 25 years old, and her year of experience was 5 years and 8 months. They polished a sample which was sprinkled metallic powder and coated by Urushi as usual.

2.2   Maki-e Specimen

Figure 1 showed a Maki-e specimen. Left image is the specimen before polishing, right image is the specimen after polishing. Size of specimen was 100 mm × 100 mm × 5 mm.

Its base was PMMA (Polymethylmethacrylate) board. Its board was polished by a sand paper, rubbed with raw Urushi. After that, black Urushi (Kuro-Roiro-Urushi, made by Shikata Yoshizo Urushi Ten) was painted on the surface of the PMMA board in twice. After hardening the black Urushi, the surface was polished by the charcoal, and rubbed with Uwazuri Urushi (Reddish clear Urushi). After that, rough design was drawn by the bengal red Urushi (E-Urushi) and gold round powder (Maru-fun, No.8, made by Asano Shoten) was sprinkled on the rough design. One large center circle and eight small circles around center circle were designed. Its design was called "Kuyo-mon" in Japan. After hardening the bengal red Urushi, sprinkled gold powder was coated by yellowish clear Urushi (Nashiji Urushi) in twice for keeping the powder on a surface of Urushi painting. Lastly black Urushi was painted on the surface of specimen in twice.

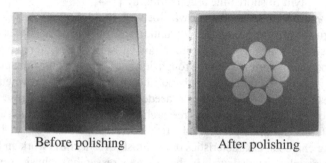

Before polishing   After polishing

Fig. 1. Maki-e specimen

2.3 Colorimetry

Colorimetric value was measured by the Spectrophotometer CM-700d (made by KONICA MINOLTA, INC.). Light source was D65. A field of view was 2 degree. Measurement diameter was 3 mm. Figure 2 showed a measurement point. L*, a* and b* values of five points were measured. This device measured by the integrating sphere, the data including a specular light data was analyzed.

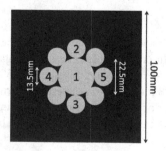

Fig. 2. Measurement points of color measurement

2.4 Gloss

Gloss value was measured by the Gloss Checker IG-331 (made by HORIBA, Ltd.). Because a surface of Urushi crafts work was high glossy, the specimen was measured with an incident and receiving angle: 20 degree. This measurement angle was convenient for measuring a high glossy subject. Light source was LED, and its wavelength was 890 nm. Measurement range was a shape of an ellipse, its major axis was 4 mm, and minor axis was 3 mm. Measurement point was the center of large circle, it was measured five times.

2.5 Surface Roughness

Surface roughness was measured by the Dektak XT (made by Bruker Corporation). Scan mode was Standard Scan, vertical measurement rage was 65.5 μm, measurement distance was 2 mm, measurement time was 10 s. Center of center large circle was measured in twice, and center of one of the small circles was measured one time. Data was analyzed by the IGOR Pro Version 6.3.4.1 (made by WaveMetrics, Inc.), and the root mean square surface roughness was calculated.

2.6 Electromyogram

Electromyogram was measured by the EMG multi-channel telemeter system WEB-1000 (made by NIHON KOHDEN CORPORATION) in the polishing process with the charcoal. Figure 3 showed the measurement muscles. Triceps brachii muscle, biceps brachii muscle, extensor muscles of the forearm, flexor muscles of the forearm, deltoid muscle, cowl muscle, pectoralis major muscle and interosseus muscle of the right arm and hand were measured in order to know the muscle activities when the subject polished a specimen with grasping the charcoal. Sampling rate was 1000 Hz. After measurement, a waveform of electromyogram was observed and compared with the movie. A difference, continuousness and pattern were analyzed. In addition, EMG of muscle activity was commuted, an average of 10 muscle activities was calculated, and was smoothed in the early, middle, final phase.

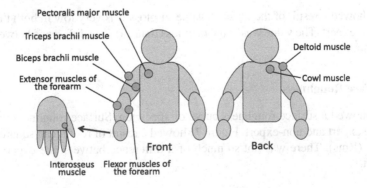

Fig. 3. Measurement muscles

3 Result

3.1 Colorimetry

Figure 4 showed a result of the colorimetry. L* value of the expert was higher than the non-expert. Specimen of expert was brighter than the non-expert. a* value of the expert was lower than the non-expert, and b* value of the expert was higher than the non-expert. Specimen of expert was more yellow than the non-expert. Specimen of the non-expert was more red than the expert.

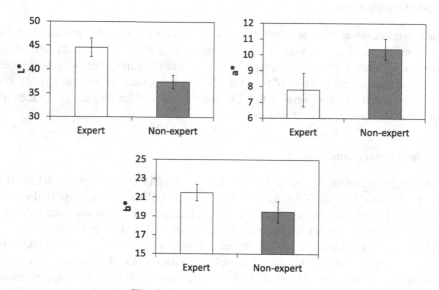

Fig. 4. Result of color measurement

3.2 Gloss

Figure 5 showed a result of the gloss. A value of gloss was very low in both the expert and the non-expert. The value was equal to or less than 1.0. The difference between them was very small.

3.3 Surface Roughness

Figure 6 showed a surface roughness curve of specimen. Surface roughness was large in both the expert and non-expert. Figure 7 showed a result of root mean square surface roughness (Rms). There was not so much of a difference between the expert and the non-expert.

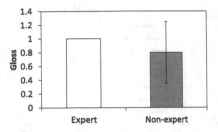

Fig. 5. Result of gloss measurement

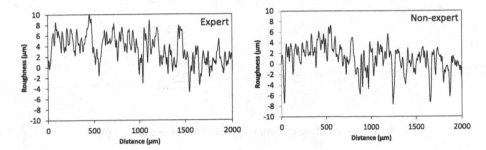

Fig. 6. Surface roughness curve

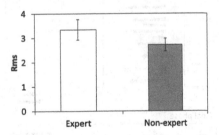

Fig. 7. Result of root mean square surface roughness

3.4 Electromyogram

Figure 8 showed the waveform of the electromyogram of the expert in each phase. Figure 9 showed the waveform of the electromyogram of the non-expert in each phase. Figure 10 showed the smoothed waveform of each muscle in the expert. Figure 11 showed the smoothed waveform of each muscle in the expert.

In the case of the expert, muscle activities except for the extensor muscles of the forearm were rhythmical in each phase. The biceps brachii muscle, flexor muscles of the forearm and interosseus muscle acted almost at the same time. Triceps brachii muscle, extensor muscles of the forearm, deltoid muscle, cowl muscle and pectoralis major muscle acted almost at the same time. It was clarified that the muscles acted and relaxed repeatedly from the complementarity of muscle. This was an alternate action of an antagonistic muscle.

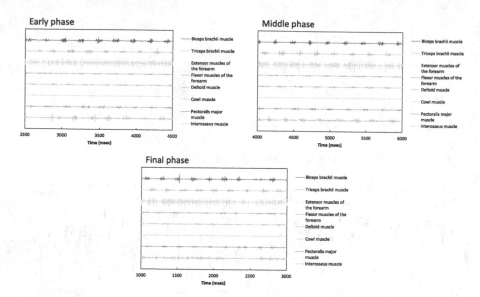

Fig. 8. Waveform of the electromyogram of the expert in each phase

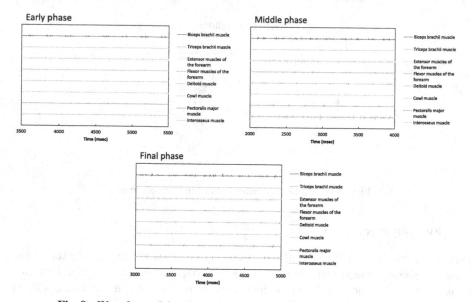

Fig. 9. Waveform of the electromyogram of the non-expert in each phase

As the results of smoothing waveform, there was so much of a difference among all phases. Constant muscle activities were shown in the polishing process. The biceps brachii muscle, triceps brachii muscle, extensor muscles of the forearm and interosseus muscle showed a high level of activities, flexor muscles of the forearm, deltoid muscle and cowl muscle showed a low level of activities. The pectoralis major muscle showed a middle level of activities. The smoothed waveforms of the biceps brachii muscle,

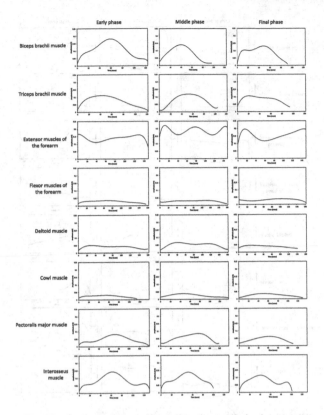

Fig. 10. Smoothed waveform of each muscle in the expert

triceps brachii muscle, pectoralis major muscle and interosseus muscle were shaped a chevron activities. The extensor muscles of the forearm showed a high level of sustained activity, and the flexor muscles of the forearm, deltoid muscle and cowl muscle showed a low level of sustained activities. The biceps brachii muscle, triceps brachii muscle, pectoralis major muscle and interosseus muscle showed high activities, and the extensor muscles of the forearm, deltoid muscle and cowl muscle showed low activities.

Muscles of the non-expert did not show the rhythmic activities. They showed the sustained arrhythmic activities. Muscle activity was increased in the second half of the polishing process. Especially, the activities of the biceps brachii muscle, extensor muscles of the forearm, pectoralis major muscle and interosseus muscle were increased in the final phase. On the other hand, the activities of the triceps brachii muscle and flexor muscles of the forearm were low. The activity of the deltoid muscle was increased from the middle phase, and it was high activity in the final phase. As the results of the smoothed waveforms, the muscle activity of non-expert was not constant like the expert.

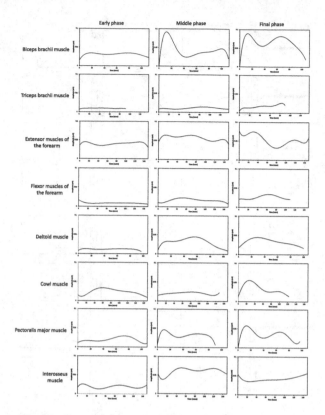

Fig. 11. Smoothed waveform of each muscle in the expert

4 Discussion

The specimen surface of the expert was more brightness than the one of the non-expert after polishing with the charcoal. There was not so much of a difference of gloss between the expert and the non-expert. Because the surface roughness was almost the same between the expert and the non-expert, an asperity of the specimen was not so much of difference. Therefore, the difference of gloss did not occur between the expert and the non-expert. As the result of the colorimetry, b* value of the expert was higher than the non-expert. Expert's specimen was more yellow than the non-expert. a* value of the expert was lower than the non-expert. Expert's specimen was less red than the non-expert. On the basis of these results, because the expert can polish the surface of Maki-e completely in the polishing process, the gold powder was seen on the Maki-e surface better than the non-expert. And then the expert specimen became more yellow. In addition to a scattering light from the asperity of the surface, the strong yellow derived from the gold powder was one of the factors that the specimen of the expert was more brightness than the non-expert.

As the result of the electromyogram, the muscles acted and relaxed repeatedly in the case of the expert because of the alternate action of an antagonistic muscle. Therefore the expert does not increase the muscle activity, and he can polish the surface of the specimen without a muscle fatigue. It is good that we get physical activity with relaxed shoulder in any work. It seemed that the expert polished the specimen without the increased muscle activity in overall trend. The activities of the biceps brachii muscle, triceps brachii muscle, pectoralis major muscle and interosseus muscle were high. It is assumed that they were needed for the rhythmic activity of muscle in the polishing process. Most efficient muscle activity pattern was shown because other muscle activities were low, the shoulder was relaxed and the back muscle of the forearm was not often needed to grasp the object. In order to keep the motion stable for a long time, it is needed that the muscle activity is not increased, a laxity time is set for muscle, the oxygen is provided to the muscle and the forming an adenosine triphosphate (ATP) promoted. From a viewpoint of the physiological mechanism, it assumed that the muscle activity pattern of the expert is very efficient. This rhythmic muscle activity pattern is the greatest characteristic of the expert.

It seemed that the non-expert felt a muscle fatigue because muscle activity was needed in the final phase. An inefficiency of the action was shown in the case of the non-expert. The non-expert raised her upper limb and shoulder strongly. The opposite activity of the forearm muscle was shown between the expert and the non-expert. It seemed that the expert polished the specimen while a functional limbs of MP flexed position and IP extended position were kept in the palmarflexion. Non-expert used the outer muscle excessively while he took a tenodesis action with the wrist dorsiflexion. Therefor it seemed that the expert grasped the charcoal with each finger pad, the non-expert flexed the interpharangeal joint. The non-expert became difficult to polish the specimen rhythmical, and the muscle activity became arrhythmic. Muscle activity was too much inefficient in comparison with the expert. The non-expert polished the specimen while the shoulder blade was elevated by the action of the cowl muscle, the shoulder joint was turned outward by the action of the deltoid muscle, the elbow joint was inflected by the overactivity of the biceps brachii muscle and the wrist was dorsiflexed excessively. It seemed that the non-expert polished the specimen without extending the elbow joint because the triceps brachii muscle was the extensor muscle of the elbow joint. This was the reason that the activities of the triceps brachii muscle and flexor muscles of the forearm were low. It seemed that the activity of the flexor muscles of the forearm for the wrist palmar flexion was low because the wrist was dorsiflexed, and the outer muscle was performed in order to grasp the object.

It was found that the finish of the surface of Maki-e is made beautiful in the case of the expert because the rhythmic action does not cause the muscle fatigue, and the expert can polish the specimen by the constant force of the muscle.

5 Conclusion

As the results of this research, it was confirmed that;

- The expert's Maki-e specimen was more brightness and yellow than the non-expert.
- There was not much difference about the gloss and surface roughness between the expert and the non-expert.

- The expert took the rhythmic activity in each muscle. Therefore it seemed that the finish of the work became more beautiful.

These results suggest that how to use the body affects the finish of the Urushi crafts work in the polishing process. The non-expert can improve the finish of the work and the level of polishing skill by training the body position and motion like the expert.

References

1. Oka, Y., Goto, A., Takai, Y., Narita, C., Hamada, H.: Motion analysis of the pounding technique used for the second lining in the fabrication of traditional japanese hanging scrolls. In: Duffy, V.G. (ed.) DHM 2014. LNCS, vol. 8529, pp. 55–65. Springer, Heidelberg (2014)
2. Furukawa, T., Takai, Y., Goto, A., Kuwahara, N., Kida, N.: Evaluation of Kyo-Yuzen-Zome fabrics with different pastes. In: Duffy, V.G. (ed.) DHM 2014. LNCS, vol. 8529, pp. 224–235. Springer, Heidelberg (2014)
3. Goto, A., Yoshida, H., Takai, Y., Zelong, W., Sato, H.: Application of E-learning system reality in Kyoto-style earthen wall training. In: Duffy, V.G. (ed.) DHM 2014. LNCS, vol. 8529, pp. 247–253. Springer, Heidelberg (2014)
4. Yamada, K., Ohgiri, M., Furukawa, T., Yuminaga, H., Goto, A., Kida, N., Hamada, H.: Visual behavior in a Japanese drum performance of *Gion* festival music. In: Duffy, V.G. (ed.) DHM 2014. LNCS, vol. 8529, pp. 301–310. Springer, Heidelberg (2014)
5. Arima, T., Maruyama, N., Hayamura, S., Okazaki, H.: Phisical properties of abrasive charcoal for Japan lacquer ware and performance in sanding. J. Soc. Mater. Sci. 37(416), 549–554 (1988)
6. Shimode, Y., Narita, C., Endo, A., Kondo, K., Yuminaga, H.: Study of fun-maki motion with surface electromygraphy. In: Proceedings of 13th Japan International SAMPE Symposium and Exhibition (JISSE-2013), Paper ID 2417, pp. 1-6 (2013)
7. Sugimoto, T., Takai, Y., Yuminaga, H., Goto, A., Hamada, H.: Analysis of expert skills in the grinding process for metallographic samples by means of monitoring finger force. J. Sci. Labour 89(6), 213–217 (2013)

Study on Method of Observing Maki-e Crafts Work in Urushi Craftspeople

Atsushi Endo[1(✉)], Noriyuki Kida[1], Yutaro Shimode[2], Isao Oda[3], Yuka Takai[4], Akihiko Goto[4], and Hiroyuki Hamada[1]

[1] Kyoto Institute of Technology, Kyoto, Japan
shootingstarofhope30@gmail.com,
{kida,hhamada}@kit.ac.jp
[2] Future-Applied Conventional Technology Centre, Kyoto Institute of Technology, Kyoto, Japan
shimode-yutaro@xa2.so-net.ne.jp
[3] Kisarazu National College of Technology, Kisarazu, Japan
oda@maple.m.kisarazu.ac.jp
[4] Osaka Sangyo University, Daito, Japan
{takai,gotoh}@ise.osaka-sandai.ac.jp

Abstract. Urushi crafts is a representative traditional crafts in Japan. Good Urushi crafts work had made in various periods in history in Japan, and it has been kept by the policymaker, shrine, temple and a person on the street. Urushi crafts work is damaged and Urushi comes off over a course of a long period of time. Urushi craftspeople need to identify the characteristics and conditions of the work when it is repaired because they can't repair the work appropriately. When the craftspeople identify the characteristics and conditions of the work, they observe the work by the naked eye. This observation technique is called "Mitate". This research aimed to know difference of a motion of the Urushi crafts work between the expert Urushi craftspeople and the non-expert Urushi craftspeople when they conduct the Mitate. The motion of the specimen and subject's head were measured when the expert and non-expert Urushi craftspeople conducted the Mitate of the Maki-e specimen. As the results, it is found that the expert can identify the change in appearance of Maki-e surface by moving the specimen up and down a little. Furthermore, he can skip the up-and-down motion and shorten the observation time by comparing one specimen with the other specimen in the case of the different number of the gold powder.

Keywords: Urushi crafts · Maki-e · Mitate · Expert · Non-expert · Motion analysis

1 Introduction

There are various traditional crafts in the world. For example, the pottery art and metal work exist in the various countries, their works and products are made in an original way based on the culture. There are many traditional crafts in the same way. Urushi crafts is a representative traditional crafts in Japan. When an alternate current between

© Springer International Publishing Switzerland 2015
V.G. Duffy (Ed.): DHM 2015, Part I, LNCS 9184, pp. 35–45, 2015.
DOI: 10.1007/978-3-319-21073-5_4

East and West had started in the Age of Discovery, the porcelain had been called "china". It was the representative traditional crafts in China. On the other hand, a lacquer ware had been called "japan". "Urushi" is a resin from Japanese lacquer tree. It has been used as a paint, artists' paint and adhesive material in Japan, China, Korea and South-East Asian countries. In the Urushi crafts, a wooden basis is made from various woods, and it was painted by Urushi resin several times. As necessary, it is decorated by a metallic powder in Japan. It is called "Maki-e". Urushi crafts work had been preferred in Europe because of its beauty and quality, the royalty and the aristocracy collected the Urushi crafts work. Many of them have been passed down as an art object in Europe now. Good Urushi crafts work had made in various periods in history in Japan, and it has been kept by the policymaker, shrine, temple and a person on the street.

Urushi crafts work is damaged and Urushi comes off over a course of a long period of time. But Urushi craft work can be repaired, and Urushi resin can be painted once again. Therefore Urushi craftspeople learn how to make and repair the Urushi crafts work. There are many Urushi crafts works in the museum and art museum. Many persons on the street keep them. These works has been repaired repeatedly by Urushi craftspeople. Urushi craftspeople need to identify the characteristics and conditions of the work when it is repaired because they can't repair the work appropriately. When the craftspeople identify the characteristics and conditions of the work, they observe the work by the naked eye. This observation technique is called "Mitate". Expert Urushi craftspeople can identify the many characteristics from the work, and use it to repair the work by conducting Mitate. It was shown that the expert Urushi craftspeople jiggle the work up and down when they conduct the Mitate in the previous research [1–3]. It seems that they can identify the characteristics by observing the change in appearance of the surface of the work with jiggling it up and down. This research aimed to know difference of a motion of the Urushi crafts work between the expert Urushi craftspeople and the non-expert Urushi craftspeople when they conduct the Mitate.

2   Measurement

2.1   Subject

There were two Urushi craftspeople as a subject in this research. They specialized on the Maki-e technique. Subject A was 59 years old, male and his year of experience was 41 years and 10 months. Subject B was 25 years old, female and her year of experience was 3 years and 10 months. Subject A was regarded as an expert because he had a high level of Meki-e technique and had many disciples. Subject B was regarded as a non-expert because she was the craftspeople under training.

2.2   Maki-e Specimen

Figure 1 showed a Maki-e specimen. Expert (Male, 58 years old, 39 years of experience) made these specimens. Size of specimen was 70 mm × 70 mm × 5 mm. Its base was PMMA (Polymethylmethacrylate) board. Its board was polished by a sand paper, rubbed with raw Urushi. After that, black Urushi (Kuro-Roiro-Urushi, made by Shikata Yoshizo Urushi

Ten) was painted on the surface of the PMMA board in twice. After hardening the black Urushi, the surface was polished by the charcoal, and rubbed with Uwazuri Urushi (Reddish clear Urushi). After that, rough design was drawn by the bengal red Urushi (E-Urushi) and gold round powder was sprinkled on the rough design. This decoration method was called "Maki-e". Maru-fun (Round shape powder, made by Asano Shoten) was used in these specimens. As the number of Maru-fun was more increased, the size of powder was bigger. The type of metal was gold, and its number was 2, 6, 8 and 14 in this research. These powders were sprinkled on the 40 mm diameter round shape.

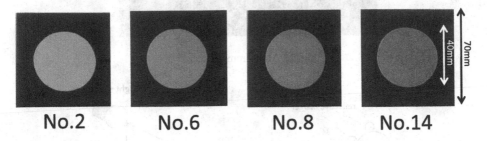

Fig. 1. Maki-e specimen

2.3 Condition of Mitate

Figure 2 showed a measurement scene. Figure 3 showed a measurement position. The light of measurement room was turned out. One light source was set in front of the subject. The light source was the TOSHIBA NEOBALL Z ReaL (EFA10EN/8-E17-S, made by TOSHIBA LIGHTING & TECHNOLOGY CORPORATION). The color was neutral white. The angle between the light source and the vertical line of specimen was 60 degrees. The distance between the light source and floor was 2000 mm. Figure 4 showed the specimen position on the frame. Four specimens were set in a straight line on the frame fixed in the tripod. The specimens were arranged in order of No.6, No.2, No.8 and No.14 from left side. The illuminance at the specimen was 768 lx (measured by Digital Lux Meter 51001 made by Yokogawa Meters & Instruments Corporation). The distance between the specimen and floor was 960 mm, and the distance between the specimen and the light source was 2420 mm. Firstly the subject sat on a chair, the angle between a subject eye and the vertical line of specimen was 60 degrees. The frame on the tripod could be made a 360-degree turn by the subject. When the subject observed each sample, they were directed to set their eye, specimen and the light source in a straight line. Observing time for each specimen was not restricted. The subject could move the specimen free. When the observation of each specimen was finished, the subject was directed to arrange them in order of the number of gold powder.

2.4 Motion Analysis

A motion of the subject and specimen was measured by the MAC3D System (made by Motion Analysis Corporation). Infrared rays were emitted by the infrared camera.

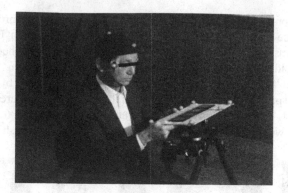

Fig. 2. Measurement scene

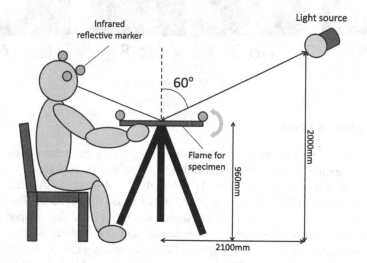

Fig. 3. Measurement position

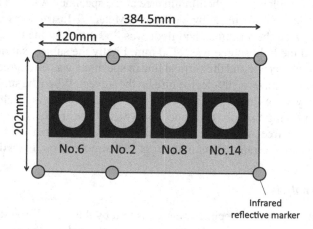

Fig. 4. Specimen position on the frame

The rays were reflected on the infrared reflective marker which set on the object, the motion of the marker was caught by the camera. The position of the marker was showed as a coordinate in the three-dimensional space. Figure 5 showed the position of the infrared camera. Four infrared cameras were set around the subject and specimen. Figure 6 showed the positon of the infrared reflective marker. There were 10 markers on the head top and, head right, head left, head front and edge of frame. The markers of head right and frame 2 were analyzed in order to know the vertical motion of the subject eye and specimen in this research.

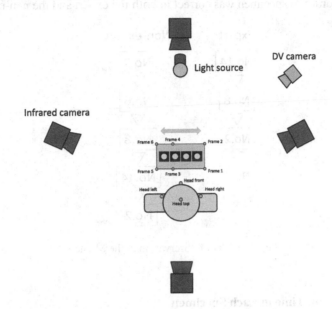

Fig. 5. Infrared camera position

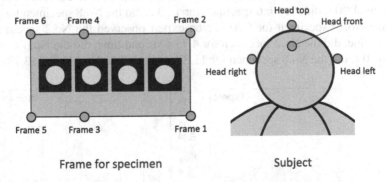

Fig. 6. Infrared reflective marker position

3 Result

3.1 Order of Observation and Arranged Order of Specimen

Figure 7 showed the observation order in each subject. Expert observed the specimen in order of No.14, No.8, No.2 and No.6 from right side of the frame. Non-expert observed the specimen in order of No.2, No.6, No.8 and No.14, and lastly observed the No.2 once again.

Arranged order of specimen was correct in both the expert and the non-expert.

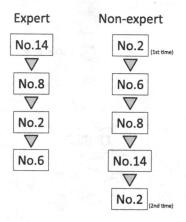

Fig. 7. Order of observation in the Mitate

3.2 Observation Time in Each Specimen

Figure 8 showed the observation time in each subject. Expert observed the No.2 specimen for 1.20 s, did the No.6 specimen for 1.23 s, did the No.8 specimen for 6.33 s and did the No.14 specimen for 5.00 s. Non-expert observed the No.2 specimen for 7.30 s first time, did the No.2 specimen for 4.73 s second time, did the No.6 specimen for the 16.10 s, did the No.8 specimen for 11.87 s and did the No.14 s for 13.73 s.

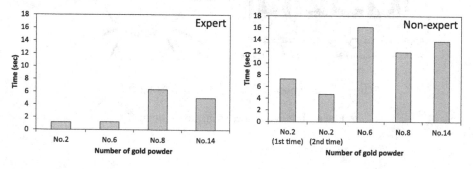

Fig. 8. Observation time in each specimen

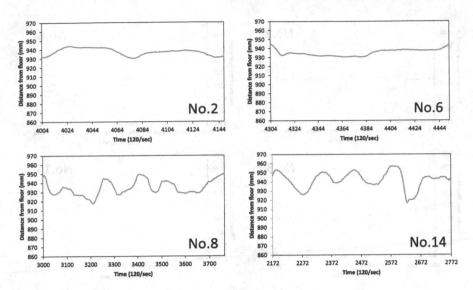

Fig. 9. Frame 2 marker position of expert in each specimen

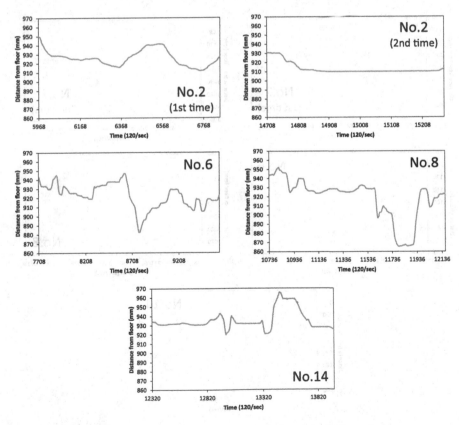

Fig. 10. Frame 2 marker position of non-expert in each specimen

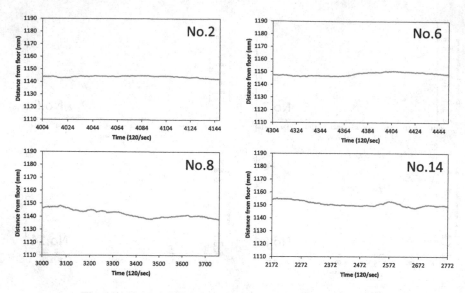

Fig. 11. Head right marker position of expert in each specimen

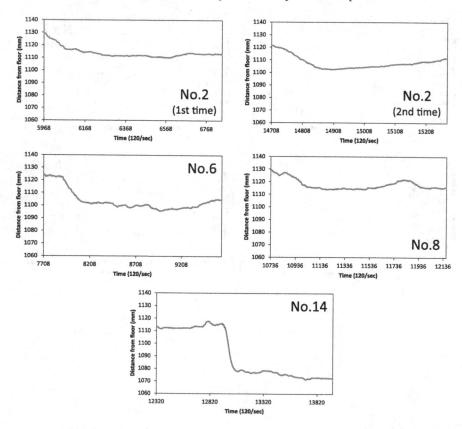

Fig. 12. Head right marker position of non-expert in each specimen

3.3   Motion of Frame 2 Marker and Head Right Marker

Figure 9 showed the position of frame 2 marker in the expert. Vertical axis showed the distance from the floor. Horizontal axis showed the time from the start of the Mitate. The marker did not much move in the case of No.2 and No.6 specimens. The marker moved up and down again and again. Figure 10 showed the position of frame 2 marker in the non-expert. The marker moved up and down strongly once time in the case of No.2 specimen of the first time. The marker did not much move in the case of No.2 specimen of the second time. The marker moved up and down strongly in the case of the No.6, No.8 and No.14 specimens. The marker also moved a little in the case of them.

Figure 11 showed the position of head right marker in the expert. The marker did not much move in the case of No.2 and No.6 specimens. The marker moved a little in the case of No.8 and No.14 specimens. Figure 12 showed the position of head right marker in the non-expert. The marker slightly moved up and down. The marker did not move up and down again and again in the case of the expert and non-expert.

Figure 13 showed the deviation of frame 2 marker position in each subject. Expert's deviation was equal to or less than 5 mm in the case of the No.2 and No.6 specimens. It was largish in the case of the No.8 and No.14 specimens, but was equal to or less than 10 mm. Non-expert's deviation was larger than the expert in each specimen. Especially, it was equal to or more than 20 mm in the case of the No.8 specimens. Figure 14 showed the deviation of head right marker position in each subject. The expert's deviation was

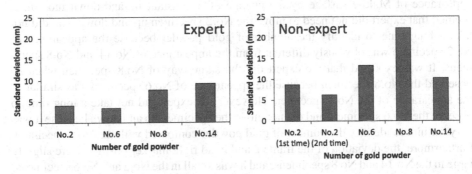

Fig. 13. Deviation of frame 2 marker position in each specimen

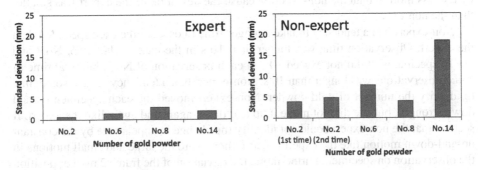

Fig. 14. Deviation of head right marker position in each specimen

equal to or less than 5 mm in each specimen. The non-expert's deviation was larger than the expert in each specimen. Especially, it was equal to or more than 20 mm in the case of the No.14 specimen.

4 Discussion

Expert observed the specimen in order from the right side. Non-expert observed the specimen in order of No.2, No.6, No.8 and No.14, lastly she observed the No.2 specimen once again. It seemed that the expert observed the specimen with an open mind, but the non-expert started observing each specimen in anticipation of the number of gold powder.

Expert's observation time of the No.14 and No.8 specimens was longer than the No.2 and No.6 specimens. Expert observed the specimen while he moved the specimen up and down again and again in the case of No.14 and No.8. It is easier to identify the size of gold powder in the case of No.14 specimen than the other specimens. It seemed that the No.14 specimen was the first specimen in this Mitate, and he identified the number of gold powder. Therefore it took a slightly long time to observe the No.14 specimen. It also took a slightly long time to observe the No.8 specimen, and he moved the specimen up and down again and again because there were many gold powders similar to No.8 like No.5, No.6, No.7, No.9 and No.10. Non-expert did not move the specimen up and down again and again. It suggests that expert identifies the change in appearance of Maki-e surface by the change of a constant up-and-down motion. It seemed that expert did not need to move the No.2 specimen up and down, and did not take a long time to identify the number of gold powder because the appearance of No.2 specimen was obviously different from the appearance of No.14 and No.8 specimens. It was expected that the expert did the same way of No.8 specimen when he observed the No.6 specimen because the appearance of No.6 specimen was similar to the appearance of the No.8 specimen. However the expert did not take a long time to observe the No.6 specimen, and did not move the specimen up and down because it was easy for him to identify the number of gold powder compared with the No.8 specimen. Furthermore, the deviation of the frame 2 and head right marker position were slightly large in the No.14 and No.8 specimens, and it was small in the No.2 and No.6 specimens. It suggests that the expert can identify the characteristics from the change in appearance by the less motion than the non-expert because the deviation of the expert was smaller than the non-expert.

Non-expert had a tendency to take a longer time to observe the each specimen than the expert. Observation time was longer than 10 s in the case of the No.6, No.8 and No.14 specimens. It did not exceed 10 s in each observation of No.2, but total time of twice observations was longer than 10 s. Non-expert had a tendency to take some time to identify the number of gold powder. Non-expert moved the each specimen up and down strongly, but she did not move it up and down again and again like the expert. It seemed that the non-expert could not identify the change in appearance by the constant up-and-down motion like the expert because there were the large and small motions in the observation on specimen. Furthermore, the deviation of the frame 2 marker position was larger than the head right marker position except for No.14 specimen, the non-expert moved the specimen more strongly than her head. However the non-expert moved her head more strongly than the expert. As these results, it suggests that the non-expert mainly moves the specimen up and down like the expert, but the non-expert makes the change in appearance of Maki-e by adding the motion of her head.

5   Conclusion

This research aimed to know difference of a motion of the Urushi crafts work between the expert Urushi craftspeople and the non-expert Urushi craftspeople when they conduct the Mitate. The motion of the specimen and subject's head were measured when the expert and non-expert Urushi craftspeople conducted the Mitate of the Maki-e specimen. As the results, it is found that the expert can identify the change in appearance of Maki-e surface by moving the specimen up and down a little. Furthermore, he can skip the up-and-down motion and shorten the observation time by comparing one specimen with the other specimen in the case of the different number of the gold powder. Non-expert needs to identify the change in appearance by constant moving the specimen up and down in order to conduct efficient, quick and accurate Mitate.

References

1. Endo, A., Narita, C., Suzuki, R., Kuroda, K., Takai, Y., Goto, A., Shimode, Y.: Study on "*Mitate*" of urushi craftspeople with different years of experiences. In: Proceedings of 13th Japan International SAMPE Symposium and Exhibition (JISSE-13), Paper ID 2416, pp. 1–5 (2013)
2. Endo, A., Narita, C., Kuroda, K., Takai, Y., Goto, A., Shimode, Y., Hamada, H.: Comparison of characteristics recognition in the "*Mitate*" of *Urushi* crafts. In: Duffy, V.G. (ed.) DHM 2014. LNCS, vol. 8529, pp. 212–223. Springer, Heidelberg (2014)
3. Endo, A., Narita, C., Kuroda, K., Takai, Y., Goto, A., Shimode, Y.: Hiroyuki hamadaeye movement analysis on observation method "Mitate" of urushi craftspeople. In: Proceedings of the 5th International Conference on Applied Human Factors and Ergonomics AHFE 2014, pp. 5198–5207 (2014)

Comparison of Description Skill on Characteristics of the Urushi Crafts Work Between Expert Craftspeople and Non-expert Craftspeople

Atsushi Endo[1(✉)], Mari Shimode[2], Yutaro Shimode[3], Seishi Namiki[1], Noriaki Kuwahara[1], and Hiroyuki Hamada[1]

[1] Kyoto Institute of Technology, Kyoto, Japan
shootingstarofhope30@gmail.com,
{namiki,nkuwahar,hhamada}@kit.ac.jp
[2] Kansai University, Suita, Japan
torima_taskurushimakie_14@yahoo.co.jp
[3] Future-Applied Conventional Technology Centre,
Kyoto Institute of Technology, Kyoto, Japan
shimode-yutaro@xa2.so-net.ne.jp

Abstract. Many of Urushi crafts works have been collected as an art in the museum and art museum. They have been treasured, but some of them spent several hundred years being made, and need to be repaired. Urushi crafts people can repair these works. Before they repair them, they need to observe the condition of the work by the naked eye. This observation is called "Mitate". Expert Urushi craftspeople can identify many characteristics by conducting the Mitate, and they can plan to repair the Urushi crafts work. This research aimed to examine how to understand the characteristics of the making process in the Urushi craftspeople. Urushi craftspeople conducted the Mitate, and they described the making process, material and so on. As the result, it is found that the Urushi craftspeople with long year of experience can identify the detail characteristics like the number of metallic powder in the Maki-e making process.

Keywords: Urushi crafts · Maki-e · Craftspeople · Expert · Non-expert · Mitate

1 Introduction

There are various traditional crafts in Japan. Urushi crafts is one of the Japanese traditional crafts, and it has about 9000-year-old history in Japan. Urushi is resin from Japanese lacquer tree, and it has been used as painting material, artists' paint and adhesive material in various life situations. A lot of good works were made in connection with Japanese culture, and many of them have been kept as the arts and craftwork. Urushi craftspeople have made these Urushi crafts works. Urushi crafts making process is divided into several processes, and there are specialized Urushi

© Springer International Publishing Switzerland 2015
V.G. Duffy (Ed.): DHM 2015, Part I, LNCS 9184, pp. 46–57, 2015.
DOI: 10.1007/978-3-319-21073-5_5

craftspeople in each process. Urushi crafts culture has been fostered in Kyoto, Japan for about 1200 years, and Urushi crafts technique has been inherited by many unknown Urushi craftspeople. However Urushi resin and Urushi crafts work do not used in present day because the lifestyle has been changed. A substitute material has been invented by the development of science and technology. In these surroundings, Urushi craftspeople continue to make the Urushi crafts work every day in order to hand on the Urushi crafts culture.

Many of Urushi crafts works have been collected as an art in the museum and art museum in Japan. There are also many Urushi crafts works in the world's museum and art museum. These Urushi crafts works have been treasured, but some of them spent several hundred years being made, and need to be repaired. Persons on the street have also kept them, and they also need to be repaired. Urushi crafts people can repair these works. Before they repair the Urushi craft work, they need to observe the condition of the work by the naked eye. This observation is called "Mitate". Expert Urushi craftspeople can identify many characteristics by conducting the Mitate, and they can plan to repair the Urushi crafts work. There are the researches on the Mitate of Urushi craftspeople in the previous researches [1–3], but the Mitate has not been analyzed with a focus on a making the Urushi crafts work.

This research aimed to examine how to understand the characteristics of the making process in the Urushi craftspeople. Urushi craftspeople conducted the Mitate, and they described the making process, material and so on. In this research, Maki-e technique was focused. Maki-e technique is one of the decoration techniques in the Urushi crafts. After painting Urushi on the basis, a design is drown by the Urushi and a metallic powder in the Maki-e technique.

2 Measurement

2.1 Subject

Table 1 showed the information of the subject. There were 8 subjects in this research. All of the subjects specialized in the Maki-e technique. The year of experience was about 60 years in the subject A and subject B. They were the

Table 1. Information of the subject

Subject	Age	Year of Urushi craft experience (Year of experience in traditional crafts technical school)	Sex
A	66	51 years and 10 months	Male
B	59	41 years and 8 months (2 years)	Male
C	33	11 years and 8 months (2 years)	Female
D	32	7 years and 8 months (2 years)	Female
E	30	6 years and 8 months (2 years)	Female
F	29	5 years and 8 months (2 years)	Female
G	25	5 years and 8 months (4 years)	Female
H	25	3 years and 8 months (2 years)	Female

expert Urushi craftspeople because they have long year of experience and have various experiences. The year of experience was about 12 years in the subject C. She was usually regarded as the full-fledged Urushi craftspeople because she has about 10 years of experience. Subject C, D, E, F, G and H were the Urushi craftspeople under training. Subject C, D, E, F, G and H learned the elementary Maki-e technique in the technical college of the traditional crafts technique. Training year was shorter than the year of experience.

2.2   Urushi Crafts Work and Condition of Mitate

Figure 1 showed the Urushi crafts work used in this research. This Urushi crafts work has been named the Makie small box with typha latifolia and butterflies (Collection ID: AN.1616), and it is a collection of the Museum and Archives, Kyoto Institute of Technology. This work was selected because the Maki-e technique, Mother-of-pearl pasting and Urushi raising were used with balance, the number of types was not large, and the work was appropriate to compare the Mitate skill of Urushi craftspeople.

Conditions of Mitate were as follows.

- Mitate was conducted in a fluorescent lighted room.
- The small box was placed on a desk.
- Allow the subject to hold and move the work in order to conduct Mitate easily.
- When the subject hold or move the work, require wear of glove in order to protect the work.
- Time limit of Mitate was 30 min.

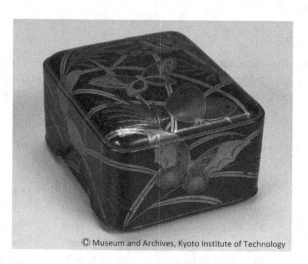

© Museum and Archives, Kyoto Institute of Technology

Fig. 1. Makie small box with typha latifolia and butterflies (Collection ID: AN.1616, Museum and Archives, Kyoto Institute of Technology).

- Subject conducted the Mitate. And then, subject describeed the order of Maki-e making process, working point, working name and working content on a paper.
- Description contents were compared among the subjects.

2.3   Maki-e Decoration of Urushi Crafts Work

Typha latifolia and butterfly were drawn in the small box by the Maki-e technique, Mother-of-pearl pasting and Urushi raising. Thin flat metallic powder (called "Nashiji-fun") was sprinkled in the back of the typha latifolia and butterfly and inside the box. This was called "Ji-maki" in Japanese, but it was named "Base Maki-e" in this research. A part of the typha latifolia and butterfly was raised by Urushi. This technique was called "Taka-age" in Japanese, but it was named "Urushi raising" in this research. Metallic powder was sprinkled flatly in a leaf and stem of the typha latifolia. This technique was called "Hira Maki-e" in Japanese, but it was named "Maki-e" in this research. Mother-of-pearl was pasted in the feather of butterfly. This technique was called "Raden" or "Aogai" in Jpanese, but it was named "Mother-of-pearl pasting" in this research. Thin line was drawn on the butterfly. This technique was called "Keuchi" in Japanese, and this name was also used in this research. Very fine gold powder was sprinkled on the edge of box. This technique was called "Ikkake" in Japanese, and this name was also used in this research.

3   Result

3.1   Order of Mitate

Typha latifolia was drawn on this small box, but all of subjects regarded it as a silver grass. Typha latifolia was described as the silver grass from this section.

Subject A conducted the Mitate in order of Base Maki-e inside and outside the small box, Mother-of-pearl pasting, Urushi raising, Top of the leaf of silver grass, Butterfly, Keuchi, Leaf and stem of silver grass. Subject B did it in order of Base Maki-e inside the small box, Base Maki-e outside the small box, Leaf and stem of silver grass, Mother-of-pearl pasting, Urushi raising, Butterfly and spike of silver grass, Keuchi, Ikkake. Subject C did it in order of Base Maki-e inside the small box, Base Maki-e outside the small box, Mother-of-pearl pasting, Urushi raising, Butterfly and spike of silver grass, Leaf and stem of silver grass, Keuchi. Subject D did it in order of Base Maki-e inside and outside the small box, Urushi raising, Mother-of-pearl pasting, Butterfly and spike of silver grass, Butterfly and Leaf and stem of silver grass, Keuchi. Subject E did it in order of Base Maki-e inside and outside the small box, Mother-of-pearl pasting, Urushi raising, Butterfly and spike of silver grass, Leaf and stem of silver grass, Keuchi, Ikkake. Subject F did not describe the order. Subject G did it in order of Base Maki-e inside and outside the small box, Mother-of-pearl pasting, Urushi raising, Butterfly and spike of silver grass, Leaf and stem of silver grass, Ikkake. Subject H did it in order of Base Maki-e inside and outside the small box, Mother-of-pearl pasting, Butterfly and silver grass.

3.2 Description Content

Description content was divided into eight positions. The positions were Base Maki-e, Leaf and stem of silver grass, Spike of silver grass, Butterfly, Keuchi, Ikkake, Urushi raising, Mother-of-pearl pasting.

In the case of Base Maki-e, when the subject B, C and G described the characteristics, they distinguished between the inside box and the outside box. Subject A, B, D, E described silver or tin about the type of metallic powder. Most of the subjects described the Nashiji-fun about the shape type of metallic powder. Only subject B pointed out a possibility of Hirame-fun. Subject A, B, C, D, E described the number of metallic powder. Most of the subjects described low amount of sprinkling metallic powder. Only subject B pointed out a specific amount. Most of the subjects described the Nashiji Urushi about the type of Urushi for coating powder. Only subject F described the clear Urushi. Most of the subjects described the 2 or 3 times about the number of coating powder.

In the case of Leaf and stem of silver grass, number of answers was very low about the type of metallic powder, but gold and silver was described. The answer of Nobe-fun or Maru-fun was large. Nobe-fun was smaller powder than the Maru-fun No.1, and it did not have the number. Number of Maru-fun was pointed out the No.1 or a smaller than the No.1. Migaki-fun was one of the Maru-fun. It was regarded as the small size of Maru-fun like No.1, No.2, No.3 and No.4. Uwazuri Urushi was described about the type of Urushi for coating powder. Number of answers was low about the number of coating powder, but the number was 1 or 2 times. Only subject C was described the sprinkling powder with separating design.

In the case of Spike of silver grass, there were the answers of gold and silver about the type of metallic powder. Only subject C pointed out a colored Urushi powder. It was the powder that the colored Urushi was hardened, and it was grinded. There were many number of the answer of Maru-fun about the shape type of metallic powder. Togi-fun was one of the Maru-fun. It was regarded as the middle and big size of Maru-fun like from No.5 to No.15. However Subject B described the Nobe-fun, and subject F did the Nashiji-fun. Four subjects described the number of metallic powder, but the number was different. The answer of the Nashiji Urushi was large number about the type of Urushi for coating powder. Subject C and F pointed out Uwazuri Urushi in addition to the Nashiji Urushi. The answer of the feathering was large number about how to sprinkle metallic powder. There was less answer about the number of coating powder, but it was 1 or 2 times.

In the case of Butterfly, most of subjects described the gold and silver, but subject B and C also pointed out bluish gold. The number of metallic powder was described by only subject A, B, C, D and E, but most of the number was small number. Subject D and E also pointed out large number. Nashiji Urushi, Black Urushi, Red Urushi, Colored Urushi and Uwazuri Urushi was described about the type of Urushi for coating powder. Feathering and sprinkling powder without space were described about how to sprinkle metallic powder. Only subject D described the 2 coatings by Uwazuri Urushi.

Keuchi was one of the Maki-e techniques. The metallic powder was sprinkled in a thin line. It was made on the butterfly. The answer of the type of metallic powder was gold. The answer of the shape type of metallic powder was Nobe-fun or Maru-fun.

The number of the metallic powder was smaller number than metallic powder No.1. The number of the type of Urushi for coating powder was Uwazuri Urushi.

In the case of Ikkake, the metallic powder was sprinkled without space. In this small box, it was made on the edge of the box. There were little descriptions in each item. The answer of the type of metallic powder was gold. The answer of the shape type of metallic powder was Nobe-fun or Maru-fun. All of subjects did not describe the number of metallic powder. The answer of the type of Urushi for coating powder was Uwazuri Urushi. Only subject F described 1 or 2 coatings by Uwazuri Urushi.

In the case of Urushi raising, an appearance of solidity was made in the design by raising Urushi. In this small box, it was made in the butterfly and spike of silver grass. Use of silver powder was described by the subject A, B and D. The number of metallic powder was No.1. Only subject D described the Maru-fun about the shape type of metallic powder. The answer of the type of Urushi was Taka-age Urushi. Only subject A pointed out the mixture of black and bengal Red Urushi.

In the case of Mother-of-pearl pasting, the mother-of-pearl was pasted on the surface of Urushi painting. In this small box, it was made in the butterfly. Most of subjects described the abalone about the type of shell. The answer of the shell thickness was thin. The answer of the type of bonding Urushi was black Urushi. Shell cutting was described by the subject A, E, F, G and H.

3.3   Number of Answer in Each Item

Figure 2 showed the description number of the item in each position. The item meant the "Material type of metallic powder", "Shape type of metallic powder", "Number of metallic powder", "Amount of sprinkling metallic powder", "Type of Urushi for coating powder" and "Number of coating powder" in the case of the Base Maki-e. For example, if there was the description in one item, it was counted one. The max of number was six in each subject in the Base Maki-e. The subjects except for the subject F could described in each item. The max of number was six in the Leaf and stem of silver grass. The number of subject D was larger than the other subject. The max of number was six in the Spike of silver grass. Subject B, C, D, E and F described in the more than half of items. The max of number was six in the Butterfly. Subject B, C, D and E described in the more than half of items. The max of number was four in the Keuchi. Subject A, B, C, D and E described in the more than half of items. The max of number was five in the Ikkake. Subject E, F and G described in many items. The max of number was four.in the Urushi raising. Subject A, B and D described in the more than half of items. The max of number was four in the Mother-of-pearl pasting. The subjects except for the subject C described in the more than half of items.

3.4   Number of Subject Described in Each Item and Each Positon

Figure 3 showed the number of subject described in each item and each positon. The number of subject describing in each item was large in the case of the Base Maki-e. The number of subject describing the type of metallic powder was six subjects, but the

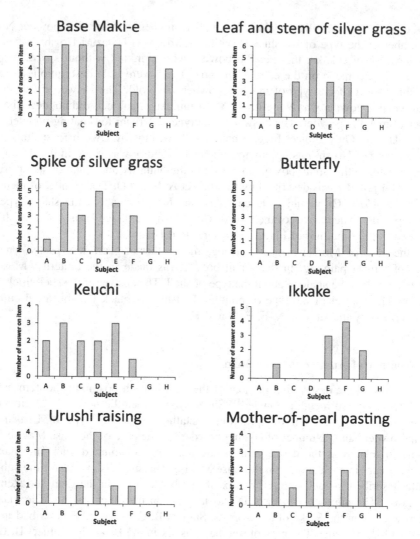

Fig. 2. Description number of the item in each position

number of subject describing the other items was small in the case of the Leaf and stem of silver grass. The number of subject describing the type of metallic powder was six subjects, the number of subject describing the shape type of metallic powder was five subjects, and the number of subject describing the other items was small in the case of the Spike of silver grass. The number of subject describing the type of metallic powder was eight subjects, and the number of subject describing the other items was slightly large in the case of the Butterfly. The number of subject describing the type of Urushi for coating powder was five subjects, but the number of subject describing the other items was small in the case of the Keuchi. The number of subject describing each item was small in the case of the Ikkake. The number of subject describing the type of Urushi was five subjects, but the number of subject describing the other items was

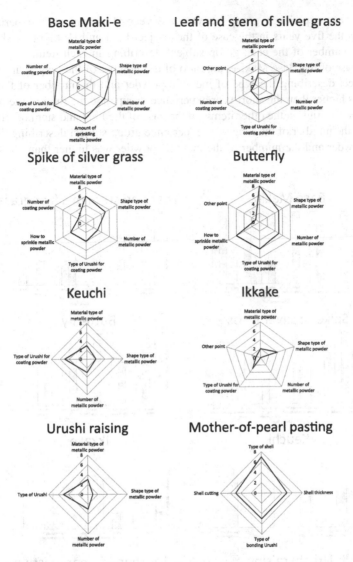

Fig. 3. Number of subject described in each item and each positon

small in the case of the Urushi raising. The number of subject describing the type of shell was seven subjects, and the number of subject describing the other items was five subjects in the case of the Mother-of-pearl pasting.

Next, the subject was divided into two groups. The year of experience in traditional crafts technical school was subtracted from the year of Urushi craft experience. Then the year of Urushi craft experience was equal to or higher than five years in the case of the subject A, B, C and D. The year of the subject E was four years and eight months, and it was close to five years. Therefore, the subject A, B, C, D and E were regarded as a long year experience group. On the other hand, the subject F, G and H were regarded as a short year experience group because the year of Urushi craft experience was shorter than the five years in the case of the subject F, G and H. Figure 4 showed the ratio of the number of the each group subject describing in each item.

In the case of the Base Maki-e, the ratio of the number of the long year experience group subject describing the type of metallic powder and the number of the metallic powder was higher than the short year experience group, and the ratio of the number of both groups was high in the other items. In the case of the Leaf and stem of silver grass, the ratio of the number of the long year experience group subject describing the type of metallic powder and the number of the metallic powder was higher than the short year

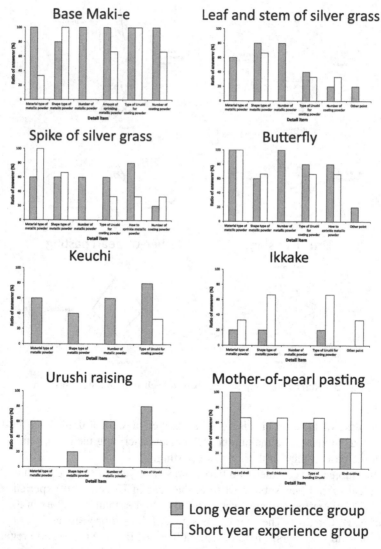

Fig. 4. Ratio of the number of the each group subject describing in each item

experience group, there wasn't so much of a difference in the other items between the long year experience group and the short year experience group, and the ratio of the number of both groups was low in the type of Urushi for coating powder and the number of coating powder. In the case of the Spike of silver grass, the ratio of the number of the long year experience group subject describing the number of the metallic powder and how to sprinkle metallic powder was higher than the short year experience group, there wasn't so much of a difference in the other items between the long year experience group and the short year experience group, and the ratio of the number of both groups was low in the number of coating powder. In the case of the Butterfly, the ratio of the number of the long year experience group subject describing the number of the metallic powder was higher than the short year experience group, there wasn't so much of a difference in the other items between the long year experience group and the short year experience group, and the ratio of the number of both groups was high in the other items. In the case of the Keuchi, only the subject of the long year experience group described in the type of metallic powder, the shape type of metallic powder and the number of the metallic powder, and the ratio of the number of the long year experience group subject describing the type of Urushi for coating powder was higher than the short year experience group. In the case of the Ikkake, the ratio of the number of the short year experience group subject describing the shape type of metallic powder and the type of Urushi for coating powder was higher than the long year experience group. In the case of the Urushi raising, the ratio of the number of the long year experience group subject describing the type of metallic powder, the number of metallic powder and the type of Urushi was higher than the short year experience group. In the case of the Mother-of-pearl pasting, the ratio of the number of both groups was high, and the ratio of the number of the short year experience group subject describing the shell cutting was higher than the long year experience group.

4 Discussion

Basic order of Mitate is the order of the Base Maki-e, Mother-of-pearl pasting, Urushi raising, Butterfly and silver grass, Keuchi, Ikkake. The order of subject except for subject F was almost the same. It is found that the subject with short year of experience can understand the basic order of making Maki-e.

Only subject B and C pointed out the order of the inside and outside of the small box in the Base Maki-e. Other subject did not distinguish between them. Especially, subject G could not the making process of the inside of the box. Most of subject pointed out the low amount in the amount of sprinkling metallic powder. Only subject B pointed out the 50 % amount inside the box, and 70 % amount outside the box. Subject B considered the amount of the powder. It is found that the subject B can set a subdivision process by identifying the Base Maki-e as two processes. Subject A, B, D and E pointed out the other metal except for gold. When the small box is observed closely, the corrosion is noticed around metallic powder. It is found that they have an experience which they identify the characteristics.

There were many characteristics pointed out by the subject B, C, D and E in the case of the Butterfly and silver grass. Especially, Subject A, B, C, D and E could point out the number of the metallic powder, but the subject F, G and H could not point out it. This result suggests it is difficult to identify the number of the metallic powder for the subject with short year of experience.

Most of subject could point out the type of shell in the case of the Mother-of-pearl pasting. Subject B, C and D did not point out the characteristics except for the type of shell. However it is difficult to think that they cannot identify the other characteristics because they can point out the number of metallic powder. It seems that they skip the description, and it is easy to identify the characteristics of the Mother-of-pearl pasting for the subject with short year of experience.

Subject with short year of experience pointed out the more characteristics than the subject with long year of experience in the case of the Ikkake. As is the case with the Mother-of-pearl pasting, it seems that the subjects with long year of experience skip the description, and it is easy to identify the characteristics of the Ikkake for the subject with short year of experience.

Subject A, C, D, E and F could pointed out the Taka-age Urushi, but only subject A,B and D could the possibility of using silver powder in the case of the Urushi raising. It is easy to point out the Taka-age Urushi. However it seems that the subject with short year of experience cannot point out the silver powder because it is not much used in the Urushi raising technique in very time.

As these results, it is found that the material type and shape type of the metallic powder are identified by most of the subjects regardless of the year of experience, and the subject with long year of experience can identify the detail characteristics like the number of metallic powder and the use of silver powder in the Urushi raising. The subject with long year of experience tends to skip the description of characteristics in the Mother-of-pearl pasting and the Ikkake. On the other hand, the subject with short year of experience identifies the characteristics of the Mother-of-pearl pasting and the Ikkake. It is assumed that it is easy to identify the characteristics of them for the subject with short year of experience because they identify many characteristics.

The subject with long year of experience can identify the many characteristics in each making process. The year of experience in traditional crafts technical school is subtracted from the year of Urushi craft experience, and the year of experience of subject C and D is equal to or higher than five years, its year of subject E is about five years. It suggests that subject A and B are regarded as the expert, subject C and D have the experience of the full-fledged Urushi craftspeople, subject E are growing into the full-fledged Urushi craftspeople, and subject F, G and H are needed to train the Maki-e technique.

5   Conclusion

This research aimed to examine how to understand the characteristics of the making process in the Urushi craftspeople. Urushi craftspeople conducted the Mitate, and they described the making process, material and so on. As the result, it is found that the Urushi craftspeople with long year of experience can identify the detail characteristics like the number of metallic powder in the Maki-e making process. Minimum of 5 years is considered appropriate for the training year as the craftspeople because the craftspeople with up to 5 years of experience in the Urushi crafts studio cannot identify the many characteristics. Moreover, the characteristics identification is important skill in the Mitate because the making process is changed when the metallic powder is changed in the Maki-e technique. Therefore, it seems that the Urushi craftspeople with short year of experience cannot identify the characteristics of the work enough, and the work is not repaired accurately. Non-expert needs to get the knowledge about characteristics in appearance based on the change of various materials and making processes in their daily training.

Acknowledgment. We express our gratitude to Miss Kanako NAKAGAWA, Technical Assistant, Museum and Archives, Kyoto Institute of Technology, and the other staff. They cooperated with us when the Makie small box with typha latifolia and butterflies was borrowed from the Museum and Archives, Kyoto Institute of Technology, and our research was made.

We also express our gratitude to the staff of Shimode Maki-e Studio. They attended this research as the subject.

References

1. Endo, A., Narita, C., Suzuki, R., Kuroda, K., Takai, Y., Goto, A., Shimode, Y.: Study on "*Mitate*" of urushi craftspeople with different years of experiences. In: Proceedings of 13th Japan International Sampe Symposium and Exhibition (JISSE 2013), Paper ID 2416, pp. 1–5 (2013)
2. Endo, A., Narita, C., Kuroda, K., Takai, Y., Goto, A., Shimode, Y., Hamada, H.: Comparison of characteristics recognition in the "*Mitate*" of *Urushi* crafts. In: Duffy, V.G. (ed.) DHM 2014. LNCS, vol. 8529, pp. 212–223. Springer, Heidelberg (2014)
3. Endo, A., Narita, C., Kuroda, K., Takai, Y., Goto, A., Shimode, Y., HamadaEye H.: Movement analysis on observation method "Mitate" of urushi craftspeople. In: Proceedings of the 5th International Conference on Applied Human Factors and Ergonomics AHFE 2014, pp. 5198–5207 (2014)

Analysis of Eye Movement of Caregiver Concerning on Transfer Operation

Akihiko Goto[1(✉)], Mengyuan Liao[2], Yuka Takai[1],
Takashi Yoshikawa[3], and Hiroyuki Hamada[2]

[1] Department of Information systems Engineering, Osaka Sangyo University,
Osaka, Japan
gotoh@ise.osaka-sandai.ac.jp
[2] Kyoto Institute of Technology, Advanced Fibro-Science, Kyoto, Japan
hhamada@kit.ac.jp
[3] National Institute of Technology, Niihama College, Niihama, Japan
yosikawa@mec.niihama-nct.ac.jp

Abstract. As well known, nowadays Japan is one of the several "super-ageing societies" all around the world. The aging of Japan is thought to outweigh all other nations, as the country is purported to have the highest proportion of elderly citizens; 33.0 % are above age 60, 25.9 % are aged 65 or above, 12.5 % aged 75 or above, as of Sep 2014. The increasing proportion of elderly people also had a major impact on increased burden for caregivers. Due to a shortage of expert nursing staff, training caregivers for long-term care facilities has also become a growing concern. Therefore, in order to help speed up training process, one of the popular care processes "transfer operation" between bed and wheelchair was examined. In this study, elder staff's eye movements during transfer was measured and compared between expert, non-expert and beginner caregiver. Comparing with beginner without experience, caregivers with occupational experience were found to pay more attention on elder's body with longer eyes rested duration according to eye movement track. Especially, expert caregiver's skillful care process was also clarified, during which he put less time than non-expert to focus the objects such as bed, wheelchair and so on. Eye moving characteristic and difference between expert and non-expert suggested that transfer care assistance could be improved by instructing the caregivers to focus on specific parts of elder's body effectively.

Keywords: Caregiver · Eye movement · Transfer operation

1 Introduction

As well known, nowadays Japan is one of the several "super-ageing societies" all around the world. The aging of Japan is thought to outweigh all other nations, as the country is purported to have the highest proportion of elderly citizens; 33.0 % are above age 60, 25.9 % are aged 65 or above, 12.5 % aged 75 or above, as of Sep 2014. The increasing proportion of elderly people also had a major impact on increased burden for caregivers. Due to a shortage of expert nursing staff, training caregivers for long-term care facilities has also become a growing concern.

© Springer International Publishing Switzerland 2015
V.G. Duffy (Ed.): DHM 2015, Part I, LNCS 9184, pp. 58–65, 2015.
DOI: 10.1007/978-3-319-21073-5_6

The behavioral responses and process analysis by visual apparatus have been of increasing interest in ergonomics. Until now, eye movement/track was widely applied in ergonomic field such as process analysis. As well known, behavioral response of sensory organs can yield relevant information about performance in visual recognition tasks, in other words record eye movement track or emphasis data would reflect following whole-body movement response in some degree. Monitoring eye movements can help identify the behavior of visual focus of experts compared with non-expert, which used to detect the detail process difference or establish a standard service procedure.

During human assistant transfer operation from bed to wheelchair, there is a high risk of injury (both acute and cumulative) and fatigue loading to both elder and caregiver assistant, especially when the height differential between transfer surfaces is greater than 75 mm or the gap between surfaces is greater than 150 mm. Therefore, it is urgent and necessary to train the beginner caregiver who employed in elder nursing facilities for a long-term effectively. A significant approach to improve young care-giver's care technique and provide safe and comfortable care environment for old patient is investigating expert caregiver's manual patient handling process. Transfer operation is one of very important and frequent old patient handling processes during daily nursing care activities [1]. Therefore, in this paper, eye movement of caregiver concerning on transfer operation was focused. In this study, beginner, non-expert and expert from the same elder nursing facility were required to conduct transfer operation for elder from bed to wheel chair. During the transfer operation process, all subject's eye movement were record and analyzed. Afterwards, eye's gazing point and move-ment track differences of caregiver with varied experience years were verified. According to the analyzed eye movement trace, it is noted to find that expert caregiver made care eye contact with old patient through good communication before and during transfer operation. However, non-expert caregiver's eye focused on the transfer instrument but not subject patient body with bad communication process. One more important point, it is deserved to find that expert caregiver pay attention to the transfer line/route to the moving destination before and during the transfer operation with eye watching movement, which ensure the safe route for transferring process and also let old patient relieved and comfortable. Based on the eye movement results, it is con-cluded that expert caregiver show thoughtful care for old patient with more eye contact and keep a safe transfer line with "Omotenashi mind" during transfer operation.

2 Experiment

2.1 Subjects

Consisting with previous study, three caregivers from the same nursing home were cooperated in current study. As shown in Table 1, caregiver's information character-istics were summarized, where two caregivers had occupational experience with 154 months and 10 months respectively, named as expert and non-expert in following discussion. One more beginner caregiver without experience also employed for com-parison. Here, a 'hypothesis' elder (caregiver guider) was determined for all subject caregiver's transfer tasks.

Table 1. Characteristic of investigated subjects

	Expert	Non-expert	Beginner
Gender	Male	Female	Male
Height(cm)	175	157	174
Work experience	154 months	10 months	–

2.2 Measuring Condition and Setting

Current research was conducted on-site in one of the real room in elderly nursing house. In order to record and analyze caregivers' eye movement, "Talk Eye II" from Takei Equipment were used. Subject caregivers were required to wear the goggles over their eyes as shown. And the goggles are equipped with CCD cameras above and beside the subjects' eyes for recording eye movement track and real gaze view field.

2.3 Predetermined Tracking Process

A. Assisted transfer of elder from bed to wheelchair.
   The caregiver entered the room with the wheelchair, approached the patient sitting on the bed, and transferred the elder o the wheelchair.
B. Assisted transfer of the patient from wheelchair to bed.
   The caregiver entered the room with the patient in the wheelchair, moved to the bed, and transferred the elder from wheelchair to the bed.

All trials of each type followed the same steps, first B-trial following with A-trial. And the trials were also carried out with the wheelchair facing the foot of the bed. Both procedures were separated into three steps and listed in following Table 2.

Table 2. Bed apparatus and transfer process

Same elder	Bed apparatus	
	Special	Normal
Subject caregiver	Expert vs. Non expert	Non-expert vs. Beginner
Process of transfer (A)		
A-1	Carry a wheelchair to bed and brake it	
A-2	Transfer assistance to wheel chair	
A-3	Place foot on the footrest	
Process of transfer (B)		
B-1	Move the requiring nursing care of the wheel chair to bed	
B-2	Brake of the wheel chair and bring one foot down from a footrest	
B-3	Transfer assistance to bed	

3   Results and Discussions

3.1   Eye Movement Track of Expert, Non-expert and Beginner

Subject caregivers' eye movement throughout transfer operation was summarized and illustrated in following black and white figures by gaze time percentage on location in sequence, which black strip represented as eye rested time percentage on corresponding location listed on left axis and white strip meant the eye focus jump to other location. As shown in Figs. 1, 2 and 3, it is obvious to find black strips nearly concentrated on objects such as assisted device, bed and floor during beginner's transfer operation, especially for long and continuous time period on floor. This phenomenon was considered as the result of without experience. Because beginner did not familiar with transfer operation process clearly so beginner always focusing on floor in order to checking a safety route during operation with nervous feeling.

As well known, both expert and non-expert have a good knowledge of transfer operation flow and steps. However, it still required to take a long-term training for non-expert to become a qualified expert. Usually even if we understand non-expert showed different performance from expert, but we did not have an evidence to prove it. Here, through comparing the expert and non-expert's eye movement, it is worthwhile to find that non-expert looked around among nearly all of elder's whole body pats with segmental time period. But expert just gazed at some parts of elder's body with continuous time and move quickly. In a word, it could be demonstrated that expert's conduct transfer operation with eye contact with elder by a longer period, but non-expert's eye movement passed through elder's body part with limited moment.

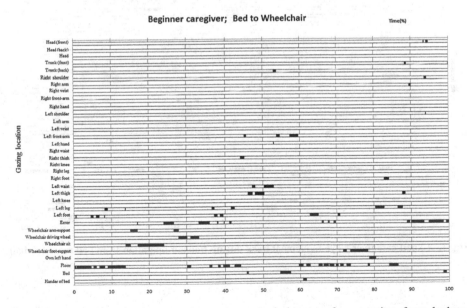

Fig. 1. Beginner caregiver's eye movement track during transfer operation from bed to wheelchair.

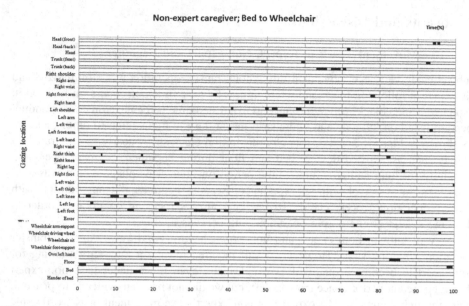

Fig. 2. Non-expert caregiver's eye movement track during transfer operation from bed to wheelchair.

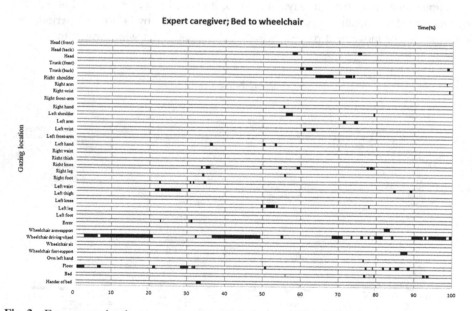

Fig. 3. Expert caregiver's eye movement track during transfer operation from bed to wheelchair

3.2   Eye Gaze Time Percentage Comparison Among Expert, Non-expert and Beginner

Eye gaze time summary was calculated from previous eye movement process and sorted into elder's body, wheelchair, own body, bed and floor five groups. Figures 4, 5 and 6 showed non-expert and beginner comparison during transfer operation from normal bed to wheelchair; Figs. 7, 8 and 9 displayed non-expert and expert comparison during transfer operation from special bed to wheelchair. As the same with previous eye movement track discussion, it was clearly to find beginner took a longest time focusing on floor following with effective gaze at wheelchair, left leg and left foot over 2 s. On the contrary, non-expert took more time for elder's body than beginner with longest time gazing at elder's trunk.

Referring to the comparison between expert and non-expert, it is notified to find that non-expert took a longer time period than expert among elder's body, wheelchair, own body, bed and floor, which suggested that expert caregiver's eyes moved more quickly than non-expert with focusing on some specific locations.

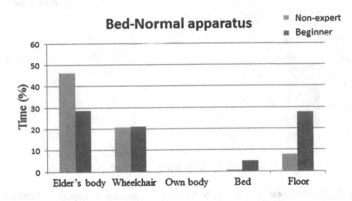

Fig. 4. Comparison of eye's gaze location between non-expert and beginner

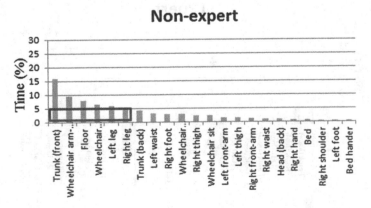

Fig. 5. Eye's gaze time rank during non-expert transfer operation

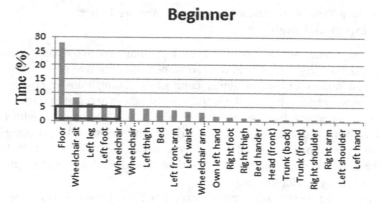

Fig. 6. Eye's gaze time rank during beginner transfer operation

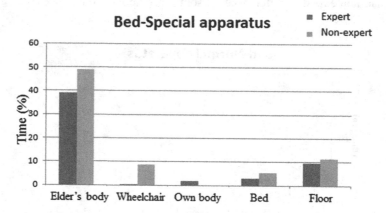

Fig. 7. Comparison of eye's gaze location between non-expert and expert

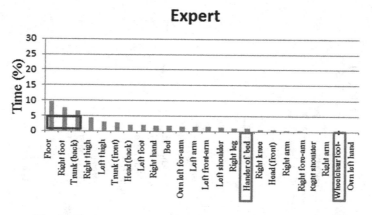

Fig. 8. Eye's gaze time rank during expert transfer operation

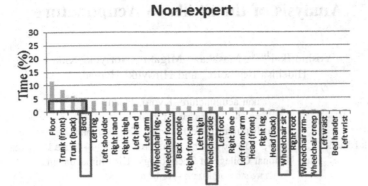

Fig. 9. Eye's gaze time rank during non-expert transfer operation

According to the eye focusing rank of expert and non-expert in Figs. 8 and 9, the experience difference was also verified, which clarified that non-expert paid more attention to assistance objects with longer eye rested period than expert.

4 Conclusions

In this research, elder caregiver's eye movements during transfer operation was measured and compared between expert, non-expert and beginner caregiver. As a result, caregivers with occupational experience were found to pay more attention on elder's body with longer eyes rested duration according to eye movement track comparing with beginner without experience. Especially, expert caregiver's skillful care process was also clarified, during which he put less time than non-expert to focus the objects such as bed, wheelchair but try to read elder's facial expressions and make related eye contact in order to release of elder's pain and uneasy. Eye moving characteristic and difference between expert and non-expert suggested that transfer care assistance could be improved by instructing the caregivers to focus on specific parts of elder's body effectively.

Reference

1. Ito, M., Endo, A., Takai, Y., Yoshikawa, T., Goto, A., Kuwahara, N.: Study on kind transfer assistance between wheelchair and bed in the case of eye movement analysis. In: Proceeding of 5th International Conference on Applied Human Factors and Ergonomics, AHFE 2014 (2014)

Analysis of the Skills to Acupuncture

Yoshio Ikai[1][✉], Masakazu Migaki[2], Noriyuki Kida[2],
Hidehisa Iwamoto[3], and Hiroyuki Hamada[2]

[1] Ikai acupuncture, Kyoto, Japan
nca01025@nifty.com
[2] Kyoto Institute of Technology, Kyoto, Japan
kida@kit.ac.jp, {iloveseta, hhamada10294}@gmail.com
[3] Kure National College of Technology, Hiroshima, Japan
iwamoto@kure-nct.ac.jp

Abstract. In Japan, health care has been carried out by Western medicine, but acupuncture has been handled in a different form from the health care system of Western medicine. Not only doctors and dental doctors, but also acupuncturists have rights to practice. Therefore, Japanese acupuncture is responsible for the treatment of disease and the health maintenance and promote. Japanese acupuncture has been widely used in a variety of diseases and symptoms in the medical field. In addition, since acupuncture be performed using a simple means, it is possible also performed in an area that does not meet the medical institutions. For acupuncture, in order to play a role in the medicine, it is necessary to academic support, and it is required the achievements and steady research. Although it has been accumulated research results with respect to the reaction of the body caused by acupuncture, there is not research relating to the operation of acupuncturists to acupuncture. Therefore, the purpose of this study is to target acupuncture with advanced technology, and it was performed motion analysis. As a result, we clarified the acupuncture motion skill of high-skilled acupuncturist.

Keywords: Acupuncture · Motion analysis · DLT method · z component · z coordinate

1 Introduction

Acupuncture and moxibustion have a history of 1500 years, and within that span Japanese acupuncture and moxibustion developed in their own unique way. In the mid-Edo period, around the 18th century, a painless method of inserting the needle (the needle-tube method, where a pipe encompasses the needle, which is inserted by tapping with the finger) was invented for acupuncture treatment [1–10]. Many years of clinical acupuncture and moxibustion led to the knowledge that if the insertion is made in the skin at high speed, then there is close to no pain. The insertion speed was never measured, but was passed on experientially. We used skin like material and a three-dimensional high-speed camera to record the motion of insertion, with the objective of quantitatively evaluating the speed of needle insertion. To investigate the factor of experience, we used as participants an experienced acupuncturist and a beginner.

© Springer International Publishing Switzerland 2015
V.G. Duffy (Ed.): DHM 2015, Part I, LNCS 9184, pp. 66–73, 2015.
DOI: 10.1007/978-3-319-21073-5_7

2   Method

2.1   Participants

The participants of the investigation were one acupuncture/moxibustion teacher (experienced: Expert) and one student enrolled at an acupuncture college (inexperienced: Non-expert). The experienced person was a 66-year-old male who had 30 years of clinical experience with acupuncture/moxibustion. The inexperienced person was a 26-year-old female who was a third-year student at the school of acupuncture and moxibustion and had just acquired foundational learning. Thorough explanations of the experiment were given to the test participants beforehand, and their consent was attained about their participation.

2.2   Environment of the Experiment and Experimental Procedure

The experiment was done indoors. A reflective marker with a diameter of 5 mm was put on the participants' right index fingernail. Four high-speed cameras (made by Dragonfly Express Point Grey Research Inc, recording speed 200 frames per second, exposure time 1/1000 s) were set in place, one each on the left side, right side, left front, and right front of the participant, to record their motions.

In the experiment, a sponge fixed atop a table was used as substitute for a human body, and the test participants were made to go through the motion of inserting a needle in it using an acupuncture tube. A reflective sheet was attached 5 mm to 15 mm from the head of the needle. To accustom the participants to the conditions of the experiment, at most three practice trials were made, and motions of 10 trials were recorded.

For the inexperienced person, after the simulated experiment using a sponge, four trials were made using an acupuncture tube to insert a needle into an actual human arm.

The images recorded were synchronized on a computer, and the coordinates were calculated using a video motion analysis system (Frame: DIAS IV, made by DKH). The time from when the index finger commenced rising to the end of the tapping and insertion was the section for analysis, and the central point of the reflective sheet attached to the needle and the reflective marker on the nail of the right index finger of the target person were digitized (Fig. 1). A three-dimensional frame of reference was made using the three-dimensional DLT method from the coordinates on the photographic images of 20 pre-recorded calibration points and the actual distances between them, and the coordinates of the index finger and needle were calculated. The direction to the right from the participant in a ready position was made the x axis, the front side of the participant the y axis, and the vertical direction the z axis.

3   Results and Discussion

Figure 2 shows the z coordinates of the reflective markers on the fingertip during the time of needle insertion. The time when the finger touched the needle was set as zero. The locations of the finger marker are shown in chronological order for the motion of insertion by the experienced person. It can be seen that the experienced person

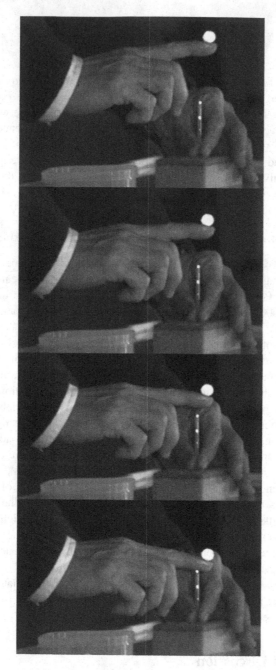

Fig. 1. Recorded images

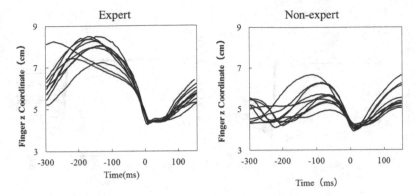

Fig. 2. Movement of the finger during needle insertion

performs the insertion from a higher point compared to the inexperienced person. The value of the difference in z coordinates from the highest point until the point of contact with the needle for the experienced person was 3.70 ± 0.41 cm, and for the inexperienced person 1.73 ± 0.35 cm; compared to the inexperienced person, the experienced person's value was significantly larger. The time required to approach the highest point for the experienced person was 170 ± 45 ms, and for the inexperienced person 150 ± 102 ms; there was no significant difference between the two (Fig. 3).

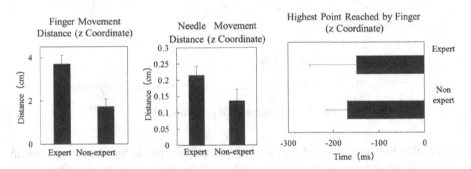

Fig. 3. Comparison of movement distance and time of highest point reached

Next, the z coordinates of the reflective sheet on the needle during the insertion are shown in chronological order (Fig. 4). The movement distance of the needle for the experienced person was 2.14 ± 0.03 mm, and for the inexperienced person it was 1.35 ± 0.04 mm; compared to the inexperienced person, the value of the experienced person was significantly longer.

Figure 5 shows the average value of the 10 trials for the movement of the needle and movement of the finger differentiated between the experienced and inexperienced persons. Figure 6 shows the average value of the 10 trials in terms of the z component of the speed of the finger differentiated between the experienced and inexperienced

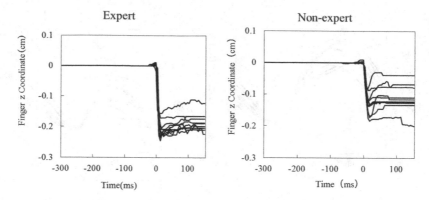

Fig. 4. Movement of needle during time of insertion

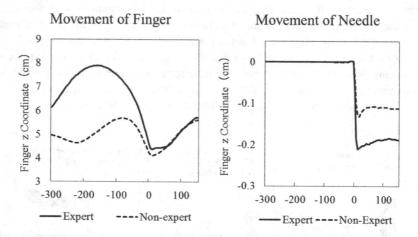

Fig. 5. Movement of finger and needle

persons. With the inexperienced person, the highest speed just before the finger came in contact with the needle was an average of −31.4 cm/s, but with the experienced person the value was at −49.5 cm/s which was 1.5 times faster. Figure 7 shows the z component in terms of the speed of the needle. The highest value of the movement speed of the needle for the inexperienced person was −11.5 cm/s, but for the experienced person it was −21.7 cm/s which was about twice as fast.

Figures 8 and 9 shows the results of the comparison of the simulation using a sponge vs actually inserting a needle into a real person. For the simulation, the average value of 10 trials is shown, but for the insertion in an actual person the average value of 4 trials is shown. Because the number of insertions in an actual person was small there is influence of noise, but as there was no great difference between the two trials, it can be said that the method used was adequate.

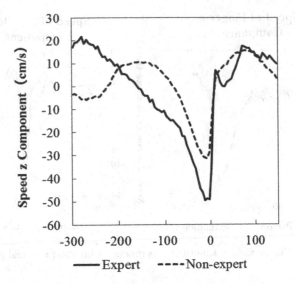

Fig. 6. Speed of finger

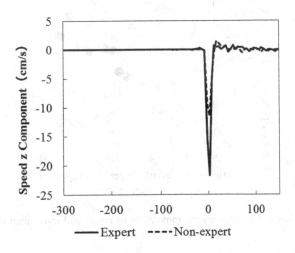

Fig. 7. Speed of needle z component

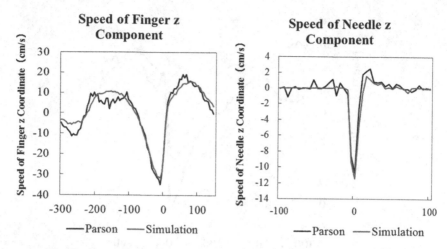

Fig. 8. Comparison of simulated experiment vs insertion into real person

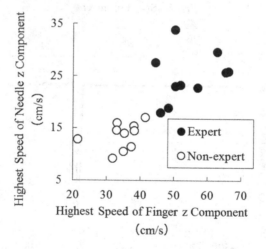

Fig. 9. Relationship between the movement of finger and movement of needle

4 Conclusion

In order to clarify the skill of acupunctures' needle insertion, we recorded the motion of insertion. As a result, the highest value of the movement speed of the needle for the Inexperienced person was −11.5 cm/s, but for the experienced person it was −21.7 cm/s which was about twice as fast. For the first time of the world, we were able to measure the movement speed of acupuncture needle.

References

1. Hinman, R.S., Pirotta, M., Bennell, K.L.: Treating chronic knee pain with acupuncture—reply. JAMA **313**(6), 628–629 (2015)
2. Chui, S.H., et al.: A case series of acupuncture treatment for female infertility with some cases supplemented with Chinese medicines. Eur. J. Integr. Med. **6**(3), 337–341 (2014)
3. Chung, K., et al.: Adverse Events Related to Acupuncture: Development and Testing of a Rating Scale. Clin. J. Pain (2015)
4. Vickers, A.J., Linde, K.: Acupuncture for chronic pain. JAMA **311**(9), 955–956 (2014)
5. Hinman, R.S., et al.: Acupuncture for chronic knee pain: a randomized clinical trial. JAMA **312**(13), 1313–1322 (2014)
6. Lao, L., Yeung, W.-F.: Treating chronic knee pain with acupuncture. JAMA **313**(6), 627–628 (2015)
7. Chiu, J.-H.: History of Acupuncture. Acupuncture for Pain Management. Springer, New York (2014)
8. Wilke, J., et al.: Short-term effects of acupuncture and stretching on myofascial trigger point pain of the neck: a blinded, placebo-controlled RCT. Complement. Ther. Med. **22**(5), 835–841 (2014)
9. Davis, R.T., Churchill, D.L., Badger, G.J., Dunn, J., Langevin, H.M.: A new method for quantifying the needling component of acupuncture treatments
10. ACUPUNCTURE IN MEDICINE 113–119. doi:10.1136/acupmed-2011-010111 (2012)

Differences in How Long an Ikebana Work Lasts Depending on the Skill Used in Cutting Floral Materials

Yuki Ikenobo[1,2], Zelong Wang[1(✉)], Yusuke Shiraishi[2(✉)],
and Akihiko Goto[3(✉)]

[1] Kyoto Institute of Technology Advanced Fibro-Science, Kyoto, Japan
hanahana@ikenobo.jp, simon.zelongwang@gmail.com
[2] Ikenobo, 248 Donomae-cho, Nakagyo-ku, Kyoto 604-8134, Japan
shiraishi@ikenobo.jp
[3] Department of Information Systems Engineering,
Faculty of Design Technology, Osaka Sangyo University,
3-1-1 Nakakakiuchi, Daito-shi, Osaka 574-8530, Japan
gotoh@ise.osaka-sandai.ac.jp

Abstract. Ikebana (Japanese flower arrangement), one of the Japanese traditional arts, requires the use of a pair of special steel scissors to compose an arrangement. Although to cut materials with the special type of scissors plays a crucial role in the composition of arrangements, the analyses of the cutting motion have not been taken so far. Comparing the cutting motion between non-experts and experts, it is found that non-experts cut in a slow speed, and on the contrary, experts cut rapidly in a short time. Normally, it is considered that the cutting strength has an effect on the duct of the material and influences the condition of the water absorption. However, there are no specific differences of the material's cut surface between non-experts and experts' cutting. The degradation of the material after cutting was not observed as well. It is assumed to be the reason that the original condition of the material was good and the material was preserved well after cutting. Therefore, we hope to analyze the original condition of the material, researching more about the different usage of the scissors and the influence brought by the usage hereafter.

Keywords: Scissor · Process analysis · Water potential · Cutting speed

1 Introduction

Ikebana (Japanese flower arrangement), one of the Japanese traditional arts, requires the use of a pair of scissors to compose an arrangement. Ikenobo (the largest school of Ikebana) advises its practitioners to use Warabite (a type of scissors). Different from usual scissors, when cutting the materials by the Warabite scissors, people have to hold one of the handles with the base of the thumb, open the scissors and cut off. According to the experience, if people cut the stem bottom at a diagonal line but not in horizon, the thick branches can be cut easily and the absorption of water can be improved. Therefore, cutting plays a crucial role not only in the composition of the arrangement

© Springer International Publishing Switzerland 2015
V.G. Duffy (Ed.): DHM 2015, Part I, LNCS 9184, pp. 74–82, 2015.
DOI: 10.1007/978-3-319-21073-5_8

but also in keeping the best condition for the materials. However, there are no analyses of the cutting motion, and the evidence-based instruction of the usage does not been taken so far.

On this experiment, focus was given to the differences between experts and non-experts with respect to the motion of cutting floral materials. By clarifying these differences, it is expected that instruction to beginners of Ikebana as to the usage of scissors will be effectively improved.

2 Methods

2.1 Outline

In order to analyze the cutting motion, FASTCAM SA4 (high-speed camera by Photoron) was set to record and observe differences in the cutting motion of the practiced and inexperienced subjects, respectively. The experiment was held in the 3 by 15 m training hall with a window facing south in a Z-shaped building. There, observations with both the naked eye and motion image analysis software were performed. For the observation with motion image analysis software, filming speed was set to 3600, and resolution was adjusted to 1024 by 1024. The screw of the scissors is "point 1," and the upper blade of the scissors is "point 2." The relative velocity of the two points was measured. All the subjects used the identical pair of scissors as shown in Fig. 1, and Ume (Japanese apricot flower) and gerbera, the common materials of ikebana arrangement, were used in the experiment. Figure 2 presented experiment setting. Each flower was prepared with three marks at the point of 15 cm, 25 cm, and 35 cm from the bottom end of the stalk, and the subjects were instructed to cut the stalk at each of these three points. After cutting, sections at each severed point were observed to measure the diameter of the stalk with a pair of vernier callipers (measurement device). Gerbera stalks were placed in a water jug for the sake of the visual degradation experiment after cutting, and the degradation was observed with the naked eye as shown in Fig. 3. Up to the 21st day from cutting, the flower conditions were checked with the naked eye once

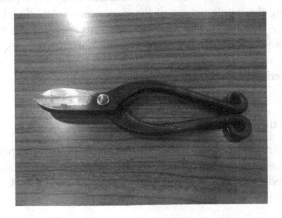

Fig. 1. Scissors (Warabite)

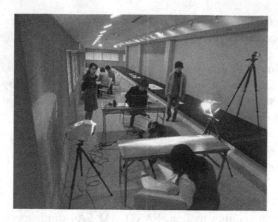

Fig. 2. Circumstances of the Experiments

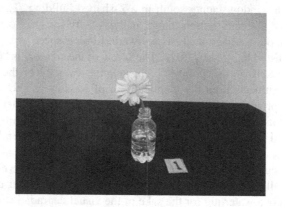

Fig. 3. Degradation Experiment

or twice daily, and recorded by camera for comparison analysis purpose. Jug water was not changed during the whole course of the experiment. Additional gerbera flowers prepared separately from the observation above were used for the measurements of water potential on sections cut by experts and non-experts, respectively. Water potential was measured on the day of the experiment, and the 1st, 2nd, 5th, and 9th days after the experiment.

2.2   Subjects of the Experiment

Fifteen subjects were chosen for the experiment, including five experts composed of staff at Ikenobo and ten non-experts of Ikebana composed of undergraduate and graduate school students of Kyoto Institute of Technology. Information on the subjects is provided as follows.

- Experts
  1. 23 years of experience (42 years old/Female)
  2. 20 years of experience (42 years old/Male)
  3. 21 years of experience (43 years old/Male)

Table 1. Differences between Experts and Non-experts

	Non-experts	Experts
Initial Angle of Scissors	• Edge line of the lower blade is horizontal	• Edge line of the lower blade faces downward (upper and lower blades face almost symmetrically across a horizontal line)
Left Hand (supporting hand)	• Left hand holds the stalk as if to grab it from above	• Left hand supports the stalk from the bottom
Right Hand (holding hand)	• Index finger lies on the outside of the handle of scissors	• Index finger lies on the inside of the handle of scissors
Initial Angle of the Stalk	• Edge of the stalk faces upward from the left hand	• Horizontal
Cutting Time	• Relatively short	• Relatively long
Cutting Angle (in relation to the stalk)	• Surface of the cutting section is almost vertical to the stalk	• Surface of the cutting section is approximately 45 degrees angled to the stalk
During Cutting	• The stalk twitches toward the blades	• The stalk is less likely to twitch
	• Left hand tends to twitch upward	• Left hand does not twitch
After Cutting	• Surrounding area of the cutting section of the remaining stalk moves like dancing	• The remaining stalk does not move a lot
Scissors After Cutting	• Upper blade and lower blade hit strongly, and then bounce	• Scissors close just to complete their sliding motion
	• Scissors (right hand) strongly move upward after cutting. Scissors held by the right hand keep moving after cutting since the right hand continues to apply power to grab them	• Scissors (right hand) leave the remaining stalk with virtually no vertical motion
Left Hand After Cutting	• Left hand tends to move upward	• Left hand does not move at all
Stalk After Cutting	• Viewed from above, stalk falls spinning counter-clockwise after cutting	• Stalk falls straight without spinning after cutting
Flow of the Motion	• Continuous motion without stop	• Before the blades hit and cut the stalk, momentary stop of motion is observed

4. 10 years of experience   (39 years old/Male)
5. 22 years of experience   (43 years old/Male)

- 10 subjects in their 20 s (male and female) account for Non-experts

3 Results

Table 1 below shows the results of the differences in the cutting motion between experts and non-experts noticed by visual observation.

Figures 4, 5, 6, 7, 8, and 9 shows the speed of the cutting process. No matter using what kinds of materials, when the experts cut, we can find that the cutting speed increases rapidly to the maximum and decelerates suddenly. On the other hand, comparing to the experts, non-experts cut in a slow-increasing speed to reach the maximum and take more time.

The following microscope images (Figs. 10 and 11) of the severed sections of gerbera do not exhibit any noticeable differences between experts and non-experts. However, those of the cutting sections of Ume flower (Figs. 12 and 13) signify that

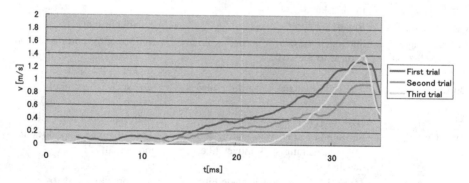

Fig. 4. Cutting speed by inexperienced person 1 (ume)

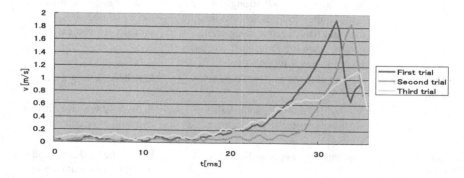

Fig. 5. Cutting speed by expert 1 (ume)

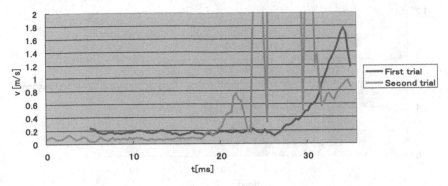

Fig. 6. Cutting speed by expert 1 (ume)

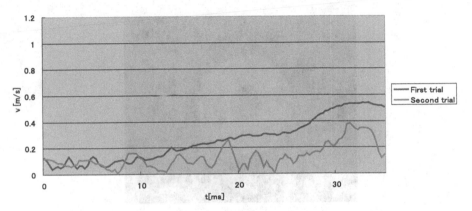

Fig. 7. Cutting speed by expert 2 (ume)

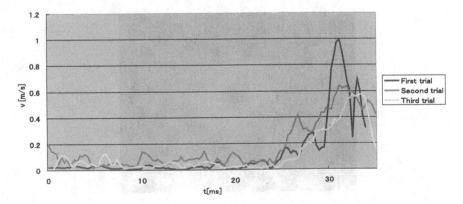

Fig. 8. Cutting speed by inexperienced person 2 (gerbera)

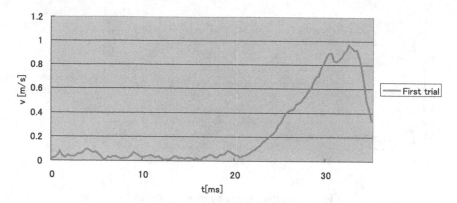

Fig. 9. Cutting speed by expert 2 (gerbera)

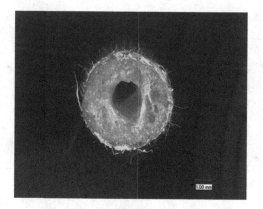

Fig. 10. Section of gerbera by expert

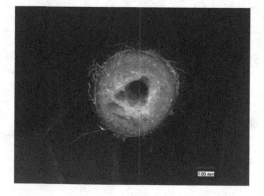

Fig. 11. Section of gerbera by non-expert

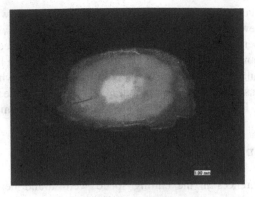

Fig. 12. Section of ume by expert

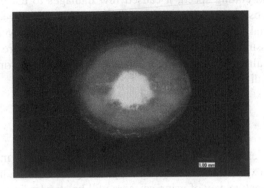

Fig. 13. Section of ume by non-expert

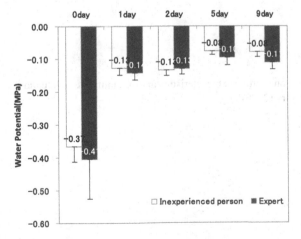

Fig. 14. Water potential of gerbera

non-experts tend to cut the flower at a vertical angle to the stalk, while all experts cut the flower at an askew angle to the stalk.

Degradation experiment on gerbera after cutting was conducted. However, visual observation with the naked eye spotted no changes caused by time lapse or differences resulting from the skills of the performer on any sample. The following Fig. 14 displays the results of the measurement of water potential of gerbera by time lapse. For the sake of the measurement, Pressure Chamber 600 (PMS Instrument Company) was used.

4   Consideration

The significant differences in the cutting speed were found between experts and non-experts. Non-experts cut in a slow-increasing speed and take more time. On the contrary, experts speed up the movement and cut in a short time. It is supposed that because of the rapid cutting speed, it caused few damages to the material stalk, providing good water absorption and kept water amount. However, the specific differences of the water potential between gerberas, cutting by experts and non-experts were not fond clearly. It is assumed that in the experiment, the materials were in good condition and preserved well after cut. Therefore, the cutting speed did not bring the influence to make the observed differences.

5   Conclusion

In the future, the research will keep investigating the cutting movement and the influence between experts and non-experts by changing the condition setting. It is expected that the effective way of using scissors will be standardized to the manuals so that beginners can quickly get used to the usage of scissors designed specifically for Ikebana and master Ikebana skills.

Reference

1. Kenji I.: Study on cutting characteristic and quantitative evaluation of sharpness for hair-cutting scissors (2006)

Study of Caregivers' Skills for Monitoring Senior Residents

Mikako Ito[1(✉)], Yuka Takai[2], Akihiko Goto[2], and Noriaki Kuwahara[3]

[1] Social Welfare Corporation Keiseikai, Osaka, Japan
Mikako_ito@kyouseikai.org
[2] Osaka Sangyo University, Daito, Japan
{takai,gotoh}@ise.osaka-sandai.ac.jp
[3] Kyoto Institute of Technology, Kyoto, Japan
nkuwahar@kit.ac.jp

Abstract. As of September, 2015, the Japanese population over 65-years old was found to be aging at a rate of 25.0 %. The results determined that the rate of aging for this sector of the Japanese population makes Japan one of the most aged societies in the world. As the aging population continues to increase in size, we anticipate that more nursing will be necessary to accommodate the future needs of seniors. Due to the complex nature and challenging field of senior care, nursing homes experience high employee turnover rates. The shortage of skillful employees is problematic, so the option of training employees without a nursing background may be an integral part of the solution. The least favorite part of nursing care among nursing-home workers is monitoring or keeping an eye on the senior residents. Caregivers are required to keep the care receivers safe, engage them in conversation, help them maintain a healthy state of mind – all while carrying out their designated routine. They have to constantly stay alert so that the elderly don't make sudden movements that make them lose their balance and fall, choke on their meals, fight with other elderly residents, or wander out of the caregivers' field of vision. There is no manual on how to best monitor the elderly. There are no pointers that come with photos – as in transfer techniques – when it comes to taking care of the elderly. Because one does not have access to visual or audio demonstrations during classes on nursing care, students who specialize in nursing care have to learn on the job. The comfort level of the elderly is largely determined by the quality of the caregivers' monitoring skill, how they use their voices and how they relate to their care receivers. The difference in experience between a skilled and a unskilled caregiver can mean the difference in the number of accidents.

Keywords: Nursing home · Skill to watch · Skill to plan

1 Introduction

1.1 Japan's Super-Aging Society

Japan is one of several "super-aging societies" in the world today, with 24.1 % of the nation's population over the age of 65. If the population continues at its current rate, the number of recipients of long-term care will likewise continue to increase (Fig. 1).

© Springer International Publishing Switzerland 2015
V.G. Duffy (Ed.): DHM 2015, Part I, LNCS 9184, pp. 83–94, 2015.
DOI: 10.1007/978-3-319-21073-5_9

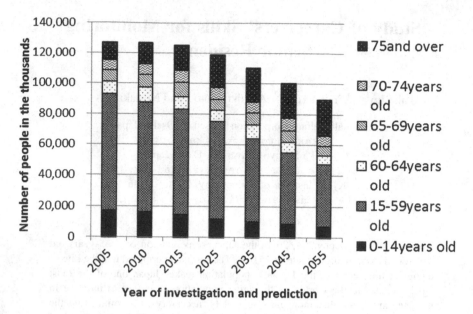

Fig. 1. Age-specific population of Japan

As the wave of elderly continues to swell, current long-term care facilities are exhausted. The turnover rate for caregivers in these facilities is also quite high compared to other occupations, causing even dedicated staff to quit from overwork (Table 1).

Table 1. Comparison of the quitting a job rate

	2006(year)	2007	2008	2009	2010	2011	2012	2013
All industry quitting a job rate	16.2%	15.4%	14.6%	16.4%	14.5%	14.4%	14.8%	14.8%
Care staff quitting a job rate	20.3%	21.6%	18.7%	17.0%	17.8%	16.1%	17.0%	16.6%

1.2   Purpose of Research

The turnover rate for caregivers in these facilities is quite high compared to other occupations, causing even dedicated staff to quit from overwork. The option of training employees without a nursing background may be an integral part of the solution.

The least favorite part of nursing care among nursing-home workers is monitoring or keeping an eye on the senior residents. There is no manual on how to best monitor the elderly. There are no pointers that come with photos – as in transfer techniques – when it comes to taking care of the elderly. Because one does not have access to visual or audio demonstrations during classes on nursing care, students who specialize in nursing care have to learn on the job.

- What is "Monitoring the Senior Residents"?

"Monitoring the senior residents" is one method to support the independence of senior residents in nursing homes. It is designed to protect the autonomy and independence of senior residents, and to prevent caregivers from limiting behaviors of elderly only based on caregivers' discretions. However, should that caregivers determine the elderly to be at risk of injury or death, the caregivers must assist the elderly immediately. (1) In this research, we checked the manual of the nursing home subjected to this experiment. It covers how to greet the elderly, daily routine work such as "assistance moving from a wheel chair to a bed or chair", "excretion assistance" and "dietary assistance". It also covers how to use large washing machines, and emergency procedure in the event of "infectious diseases", but it doesn't include "monitoring the senior residents". There is the close item titled "Communication", but it refers only the basic knowledge about appropriate words and dialogues when speaking to elderly. (2) We wondered how nursing homes train new staff for "monitoring the senior residents" without any solid educational tools. In this study, we evaluate the difference in monitoring assistance skills between skilled and non-skilled caregivers.

2 Questionnaire Survey and Results

2.1 Survey Subjects

The subjects were 16 regularly employed caregivers working on the same floor in the nursing home where the experiment was conducted.

Table 2 shows how many years of experience the 16 subjects had as caregivers.

Table 2. The list of caregivers

Years of experience	First year	Two ~ three year	Four ~ five year	Six ~ seven year	Eight year ~
Number	3	7	2	3	1

2.2 Questionnaire Survey

The purpose of this survey was to comprehend the caregivers' senses when monitoring the senior residents. We conducted the survey on 16 caregivers: 10 unskilled workers with 1–3 years of experience, and 6 skilled workers with more than 4 years of experience. We clarified the survey results according to the length of working experience.

The Survey items are as shown below:

- What do you think of your ability to "monitor the senior residents"?
  Very Poor, Poor, Okay, Good, Excellent
- Are there any particular times during the day or days of the week when you find monitoring the senior residents to be most difficult? (Please write the exact day, time and reason)

2.3 Survey Results

Figure 2 shows the survey results of how the 10 unskilled workers with 1–3 years' experience felt about monitoring the senior residents. Figure 3 shows the results of 6 skilled workers with over 4 years' experience.

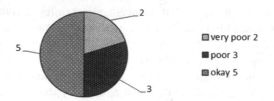

Fig. 2. The conscious of caregivers to monitoring senior residents (unskilled workers)

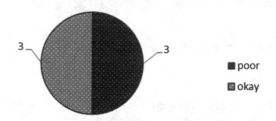

Fig. 3. The conscious of caregivers to monitoring senior residents (skilled workers)

Listed below are the reasons why the 10 unskilled workers with 1–3 years' experience found it difficult to monitor the senior residents:

- They have to engage in routine work while watching the senior residents.
- They sometimes do not notice a change in the senior residents.
- They need to concentrate on paying attention to the senior residents
- It is very stressful when engaged in monitoring work by themselves.
- They are rushed to handle many hyperactive seniors but enjoy communicating with the senior residents.
- Hyperactive seniors cause a mental burden.

Listed below are the reasons why the 6 skilled workers with over 4 years' experience found it difficult to monitor the senior residents.

- Monitoring 30 to 40 senior residents places a mental burden on them.
- They becomes sensitive to little sounds and voices.
- They find it difficult to handle hyperactive senior residents

Figures 4 and 7 respectively show particular times of day when the 10 unskilled workers and 6 skilled workers found it difficult senior residents (Fig. 5).

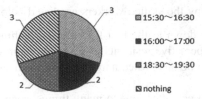

Fig. 4. Most difficult time to monitor senior residents (unskilled caregivers)

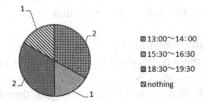

Fig. 5. Most difficult time to monitor senior residents (skilled caregivers)

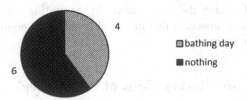

Fig. 6. Most difficult day of a week to monitor senior residents (unskilled caregivers)

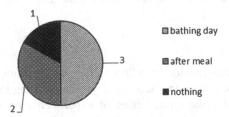

Fig. 7. Most difficult day of a week to monitor senior residents (skilled caregivers)

The reasons put forward by the unskilled workers are listed below:

- All caregivers are busy during bathing time.
- With taking senior residents to tables and preparing their meals after bathing time, they do not have time to do other tasks.
- When cleaning up tables after meals and administering medicine dosages, the senior residents tend to be hyperactive.

The reasons put forward by the skilled workers are listed below:

- Most caregivers come down to the first floor during bathing time and cannot take immediately assist hyperactive residents or residents requesting toilets.
- The caregivers have to be alert when administering medication doses and cleaning up tables.
- The caregivers need to pay attentions to many things, such as taking seniors to the toilet or bed.

As shown in Fig. 2, only two new staff selected "very poor" in response to the first question. Half of the new staff and skilled workers answered "okay". This is an unexpected result, because the author expected that most caregivers would answer "poor".

Considering these results, monitoring does not include physical contact with senior residents. This means that there is less risk of care-induced mistakes. We presumed that most caregivers feel that they must be careful only if the senior residents tend to be active. As shown in Fig. 4, some new staff answered that they have no particular time of day when they feel challenged monitoring the senior residents. Comparing the results in Figs. 6 and 7, more new staff answered that they do not have any particular day or time that they feel challenged monitoring the senior residents. This means that the new staff cannot predict the risks caused by neglecting "monitoring the senior residents". 44 % of staff answered that they feel challenged monitoring the senior on days when they bathe them.

3 Verifying the Monitoring Skills of New Caregivers

3.1 Subjects

The subjects were four new caregivers working on the same floor in the nursing home. The average age was 22.3 years old. 3 were male and 1 was female.

3.2 Survey Method

The survey was conducted in a hall on a floor in the nursing home from 3:30 – 4:30 pm on a bathing day. We observed the new caregivers monitoring the senior residents by themselves. We recorded the entire series of experiments on a video camera. We repeated the same procedure for each of the four subjects. After recording, we conducted individual interviews with each of the subjects.

Figure 8 shows the allocation in a hall where a new caregiver is engaged in monitoring the senior residents by him/herself.

Although there were differences in the numbers of senior residents during the four survey times, an average number of 26 senior residents in wheel chairs spent time around the tables. The new staff member was engaged in monitoring the senior residents by him/herself.

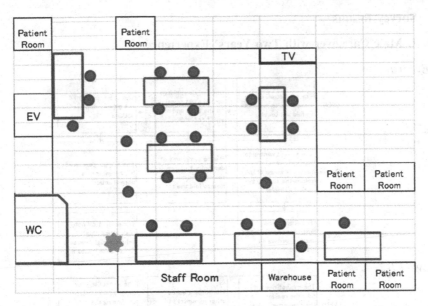

Fig. 8. The allocation in a hall in the nursing home (★ New staff ● Senior residents in wheel chairs spending time near tables)

All events which happened when the staff member was monitoring were clarified using an "event flow chart" based on the RCA (Root Cause Analysis). We also evaluated their "monitoring skills" based on their interviews. The author experienced both the old and the new admission systems; in the old system, administrative institutions allocated the elderly to nursing homes, and in the new system, the admission contract can be made directly between the elderly and the nursing home. The author observed the survey from the viewpoint of an administrator; thus, the evaluation results had the potential to bias.

In order to evaluate objectively, we asked two care managers with more than 5 years working experiences, who are now engaged in different tasks in care service, to observe and evaluate the survey.

Care Manage 1: Male, 29 years old. After 6 years of work experience, he obtained a care manager license and now has two years' experience working as a care manager.

Care Manager 2: Female, 49 years old, has nursing license. After 5 years of work experience, she obtained a care manager license and now has more than 10 years' experience working as a care manager.

*Care Manager 2 has experienced both the old and the new admission systems, just like the author.

3.3 Survey Results

Case 1: Male Caregiver with Two Years' Experience

Event 1-1

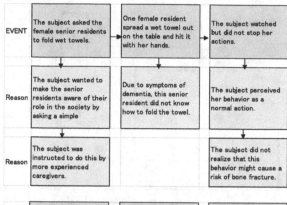

Event 1-2

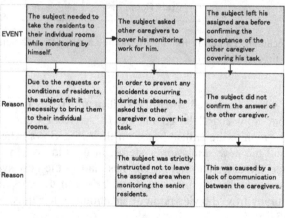

Event 1-3

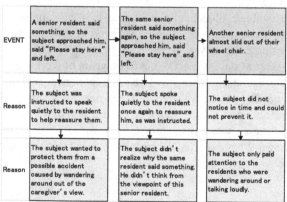

(Case 1 (Evaluation of Monitoring Skills assessed by Interviewing the Subject))

- The subject can react based on the rules specified in the manuals. His intellectual level is high.
- The subject does not think about "Why senior residents take these actions", or "Why they say such things."

He is not accustomed to think from the viewpoint of the senior residents.

- The subject is less skilled and less experienced at predicting the occurrence of risks.

CM1

- Without thinking about the reason, the subject said "Please stay here" in a nonchalant attitude.
- The subject just followed the method of the skilled caregivers, but he is not accustomed to thinking why the senior residents wanted to move.

CM2

- The subject was less considerate to the behavior or comments of the senior residents. He just reacted in an impromptu manners, so he could not predict accidents.

Case 2: Female Caregiver with Two Years' Experience

Event 2-1

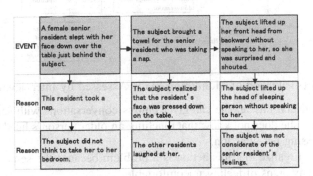

(Case 2 (Evaluation of Monitoring Skills assessed by Interviewing the Subject))

- The subject could not think from the viewpoint of the senior residents.
- The subject can react based on the rules specified in the manuals, but she was less conscious of predicting risks.

CM1

- Lifting a head of sleeping person without speaking to them is prohibited. I feel that it is necessary to teach this subject "common sense actions".
- The reasons that this subject failed to speak to the elderly residents is because she does not know the importance of these rules and words.

CM2

- Of course, anybody would be surprised or upset if someone touched their face while they were sleeping. She is less considerate of other's feeling. This makes me very uneasy because this action is not appropriate for a caregiver.
- The subject lacks the skills to predict risks. She also lacks the ability to think from another person's perspective.

Case 3: Male Caregiver with One Year of Experience
No event happened when this subject was monitoring the senior residents. We picked up this event when the female caregiver with two years' working experience went through the hall.

Event 3-1

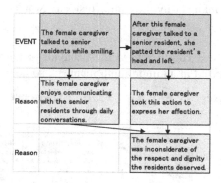

(Case 3 (Evaluation of Monitoring Skills Assessed by Interviewing the Subject))

- It is good that this female caregiver enjoys conversations with senior residents.
- However, she does not know that touching an older person's head is rude, even if it is expressing her affection.
- She didn't realize that this action is a problem because the senior resident did not display any signs of feeling uncomfortable.

CM1

- I understand that she likes residents, but she should refrain from acting like this in front of others.

CM2

- She was not offensive, but she does not know the rules for how to appropriately communicate with the residents.
- She was inconsiderate of the respect and dignity the residents deserved. These kinds of staff exist in every elderly care facility, not just this nursing home.

Case 4: Male Caregiver with One Year of Experience

Event 4-1

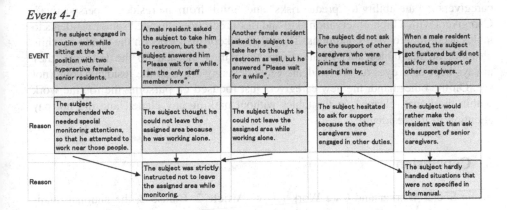

(Case 4 (Evaluation of Monitoring Skills Assessed by Interviewing the Subject))

- The subject has a high awareness for pursuing the assignments according to the manual, but he has less applied skill.
- The subject did not think from the perspective of "If I were him/her".
- The subject knows the philosophy to prioritize senior residents always, but he was overwhelmed by hesitance to ask for the support of senior caregivers.

CM1

- It is understandable that the subject would rather cause trouble for the residents than bother his senior caregivers. But considering the feeling of the residents, there were other solutions. For example, if the senior caregivers told the new staff "Please call us anytime when you need help", the new caregiver should feel it easy to monitor by himself.

CM2

- Caregivers feel stress when using the word "Please wait for a while". Having firm emotional strength to handle any irregular situations is necessary.

4 Discussion and Results

In modern nursing homes, people in more severe states are given priority when admitted to facilities. Thus, the contents of care services becomes more complex and multiplied, and "end of life" care service is also required of the facilities. In such situations, caregivers engage in daily work with a lot of pressure. Every caregiver bears the risk of a fall occurring when they are on monitoring duty by him/herself. While caregivers say "We are anxious about preventing accidents from happening", we did not feel any sense of crisis from all the new staff who engaged in monitoring in this research. In fact, one resident had a fall occur during the research.

We observed skilled caregivers engaged in monitoring in the same hall on different days, and we realized that the obvious differences between skilled and unskilled caregivers are the ability to "predict risks" and "think from the residents' perspective". Caregivers with a high observation skill and risk prediction allocated senior residents to tables according to their conditions. They always kept their eyes on the residents while cleaning up the tables after meals. Even when they cleaned up the leftovers, they always kept their eyes on the residents while devising ways so the residents could not see. On the other hand, the new caregivers just focused on pursuing the routine work within the hours, cleaned up the tables without making any clatter, and did not pay attention to the residents.

5 Conclusion

In the Social Worker and Care Worker Law, Article 2, Clause 2, the national qualification for care workers is defined as; "Under the name of care worker, care worker means a person with special knowledge and techniques who provides care services for bathing, excretion and diet to persons who are unable to engage in daily life due to physical or mental disabilities, or who engages in the instruction of care services to caregivers". The legal definition of nursing care is sufficient with this definition. However, the author feels the importance to take more time to teach new caregivers about the comprehensive knowledge concerning diseases and dementia when hiring. We proposed to give the opportunity to new caregivers to learn "Why this care service is necessary", and "How to devise a care method according to the symptoms of diseases". In order to improve their skills in monitoring senior residents, it is necessary to provide more educational opportunities in considering the feelings of senior residents from their perspective.

References

1. The 2012 White Paper on Aged Society, in the page 2, Cabinet Office
2. Turnover Rates of Nursing Care Staff and Home Visit Care Staff from "Care Work Factual Investigation", Care Work Foundation
3. The Self-Evaluation Implementation Status of Each Facility base on "Common Evaluation Standards for the Facilities for Disabled and Juvenile" of 2012 version, in P141 in Appendix 3
4. The Operation Manual of the special elderly nursing home, Zuikouen, clause "Communications" in P12-1
5. The New Dementia Care – Practical Version-P9, Dementia Care Information Network, Tokyo Research Center, Chuohoki Publishing Co., Ltd
6. The Practical Manual for RCA Fundamental Reason Analysis, Use of Recurrence Prevention and Medical Safety Educaton, Igaku-Shoin
7. Factor Analysis of Incident/Accident Case – Case Analysis Exercise, Medical Risk Management Division, Sompo Japan Nipponkoa Insurance Inc
8. Medical Safety Administrator Training Course Seminar Material in 2014, All Japan Hospital Association

Research on the Performance of Three Tea Whisks of "The Way of Tea" with Different Experience

Soutatsu Kanazawa[1], Tomoko Ota[2], Zelong Wang[3(✉)], Akihiro Tada[3],
Yuka Takai[4], Akihiko Goto[4], and Hiroyuki Hamada[3]

[1] Urasenke Konnichian, Kyoto, Japan
kanazawa.kuromon.1352.gentatsu@docomo.ne.jp
[2] Chuo Business Group, Osaka, Japan
Tomoko.ota@k.vodafone.ne.jp
[3] Advanced Fibro-Science, Kyoto Institute of Technology, Kyoto, Japan
simon.zelongwang@gmail.com
[4] Department of Information Systems Engineering, Osaka Sangyo University, Osaka, Japan
gotoh@ise.osaka-sandai.ac.jp

Abstract. In this paper, three kinds of Japanese tea whisks' influence on bubble form in "the way of tea" process were investigated. The bubble form and distribution state by each whisk after 30 %, 50 %, 80 % and 100 % of tea making finishing time were recorded and analyzed through numerical processing. In order to verify the quality of tea whisk, two tea masters were employed as expert and non-expert, and three kinds of tea whisks' performance were evaluated and compared during the whole tea making process. The expert can controlled three tea whisks very well.

Keywords: The way of tea · Tea whisk · Bubble form · Japanese tea

1 Introduction

Japanese tea ceremony is developed based on "daily after-meal". "The Way of Tea", also called the "Japanese tea ceremony", is a special ceremonial art preparation and presentation of "Matcha" (a kind of green tea powder) to entertain the guests, through the tea ceremony people will achieve temperament, improve the cultural quality and aesthetic view. The essence of "The Way of Tea" is meant to demonstrate reverence and respect between host and guest, both of them can truly experience the artistic conception and taste the most primitive taste of green tea during tea-tasting activity and service process with the tallest state of the etiquette.

"The Way of Tea" is consisted of many specific and strict procedures, whose basic skill just only handed over by oral instructions by expert. Furthermore, the spirit of modern Japanese tea ceremony extends to the exterior and interior decoration of the "Tea house". Appreciating the painting and calligraphy decorated in the "Tea house", enjoying the gardening design and tea pottery are also the important parts in the "The Way of Tea". Among them, using Japanese Tea-whisks stir the tea powder to mixing uniformity and make sure the infusion of the tea leaves combined with the water is the

© Springer International Publishing Switzerland 2015
V.G. Duffy (Ed.): DHM 2015, Part I, LNCS 9184, pp. 95–103, 2015.
DOI: 10.1007/978-3-319-21073-5_10

highest technique and important process, which directly affected was directly affected the taste of tea.

As a an important tool for "The Way of Tea", there appeared some genre of tea whisks with distinguishing shape features and many representative "The Way of Tea" arts masters during the long course of its development. Different genre of tea whisks exhibit has great influence on the development of Japanese tea ceremony. However, the different shapes of tea whisks have different mixing effects and impacts in the whole process of tea making. Basically, tea's mixing uniformity is characteristic by bubble size and distribution attached on the tea surface.

Different tea whisks have different use skills caused by its special shape. Therefore, in order to obtain a delicious cup of tea mixed homogeneously between the green tea power and the hot water the tea masters have to study and practice for a long time to master and understand the performance of tea whisk very well. However, until now the scientific evaluation for the quality of tea whisk is limited. But above all, it's very difficult for every master to inherit the essentials of tea whisks using method to the next generation without an effective way.

In previous research, an excellent tea master from Kyoto was selected as a unique participator called expert. 3 types tea whisks with different shape were investigated as the subject, they were called "Yabunouchi", "Kankyuan", "Ensyu". According to the record of investigation during tea ceremony process, each process's point of degree of mixing and bubble distribution were focused, relationship between timeliness and different tea whisks were extracted and analyzed according to each process, 30 %, 50 %, 80 % and 100 % of tea making finishing time.

In this research, expert and non-expert with different experience years were employed as the behavior subject. The three types of different tea whisks as the same with previous research, "Yabunouchi", "Kankyuan", "Ensyu" were paid attention. During test performance, the difference of formed bubbles distribution on the tea surface and temperature variation with different 3 types were inspected and recorded. The characteristic of bubble distribution and the performance of tea whisks were discussed. The bubble form and distribution state after 30 %, 50 %, 80 % and 100 % of tea making finishing time described by recording photos were transferred by numerical processing. Finally, understanding and knowledge of three types of tea whisks by expert and non-expert were observed and compared according to the bubble distribution situation.

As well known, no matter use what kind of tea whisks, the final bubble distribution was one of most important features for a tasty tea, which depend on the bubble size, distribution and so on. On the other hand, the bubble forming process was also reflected the characteristics of the tea whisks' performance.

In a word, this study was focus on the bubble distribution situations of three types tea whisks between expert and non-expert. Through numerical processing and analyzing, the performance characteristics of three types tea whisks during the whole making process were summarized and compared. It is notify that expert can master the performance of three types of tea compared with non-expert, and made excellent cups of tea with small bubble. The expert's differences and characteristic of bubble forming process on the way of tea were revealed and also delivered to non-experts and beginners consequently (Fig. 1).

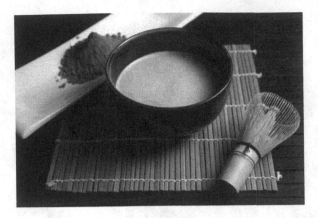

Fig. 1. The way of tea

2 Experiment

2.1 Participants

Two Japanese tea masters from Kyoto were employed as the participants. One of the participants had more than 30 years experience in "the way of tea", who can keep the motion of scooping water and ensure the added water weight in the bowl nearly the same for each tea making process, which was called as expert in this paper. Other participant had 20 years experience as called non-expert.

2.2 Subjects

Three types of Japanese tea whisks were selected for proceeding the experiment called as "Yabunochi", "Kankyuan", "Ensyu", which were the three tea whisks in Japan as shown in Fig. 2.

2.3 Experimental Process

1.5 g of "Matcha" tea power and approximate 56 g of hot water were dumped into the bowl, and the moisture content of tea was controlled at approximately 97 % steadily.

Four time stages including 30 %, 50 %, 80 % and 100 % of tea making finishing time were focused and investigated for the tea made by three kinds of tea whisks. And bubble form and distribution state after 30 %, 50 %, 80 % and 100 % of tea making procedure were also recorded and illustrated by single-lens reflex camera (D40x Nikon CO. Ltd). Especially, in order to obtain high-quality photographs a camera device was employed to support and fix the camera as shown in Fig. 3.

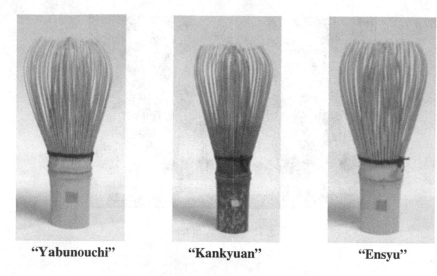

"Yabunouchi"   "Kankyuan"   "Ensyu"

Fig. 2. Three types of Japanese tea whisks

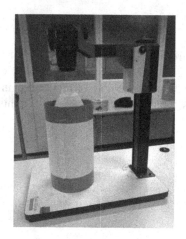

Fig. 3. Camera device

2.4 Image Processing

In this research, all the photos were transformed into the same size as the size of the bowl (Diameter: 12.6 cm) firstly. Afterwards, circle region of all bowl were analyzed and transferred by numerical processing from Fig. 4(a) to (b). It should be mentioned that only bubble forms larger than 0.02 mm^2 area was marked. Furthermore, marked bubbles were transformed by the binarization processing method into a white and black two colors as shown in Fig. 4(c). The outlines of bubble form and bubbles' distribution state were also sketched on the processed image. Finally, the areas of the bubbles were calculated and converted to the area unit.

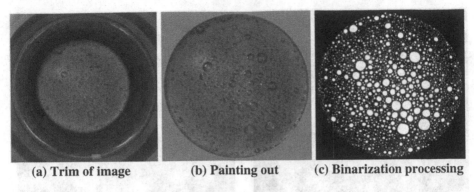

(a) Trim of image   (b) Painting out   (c) Binarization processing

Fig. 4. Procedure of image processing

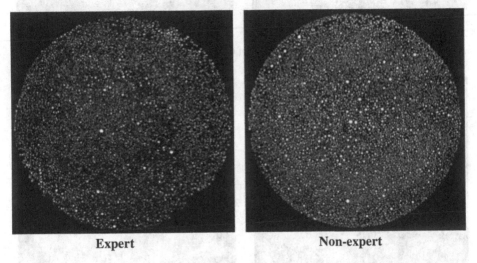

Expert   Non-expert

Fig. 5. The 100 % stage bubble distribution of expert and non-expert made by "Yabunouchi"

3 Results and Discussions

The final proceeded products of expert and non-expert at 100 % stage by expert and non-expert was illustrated on Figs. 5, 6 and 7. The bubbles sizes of expert and non-expert after mixing by three tea whisks were concentrated in the 1 mm^2. However, all the bubbles of expert made by three tea whisks were presented smaller sizes, which had more bubble's size closed to the range of 0.02 mm^2 – 0.1 mm^2. On the contrast, the non-expert's bubbles showed few larger sizes after mixing by applying "Ensyu" tea whisk.

Because expert can controlled the three types tea whisks to obtain the excellent final tea products. Therefore, the Bubbles' size and the distribution made by expert for "Yabunouchi" tea whisks in four time stages including 30 %, 50 %, 80 % and 100 % of tea making process were presented as example in Fig. 8. The Bubbles' size and the distribution made by non-expert for three tea whisks, "Yabunouchi", "Kankyuan",

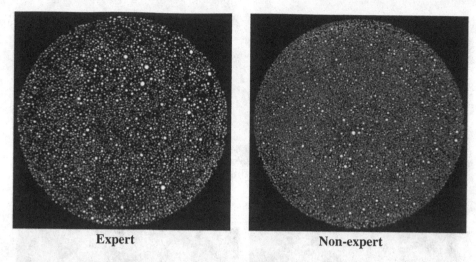

Expert   Non-expert

Fig. 6. The 100 % stage bubble distribution of expert and non-expert made by "Kankyuan"

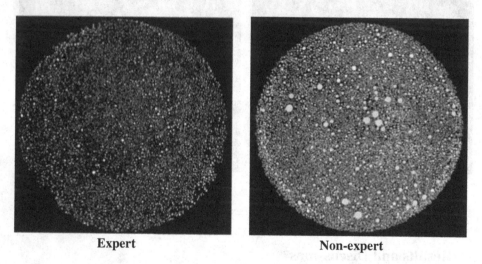

Expert   Non-expert

Fig. 7. The 100 % stage bubble distribution of expert and non-expert made by "Ensyu"

"Ensyu", in four time stages including 30 %, 50 %, 80 % and 100 % of tea making process were presented in Figs. 9, 10 and 11.

In following figure, the horizontal axis shows the area of the bubble by the logarithm scale and the vertical axis shows the bubble size frequency. According to Fig. 5, in case of expert, it can be found that expert was able to produce larger area of bubble at the beginning of tea making procedure as shown in the case of 30 % time. And areas of bubble produced by three kinds of tea whisks were showed similar distribution in the case of 50 %. And it is easy to find that the bubbles existed in the 50 % case was decreased significantly compared with 30 % case. All bubble size was concentrated in less then 1 mm^2.

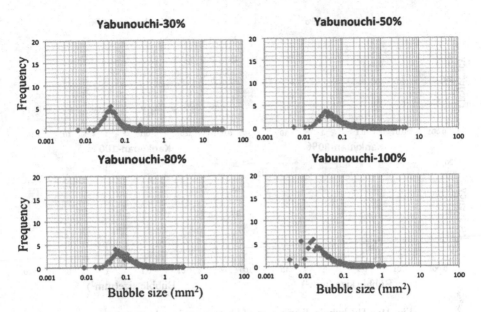

Fig. 8. The bubble distribution of "Yabunouchi" made by expert

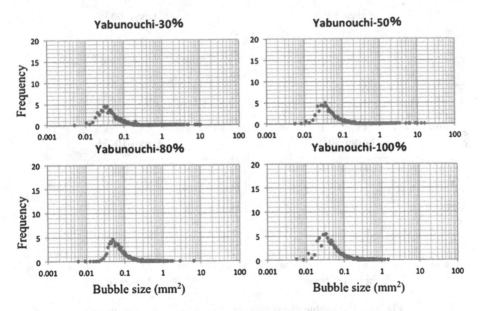

Fig. 9. The bubble distribution of "Yabunouchi" made by non-expert

However, in case of non-expert, the large bubble only can produce by tea whisk of "Ensyu". And the medium sized bubbles were appeared intensively for the same 30 % time case for "Yabunouchi" and "Kankyuan" as shown in Figs. 6 and 7. In additionally, the areas of bubble by all tea whisks, "Yabunouchi", "Kankyuan" and "Ensyu", were

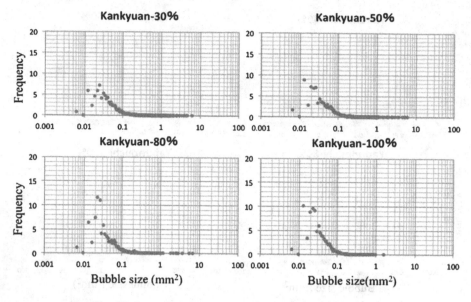

Fig. 10. The bubble distribution of "Kankyuan" made by non-expert

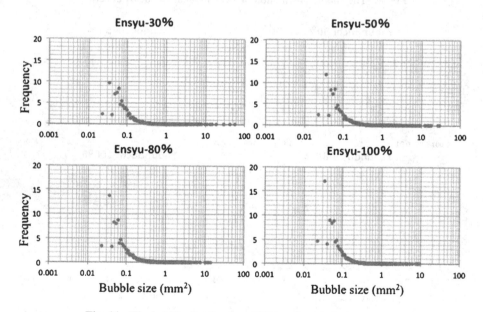

Fig. 11. The bubble distribution of "Ensyu" made by non-expert

just showed a slight decreasing trend in the case of 50 % and 80 %. It is deserved to find that the majority of bubbles existed in the non-expert's tea whisk produced by all three kinds of tea whisks are almost below 1 mm^2 when time stage increased to 100 %. Comparing non-expert's final product made by three tea whisks, the tea whisk of "Yabunochi" was presented the wider distribution of small bubbles even if can not reach the level of expert. The performance of "Kankyuan" was close to "Yabunouchi", which the tendency of 100 % stage was similar with "Yabunouchi".

4 Conclusions

In a word, the expert can controlled the three tea whisks very well, which all the bubble distribution of final products was concentrated on the small size. All final tea products were better than non-expert. However, expert can obtain the ideal final tea products by tea whisks of "Yabunouchi" and "Kankyuan". The final tea product of non-expert made by tea whisk of "Ensyu" was not shown a good surface in the end.

References

1. Tujimoto, N., Ichihashi, Y., Iue, M., Ota, T., Hamasaki, K., Nakai, A., Goto, A.: Comparison of bubble forming in a bowl of thin tea between expert and non-expert. In: Proceedings of the 11 th Japan International Sampe Symposium and Exhibiton (2009)
2. Goto, A., Endo, A., Narita, C., Takai, Y., Shimodeand, Y., Hamada, H.: Comparison of painting technique of Urushi products between expert and non-expert. In: Trzcielinski, S., Karwowski, W. (eds.) Advances in Ergonomics in Manufacturing, pp. 160–167. CRC Press, USA (2012). ISBN 978-1-4398-7039-6
3. Aiba, E., Kanazawa, S., Ota, T., Kuroda, K., Takai, Y., Goto, A., Hamada, H.: Developing a system to assess the skills of Japanese way of tea by analyzing the forming sound: A case study. In: Proceedings of the Human Factors and Ergonomics Society International Meeting (2013)

Effects of Quantified Instructional Tool on Spray-up Fabrication Method

Tetsuo Kikuchi[1,2(✉)], Erika Suzuki[1], Yiyi Zhang[2], Yuka Takai[3], Akihiko Goto[3], and Hiroyuki Hamada[2]

[1] Toyugiken Co., Ltd., Kanagwa, Japan
{tetuo-kikuchi, erika-suzuki}@toyugiken.co.jp
[2] Department of Advanced Fibro-Science, Kyoto Institute of Technology, Kyoto, Japan
choii0lll@yahoo.co.jp, hhamada@kit.ac.jp
[3] Osaka Sangyo University, Osaka, Japan
{takai,gotoh}@ise.osaka-sandai.ac.jp

Abstract. Spray up fabrication has been used for forming composite structures since ancient times as it can be performed as long as the mold, skills, and materials are available. Hence highly specialized control technique and the tradition of skill are required to ensure the consistent stability of product quality. In this study, the authors thus conducted a motion analysis experiment using spray-up fabrication experts as subjects. The experiment, seemingly a new and only attempt in Japan, quantified techniques that are not visibly apparent and considered to be tacit knowledge. The dimension stability of samples was measured, and their relationships with the motions of experts were also evaluated. It was also suggested that highly specialized control techniques, the appropriate training of non-experts, and technical tradition are possible.

Keywords: Spray up fabrication · Dimension stability · Motion analysis · Composites · Explicit knowledge

1 Introduction

In Spray up fabrication work, the characteristics of the composite material will be usually the same regardless of which forming method is used as long as the reinforced substrate, reinforcement morphology, matrix resin, and volume content of reinforcing material are the same. Composite materials, particularly fiber reinforced plastics (FRP) made of fibers and resins, are basically formed by impregnating fibers with resin, i.e., replacing the air contained in fibers with resin. Consequently, the impregnation method is expected to contribute to changes in the properties of the interface formed. To review the effects of different spray up technique on the mechanical properties of the composite structure, an experiment was conducted to analyze the process of work and investigate the relationships with mechanical strength and dimension stability of the structures built in craftsmen (experts and non-experts) specializing in making bathtubs using the spray up technique, who were asked to create FRP structures.

© Springer International Publishing Switzerland 2015
V.G. Duffy (Ed.): DHM 2015, Part I, LNCS 9184, pp. 104–113, 2015.
DOI: 10.1007/978-3-319-21073-5_11

2 Methodology

2.1 Subject Persons

In this study, two people were tested: an expert spray up craftsman (male, 42 years old, 19-year work career) and a non-expert (male, 37 years old, 1-year work career). The biological data of the subjects is shown in Table 1. Both subjects were right handed, and didn't have physical handicaps or a disease that restricted their work. The purpose and method of this study were explained in advance to the subjects. Their consent to participate was obtained.

Table 1. Biological data of subjects

Subject	Age	Years experience	Height (cm)	Weight (kg)	Dominant- hand
Expert	42	19	162	65	right
Non-expert	37	1	166	70	right

2.2 Measurement Techniques

Motion analysis and eye movement measuring were done from start to finish for the entire work process. The experiment was performed under the same circumstances as their usual workplace so that the subjects could work as normal. Moreover, instructions—except restrictions for measurement—were omitted so that the subjects could work at their own pace. In addition, three-dimensional motion and eye movements were measured separately.

2.3 Analysis Objective

The object of the analysis was to evaluate the work done for fabricated composites using the spray up method. The size of the mold was 1820 mm high and 910 mm wide. A blue rectangle (1250 mm × 800 mm) was drawn on the 1 square meter spray region. In addition, in this experiment, it was presupposed that the process of degassing (pressing down with a roller after completely spraying on the resin and the roving) would not be done. Since the surface smoothness and thickness distribution vary greatly through control of a roller, in this research only spray up skills were evaluated (Fig. 1).

2.4 Spray up Method

The spray up machine that was used was made in Japan. The quantities and conditions of the spray up method were:
    Amount of resin sprayed on : 2044 [g/min].
    Amount of glass fiber sprayed on : 1080 [g/min].

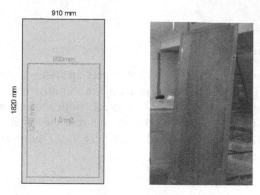

Fig. 1. Mold used in this study (1820 mm high, 910 mm wide)

Spread angle of resin : 200 mm / 500 mm.

Here, the glass fiber was in a continuation filament cut into 4 or 25 mm strands, and then sprayed on. As a base material, glass roving was used, as well as isophthalic unsaturated polyester resin.

2.5   Three-Dimensional Motion Measurement

Three-dimensional motion measurement was performed using an optical real-time motion capturing system, the MAC 3D System (manufactured by Motion Analysis Corporation). Before measurements were taken, in order to acquire the three-dimensional coordinates of markers, an L-shaped frame (with infrared markers attached) was shot and the calibration of the shooting range was performed using a T-shaped wand (with two infrared markers attached). A total of 19 infrared reflective markers were attached to the subjects' bodies. Similarly, three markers were attached to the tool. The position of each marker was captured with six cameras (manufactured by Motion Analysis Corporation), and the three-dimensional position data of all the markers was synchronously downloaded to a PC (sampling rate: 120 Hz). Moreover, the data from one digital video camera was also simultaneously synchronized. Here, the x axis was defined as perpendicular to the spray direction. The y axis was defined as the spray direction and the z axis was defined as the height. For data processing, the coordinate data from the 19 markers attached to each joint was obtained using EvaRT Ver. 5.0.4 software (manufactured by Motion Analysis Corporation).

2.6   Eye Movement Measurement

Eye movement measurement was performed using TalkEyeII (manufactured by Takei Scientific Instruments Co., Ltd.) for analyzing eye movement. A goggle-like apparatus was worn by the subjects. The subjects' point of view was captured with the camera from the center of both eyes, and two cameras detected the point of view. The sampling rate was 30 Hz. Moreover, a digital video camera was used to record the motion of objects. Cameras were arranged so that the motion could be captured clearly.

2.7   Dimensional Stability

To compare the dimensional stability of the expert and non-expert, the surface coarseness of the plane of the acquired molded product was measured. A micrometer was used for measuring thickness. All samples (1250 mm × 800 mm) obtained in the experiment were cut and divided into 16 sections. Moreover, the thickness of the cross section of each area was measured every 10 mm. About 1,110 data points were obtained per subject.

3   Results and Considerations

3.1   Dimensional Stability

The dimensional stability (thickness distribution) of the expert and non-expert are shown in Fig. 2. The classification by color in the figure is every 1.0 mm.

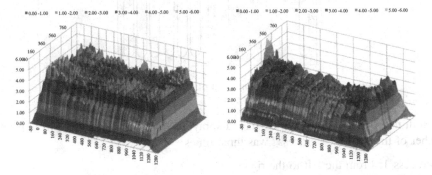

Fig. 2. Comparison of thickness distribution (left: expert, right: non-expert)

The expert's average thickness was 3.52 mm and the coefficient of variation (CV) value was 11.4 %. On the other hand, the average thickness for the non-expert was 2.47 mm and the CV value was 16.2 %. As the theoretical thickness of this study was 3.50 mm, the non-expert's thickness distribution was thin and the CV value was also large. The CV value of the horizontal cross-sectional thickness for the non-expert was especially high. This thickness came from overlapping strokes or an inconsistent speed. Moreover, the ends of the horizontal sections were extremely thin.

The thickness distribution of the superior extremity and the lower end shows that the expert had precise thickness control. Therefore, the expert's loss of spray also decreased. In addition, to refine the spray up method, there needs to be a consistent coefficient of variation of less than 10 %. Improving the spray up technology would substantially contribute to dimensional stability and reduced waste.

3.2   Process Analysis

First, each motion under work was defined, and could be divide into two motions: first the "stroke" and second the "process." The "stroke" was defined as the reciprocating movement of the spray in the height direction of the mold and the "process" was defined as the movement one way in the horizontal direction of the mold by repetitive "strokes" (Fig. 3).

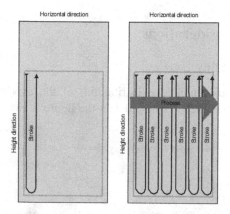

Fig. 3. Definition of "stroke" and "process"

Both the expert and non-expert started spraying from the upper left. For both, the number of times of the "process" was three times.

Process 1: From the left to the right.
Process 2: From the right to the left.
Process 3: From the left to the right.

The number of "strokes" in each process is compared (Table 2).

In process 1 and 2, the expert took seven strokes. On the other hand, the non-expert took five and six strokes. In process 3, the expert took six strokes, and the non-expert took nine. The number of strokes made by the non-expert in each process varied although the number of strokes made by the expert was consistent.

Table 2. The number of strokes

	Expert	Non-expert
Process 1	7	6
Process 2	7	5
Process 3	6	9

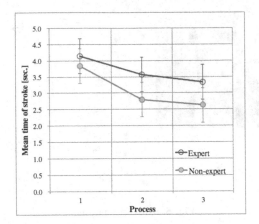

Fig. 4. The mean work time per stroke for each process

Next, the mean work time of the stroke in each process was compared (Fig. 4). The mean work time of the expert and non-expert shortened with the increase in process. The expert's mean work time was short by 19.5 %. On the other hand, the non-expert was short by no less than 31.5 %. That is, the spray per stroke gradually became faster.

3.3 Motion Analysis

The operations at the time of the spraying by the expert and non-expert were compared. Attention was paid to the motion of the lower half of the body. The difference in motion was especially noted. Here, the x axis is defined as the direction perpendicular to the spray. The y axis is defined as the spray direction. And the z axis is defined as the height direction (Fig. 5).

First, the change in the position of the knees in the y-z coordinates is shown in Fig. 6.

This figure shows the displacement of the knees from start to finish. The expert was moving his right knee smoothly. The non-expert showed no such movement during the spray-up

Next, the angle variations between the knee, greater trochanter and shoulder (right side) are shown in Fig. 7.

The expert had a wide angle variation (wide arc) and it turns out that this is the stable angle variation. Moreover, it is clear that the expert is further "crooked" by about 20 degrees, and it turns out that the "crookedness expansion movement" for each stroke by the expert was performed smoothly. That is, the expert is performing the "crookedness expansion movement" efficiently while on tiptoes. An image of an angle variation is shown in Fig. 8.

The difference in the angle variation can be clearly seen from this figure. Moreover, the motion of the non-expert placed a burden on the body, preventing a smooth motion.

Next, the change in the position in the x-z coordinates for the top of the spray-gun (Fig. 9).

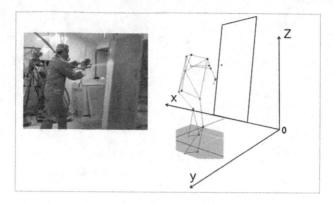

Fig. 5. Motion analysis

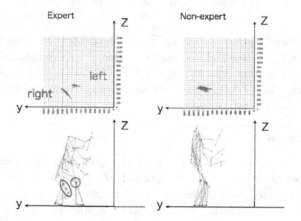

Fig. 6. Motion analysis (left : Expert, Right :Non-expert)

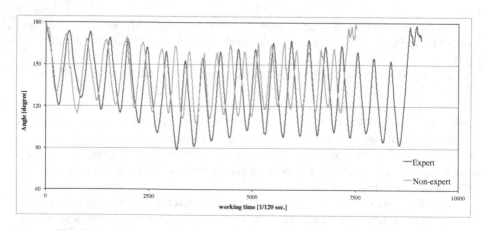

Fig. 7. Angle between the knee, greater trochanter and shoulder (right side)

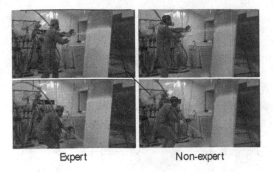

Expert   Non-expert

Fig. 8. Image of angle variation

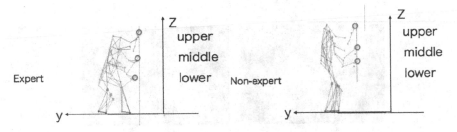

Fig. 9. Trace of spray-gun

Here, maintaining constant distance from the mold was thought to be a basic part of producing FRP with consistent thickness. On the other hand, as a result of motion analysis, we found that the non-expert followed the basic rules in all processes, while the expert went against this guideline. The expert visually checked the thickness and areas of the spray on the mold and adjusted his distance accordingly. A uniform thickness distribution is only possible by adjusting the distance from the mold in real time. The non-expert, on the other hand, paid too much attention to keeping his distance from the mold constant, and missed his mark. The trace and thickness of his resulting product were not consistent. Also, the amount of discharged resin from spray-gun varies significantly depending on temperature, humidity and production lot and so on. The expert was able to adjust to these tiny changes and precisely change his technique. This is what we consider expert spray-up technique (Fig. 10).

3.4 Eye Movement Analysis

A comparison of the points of view of the expert and non-expert is shown in Fig. 11. The expert's point of view was stable and the path of the point of view matches the path of the stroke. On the other hand, it is clear that the non-expert's eye movement is not smooth.

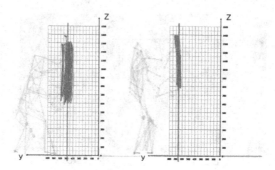

Fig. 10. Comparison of the change in the position in the y-z coordinates for the top of the spray-gun (left: expert, right: non-expert).

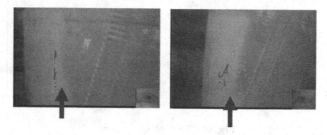

Fig. 11. Comparison of points of view (left: expert, right: non-expert)

4 Conclusions

Analysis of the spray up method revealed the following:

1. The expert smoothly bent and extended his body with each stroke.
2. The "bend and extend movement" was more efficient because the operator was standing on his tiptoes, allowing greater reach and flexibility.
3. The expert always observed the thickness of resin on the mold. He produced a uniform thickness distribution by adjusting the distance between the gun and mold in real time.
4. The expert's point of regard was stable, and the path of the point of regard matched the path of the stroke.
5. Moreover, the expert's motion data could be fed to a spray up robot, resulting in minimal errors during fabrication of composite.

Acknowledgements. Special thanks to KIT members.

References

1. Kikuchi, T., Koyanagi, T., Hamada, H., Nakai, A., Takai, Y., Goto, A., Fujii, Y., Narita, C., Endo, A., Koshino, T.: Biomechanics investigation of skillful technician in hand lay up fabrication method. In: ASME 2012 International Mechanical Engineering Congress & Exposition, Houston, Texas, USA, IMECE2012-86270, pp. 288 (2012)
2. Karimi, A., Manteufel, R.: Understanding why engineering students take too long to garaduate. In: ASME 2013 International Mechanical Engineering Congress & Exposition, San Diego, California, USA, IMECE2013-65367 (2013)
3. Miller, A., Samples, J.: Building a community – how to enrich an engineering technology program whith identity, presence and pride. In: ASME 2013 International Mechanical Engineering Congress & Exposition, San Diego, California, USA, IMECE2013-65034 (2013)
4. Kobus, C.J.: Storytelling – a most powerful tool in shaping lesson plans in engineering education. In: ASME 2013 International Mechanical Engineering Congress & Exposition, San Diego, California, USA, IMECE2013-65604 (2013)
5. Zhang, Z., Yang, Y., Hamada, H.: Mechanical property of glass mat composite with open hole. In: ASME 2012 International Mechanical Engineering Congress & Exposition, Houston, Texas, USA, IMECE2012-87270, pp. 79 (2012)
6. Shirato, M., Kume, M., Ohnishi, A., Nakai, A., Sato, H., Maki, M., Yoshida, T.: Analysis of daubing motion in the clay wall craftsman: Influence on several kinds of clay with different fermentation period on the daubing motion properties. In: Symposium on Sports Engineering: Symposium on Human Dynamics 2007, Japan, pp. 254–257 (2007)
7. Kikuchi, T., Fudauchi, A., Koshino, T., Narita, C., Endo, A., Hamada, H.: Mechanical property of CFRP by carbon spray up method. In: ASME 2013 International Mechanical Engineering Congress & Exposition, San Diego, California, USA, IMECE2013-64144, pp. 63 (2013)
8. Kikuchi, T., Hamada, H., Nakai, A., Ohtani, A., Goto, A., Takai, Y., Endo, A., Narita, C., Koshino, T., Fudauchi, A.: Relationships between degree of skill, dimension stability and mechanical properties of composites structure in hand lay-up method. In: 19th International Conference on Composite Materials, Montreal, Canada, pp. 8034–8042 (2013)

An Investigation on Conversion from Tacit Knowledge to Explicit Knowledge in Hand Lay-Up Fabrication Method

Tetsuo Kikuchi[1,2(✉)], Erika Suzuki[1], Yuka Takai[3], Akihiko Goto[3], and Hiroyuki Hamada[2]

[1] Toyugiken Co., Ltd., Kanagwa, Japan
{tetuo-kikuchi, erika-suzuki}@toyugiken.co.jp
[2] Department of Advanced Fibro-Science, Kyoto Institute of Technology, Kyoto, Japan
hhamada@kit.ac.jp
[3] Osaka Sangyo University, Osaka, Japan
{takai,gotoh}@ise.osaka-sandai.ac.jp

Abstract. Hand lay-up fabrication has been used for forming composite structures since ancient times as it can be performed as long as the mold, skills, and materials are available. Hence highly specialized control technique and the tradition of skill are required to ensure the consistent stability of product quality. In this study, the authors thus conducted a motion analysis experiment using hand lay-up fabrication experts as subjects. The experiment, seemingly a new and only attempt in Japan, quantified techniques that are not visibly apparent and considered to be tacit knowledge. The mechanical properties and dimension stability of samples were measured, and their relationships with the motions of experts were also evaluated. It was also suggested that highly specialized control techniques, the appropriate training of non-experts, and technical tradition are possible.

Keywords: Hand lay-up · Dimension stability · Motion analysis · Composites · Explicit knowledge

1 Introduction

In hand lay-up (HLU) fabrication work, the characteristics of the composite material will be usually the same regardless of which forming method is used as long as the reinforced substrate, reinforcement morphology, matrix resin, and volume content of reinforcing material are the same. Composite materials, particularly fiber reinforced plastics (FRP) made of fibers and resins, are basically formed by impregnating fibers with resin, i.e., replacing the air contained in fibers with resin. With the HLU technique, rollers are used to impregnate reinforced fibers with resin. Consequently, the impregnation method is expected to contribute to changes in the properties of the interface formed. To review the effects of different roller use in the HLU technique on the mechanical properties of the composite structure, an experiment was conducted to analyze the process of work and investigate the relationships with mechanical strength and dimension stability of the structures built in craftsmen (experts, intermediates, and

© Springer International Publishing Switzerland 2015
V.G. Duffy (Ed.): DHM 2015, Part I, LNCS 9184, pp. 114–123, 2015.
DOI: 10.1007/978-3-319-21073-5_12

non-experts) specializing in making bathtubs using the HLU technique, who were asked to create FRP structures.

2 Methodology

2.1 Subject Persons

The subjects consisted of a total of five craftsmen ranging from an expert with 25 years of experience to one with only one year of experience. In this experiment, the craftsman with 25 years of experience is defined as expert, one with only one year of experience as non-expert, and those in between as intermediates. Table 1 shows the biological data of the subjects.

2.2 Experimental Protocol

FRP laminate molding using the HLU technique was analyzed. Figure 1 shows the size of the mold used in this experiment: length of 415 mm, width of 1,600 mm, and height of 50 mm.

2.3 Materials

The mold surface was pre-coated with a gel coat (white) of 0.5 mm in thickness, after which lamination was carried out using the HLU technique. Glass fiber chopped strand mat (380 g/m2) was used as the reinforced substrate, and isophthalic unsaturated

Table 1. Biological data of subjects

Subject	Age	Career (year)	Height (cm)	Weight (kg)	Dominant-hand
Expert	48	25	171	52	Right
Intermediate-1	41	18	163	61	Right
Intermediate-2	45	15	175	63	Right
Intermediate-3	28	4	163	60	Right
Non-expert	29	1	164	52	Right

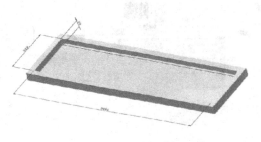

Fig. 1. Mold used in this study

polyester resin was used as the matrix. Cutting agent (MEKPO) was added to the resin at the ratio of 100 to 1.0. Two sheets of glass fiber chopped strand mats were used in the forming process.

2.4 Motion Analysis and Eye Movement Analysis

To measure the motion of the subjects, the MAC3D System (Motion Analysis Corporation) was used. The left side of Fig. 2 shows the motion analysis system. The infrared markers attached to the body of the subjects were captured using five cameras, and the collected information was sent to the PC as the 3D positional data of all the markers. The sampling frequency was set at 60 Hz. For eye movement, eye movement detector Talk Eye II (Takei Scientific Instruments Co., Ltd.) was used. The sampling frequency was set at 30 Hz. The right side of Fig. 2 shows the eye movement analysis system. The center camera was used to capture the field of vision of the subjects, while the cameras on both sides were used to capture eye movements.

2.5 Dimension Stability

To compare dimension stability between the expert and non-experts, the planar section and cross-sectional surface of the molded product obtained were observed (Fig. 3). A micrometer was used to measure the thickness. To compare the roughness of the surface of planar section, the 300 mm × 300 mm area in the center of the sample was measured. Subsequently, eight sections on the short side of the samples were cut out to observe the thickness distribution of the cross-section.

2.6 Mechanical Property

To evaluate mechanical property, twenty 150 mm × 30 mm specimens were sampled from the FRP molded product alternately in the lengthwise direction, as shown in Fig. 4. Two types of specimens were prepared: 10 with a drilled hole ($\varphi = 10$ mm) and 10 without a drilled hole. Because the drilled hole is easily damaged due to the

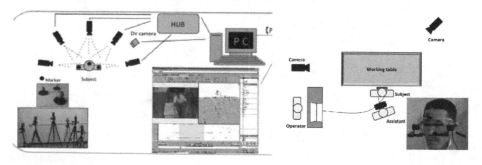

Fig. 2. Motion analysis and eye movement measurement systems in this experiment

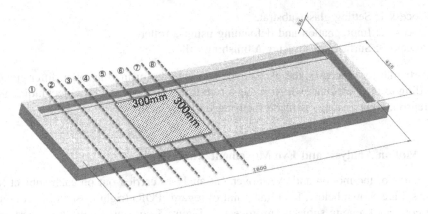

Fig. 3. Observation of dimension stability

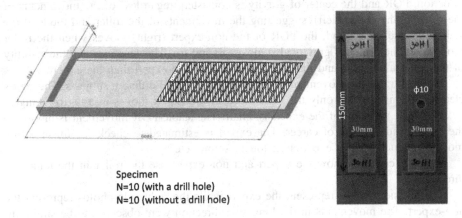

Specimen
N=10 (with a drill hole)
N=10 (without a drill hole)

Fig. 4. Sampling of specimens for tensile testing

concentration of stress, there existed some difference from the data of the non-porous specimens. However, punching must be carried out for attaching parts, etc. for products in the actual uses of FRP structures in the automotive and aerospace areas. In this experiment, strength tests using porous specimens were also conducted to evaluate the actual uses of FRP structures. The test conditions were inter-chuck distance of 80 mm, and crosshead speed of 1 mm/min.

3   Results and Considerations

3.1   Process Analysis

The analysis of the work process of HLU molding among craftsmen with different careers found that the work process can broadly be divided into three:

Process 1: Setting glass substrate.
Process 2: Impregnation and defoaming using a roller.
Process 3: Surface finish using a finishing roller.

Particular for process 3, the work time and method of using the roller differ greatly according to the craftsman, which is suggested to characterize the HLU technique. For this reason, comparison was made focusing on process 3.

3.2 Motion Analysis and Eye Movement Analysis

The results of the motion and eye movement analyses carried out on each subject for process 3 are shown below. First, the point of regard (POR) (right eye) and operations were compared among subjects in process 3. Figure 5 compares how the expert and non-expert use the roller in the short-side direction. The left photos represent the expert while the right photos represent a non-expert. During the movement in the short-side direction, POR and the center of gravity is consistent regardless of the movements of the roller in the expert (left), suggesting the movements of the roller and the load are stable. On the other hand, the POR of the non-expert (right) moves when the roller moves, and the center of gravity also moves to and fro. This suggests that the stability of the roller movement and load are poorer in the non-expert than the expert.

Figure 6 traces the movements of the right eye POR of different subjects. The charts clearly demonstrate that only the POR locus of the expert moves in a narrow range.

The POR variation of the expert is small. The stable-POR movement is unique to the expert, independent of career. The expert is estimated to check the finish of the molded product through experience, touch, sound, etc.

Figure 7 compares how the expert and non-expert use the roller in the long-side direction.

The left side photos represent the expert while the right side photos represent the non-expert. The movements in the long-side direction were observed to be similar to those in the short-side direction. Instead of following the movement of the roller, the expert (left) constantly looked ahead, and the to and fro variations of the center of gravity were limited. In contrast, the POR of the non-expert (right) moved together

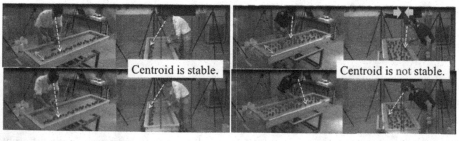

Expert   Non-expert

Fig. 5. How to use a roller between expert (left) and non-expert (right): short-side direction

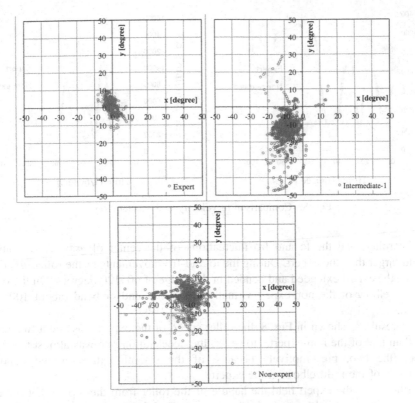

Fig. 6. Right-eye POR movements in subjects (process 3: during the motion in the short-side direction)

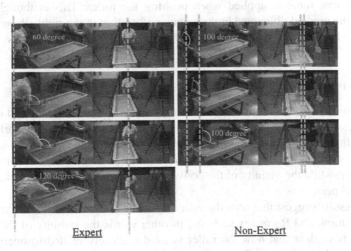

Fig. 7. How to use a roller between expert (left) and non-expert (right): long-side direction

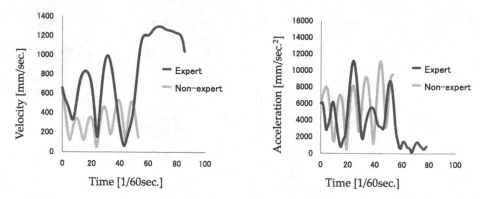

Fig. 8. Comparison of velocity and acceleration

with the roller, and the to and fro fluctuations of the center of gravity were about 2.5-fold larger than the expert. During the to-and-fro movements of the roller, the right elbow of the expert extended and bended in the range of 60–120 degrees. On the other hand, the elbow of the non-expert virtually did not extend or bend (about 100–110 degrees).

As a result, as shown in Fig. 8, the roller speed of the expert was about two times faster than that of the non-expert. However, the acceleration rate was almost the same between the two, presumptively because of the smooth extension and bending movements of the right elbow in the expert.

Furthermore, the expert held the handle of the roller from the top so that force is applied when pulling the roller. In fact, it was found later in interviews with the subjects that the expert tend to concentrate more on pulling than pushing the roller. On the other hand, the non-expert was found to hold the handle of the roller from below upwards so that force is applied when pushing the roller. This is thought to have resulted in the marked difference in the extension/bending of the right elbow and speed of the roller between the expert and non-expert.

3.3   Dimension Stability

Figure 9 shows the distribution of the thickness in the short-side direction. It is apparent that thickness is consistent (1.9 mm) for the expert even in the elevation surface and R convex section, while it is not consistent for the non-expert in the convex section and its vicinity, which are thought to be difficult to form. The convex section was about 15 % thinner, while the vicinity of the convex section was about 15 % thicker than the average thickness.

These results suggest that how the roller is used clearly affects the thickness of the planar, elevation, and R convex sections, in other words the stability of the shape. In addition, it is evident that how the roller is used is closely related to operations that define "career," as shown in Fig. 10.

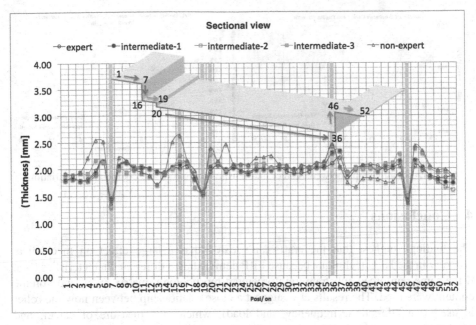

Fig. 9. Sectional view

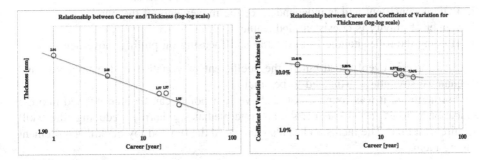

Fig. 10. Relationships between career and thickness or the coefficient of variation

3.4 Mechanical Property

The effects of career on mechanical property were investigated. Figure 11 shows the tensile strength and coefficient of variation, with respect to career, in specimens with and without drilled holes.

First, comparison of the tensile strength of specimens between the expert and non-expert indicates that it is about 15 % higher in the expert's specimen. In addition, a strong correlation was found between career and tensile strength (coefficient of correlation: 0.99 (NHT), 0.92 (OHT)). On the other hand, correlation was weak in the coefficient of variation (coefficient of correlation: −0.87 (NHT), −0.65 (OHT)).

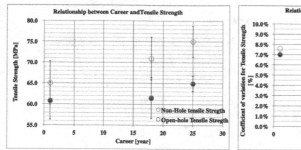
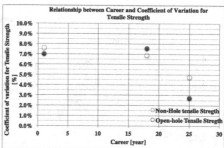

Fig. 11. Relationships between career and tensile strength or the coefficient of variation

4 Conclusions

The findings suggest that the craftsman's career has a large effect on mechanical property in the HLU technique because FRP demonstrated different characteristics even if the same reinforced substrate, reinforcement morphology, matrix resin, and volume content were used. The results also suggest a close relationship between how the roller is used (e.g., direction, frequency, and load), which is a measure of career, and mechanical property.

Characteristics of the expert can be summarized as follows:

1. Smooth movement of the right elbow during roller movements*.
2. POR is consistent and is independent of the movements of the hand.
3. Center of gravity is consistent and stable.
4. Holding the roller handle from the top and focusing on pulling movements.

*As force is evenly distributed, the coefficient of variation of the thickness and mechanical strength is estimated to be small.

Furthermore, it was found that the above four points can be incorporated into the educational tools of non-experts and intermediates, sharply reducing the skill acquirement time. The inclusion has also increased the fun and joy of skill acquirement among them.

Acknowledgements. Special thanks to KIT members.

References

1. Kikuchi, T., Koyanagi, T., Hamada, H., Nakai, A., Takai, Y., Goto, A., Fujii, Y., Narita, C., Endo, A., Koshino, T.: Biomechanics investigation of skillful technician in hand lay up fabrication method. In: The ASME 2012 International Mechanical Engineering Congress and Exposition, Houston, Texas, USA, IMECE2012-86270, pp. 288 (2012)
2. Karimi, A., Manteufel, R.: Understanding why engineering students take too long to graduate. In: The ASME 2013 International Mechanical Engineering Congress and Exposition, San Diego, California, USA, IMECE2013-65367 (2013)

3. Miller, A., Samples, J.: Building a community – how to enrich an engineering technology program with identity, presence and pride. In: The ASME 2013 International Mechanical Engineering Congress and Exposition, San Diego, California, USA, IMECE2013-65034 (2013)
4. Kobus, C.J.: Storytelling – a most powerful tool in shaping lesson plans in engineering education. In: The ASME 2013 International Mechanical Engineering Congress and Exposition, San Diego, California, USA, IMECE2013-65604 (2013)
5. Zhang, Z., Yang, Y., Hamada, H.: Mechanical property of glass mat composite with open hole. In: The ASME 2012 International Mechanical Engineering Congress and Exposition, Houston, Texas, USA, IMECE2012-87270, pp. 79 (2012)
6. Shirato, M., Kume, M., Ohnishi, A., Nakai, A., Sato, H., Maki, M., Yoshida, T.: Analysis of daubing motion in the clay wall craftsman: influence on several kinds of clay with different fermentation period on the daubing motion properties. In: Symposium on Sports Engineering: Symposium on Human Dynamics 2007, Japan, pp. 254–257 (2007)
7. Kikuchi, T., Fudauchi, A., Koshino, T., Narita, C., Endo, A., Hamada, H.: Mechanical property of CFRP by carbon spray up method. In: The ASME 2013 International Mechanical Engineering Congress and Exposition, San Diego, California, USA, IMECE2013-64144, pp. 63 (2013)
8. Kikuchi, T., Hamada, H., Nakai, A., Ohtani, A., Goto, A., Takai, Y., Endo, A., Narita, C., Koshino, T., Fudauchi, A.: Relationships between degree of skill, dimension stability and mechanical properties of composites structure in hand lay-up method. In: The 19th International Conference on Composite Materials, Montreal, Canada, pp. 8034–8042 (2013)

Process Analysis of Manufacturing of Sewing Scissors by All Forging Process and Understanding of Its Sharpness

Yasuko Kitajima[1(✉)], Kazuki Kito[2], Masakazu Migaki[3],
Kanji Matsumuro[3], Yasuhiko Murata[2], and Hiroyuki Hamada[3]

[1] Tokyo Ariake University of Medical and Health Sciences, Tokyo, Japan
kitajima@tau.ac.jp
[2] Nippon Institute of Technology, Saitama, Japan
kito_kazuki@yahoo.co.jp, ymurata@nit.ac.jp
[3] Kyoto Institute of Technology, Kyoto, Japan
{iloveseta, hhamada10294}@gmail.com,
kmatsumu@kit.ac.jp

Abstract. In Japan there are several types of scissors such as pruning scissors, flower scissors, U-shaped scissors, and sewing scissors and so on. Among them sewing scissors was introduced when the black ships of Commodore Perry came from the United States in the last Edo period almost 160 years ago. The shape and size of sewing scissors have been changed to fit Japanese people. Yakichi Yoshida started Japanese sewing scissors by his own manufacturing process; all a forging process. His technique was distributed to many persons who learned his process through implicit knowledge base. According to the family tree starting with Yakichi, there has been a spread to the manufacturing family of 23. However at present only one person is remained. He is still making the cutlery which has very good reputation among high ranking wear making persons and other high quality manufacturing persons. In order to preserve this manufacturing technique the process analysis was performed through video recording and the records were put in this paper. The process was divided into 9 steps such as Preparation, Making the ring, Making part of the blade, Making the neck part, Grinding, Finishing machinery, Quenching, Finish grinding, Post finishing, Normally the expert needs dozens of years for the whole process, therefore the number of products per day is very small. In the case of cutting some materials two blades contact each other at very small part. Small as possible makes sharp cutting because of stress concentration at the cutting point. In order to create this phenomenon the inside of the blade should not be a flat surface; instead the surface is required to be dented. This dented surface was made at the third step, and particularly only one sub process can make it. Our further study will be made for more accurate time analysis and also the bending process will be focused to understanding the secret of sharp cutting.

Keywords: Sewing scissors · Process analysis · Skill succession

© Springer International Publishing Switzerland 2015
V.G. Duffy (Ed.): DHM 2015, Part I, LNCS 9184, pp. 124–132, 2015.
DOI: 10.1007/978-3-319-21073-5_13

1   Introduction

There are two types of scissors in Japan. One type is Japanese and the other is western. It is said that the western style scissors were brought from the United States in the late Edo period. Its history is described in the next section. As improvements were made on the scissors that were brought in, they have become part of ordinary life for the Japanese. There are various forms of manufacturing methods such as using pressing machines for mass production and hand-made. Among the various types of scissors there is one that is used by a craftsman specifically for high-class men's clothing. It is made by the blacksmith's method that was started by Yoshida Yajuuro. However, there is now only one craftsman who makes this type of scissors using the method and the craftsman is in his old age.

So we began the research in to the secrets of scissors blade that are loved, and took records of how it is made with hope that it will lead to a succession of the techniques. In this thesis first the history of scissors is described, and through observation with video, each important scene of the manufacturing process is shown. By doing this the holistic perspective of the process can be captured, and simultaneously there can be data left for the next generation. Also, to understand the secret of the sharp quality of the scissors, it was found that there was contact between the two blade in a small range in the case of opening or closing. Furthermore, we state about the form of the blade of the scissors that allows there to be contact at one point. These are the first step of our research report.

2   Methods

A pair of scissors is a tool that cuts an object by crossing two blades. Scissors that exist from ancient times in Japan are U-shaped and called "grip scissors." Japanese scissors have a long and thin metal board on both sides with a blade, and are designed to cut an object by bending it into a U-shape and having the blade of the two sides cross. Japanese scissors have an old history, and the oldest ones have been excavated from the ancient tombs in Shuyama Castle (Nara Prefecture) and Notsuke (Gunma Prefecture).

Currently, in Japan the scissors that are mainly used are the western-style X-shaped scissors (Rasha scissors, sewing scissors). Compared to the U-shaped Japanese scissors the X-shaped western scissors have a blade in the inside of both metal boards, and it is designed for the blades to come together and cut an object by crossing the two blades with the supporting point as central axis. Rasha scissors have the characteristics of the blade being long from the point where the screw is, and the finger rings are different in size because one is a ring for the thumb and the other is the ring for the rest of the fingers.

Western scissors are said to have been brought in at the time when Matthew Perry landed his black ship at Uraga in 1853. At the time the scissors were called "Meriken scissors (American scissors)," and they were scissors for cutting thick fabric such as Rasha. The scissors were big and heavy, having a total length of about 330 to 360 mm, and the weight being about 1 kg. They were not suitable for the hands of Japanese people. The beginning of Rasha scissors was in 1877 based on "Meriken scissors." And in 1892 the first original Japanese pair of Rasha scissors was made by Yoshida Yajura (later renamed Yakichi). Yakichi was called the "founder of sewing scissors," and made use of the sword smith techniques at the time and repeated many trials and finally produced what is now the scissors of modern time. The characteristic of Japanese Rasha scissors is that compared to Meriken scissors they are small and light, and do not require support from a tailor stand and can be controlled freely with only the hands. The function of the scissors gained precision and mobility. The characteristics of shape were that ridges were put on the blade peak and the hit point was lengthened. Meriken scissors were made entirely by bronze, but the Japanese Rasha scissors were "chakko-zukuri" (a unique Japanese forge welding method based on the traditional Japanese sword smith method) which is based on the ancient ways of Japanese sword smith. The entire shape of Rasha scissors were made by extra-mild steel, but hard steel was applied only for the blade portion. The manufacturing method for sewing scissors designed by Yakichi is called "so-hizukuri," not like the casting method of pouring into a model but to heat extra-mild steel and rofge by hitting a hammer to form the shape. The "so-hizukuri" technique has been taught to many people. According to the geneaology of scissors craftsmen with Yakichi at the top, this technique has been spread to 23 different systems. However, the systems gradually vanished, and now there only one craftsman who uses the "so-hizukuri" technique.

3   Manufacturing Scissors

Figure 2 shows the photo of the shape in the middle of manufacturing scissors. The blades for the "thumb ring" and for the "lower fingers ring" are made respectively. They are combined after completion. We introduce the process in the following eight steps for manufacturing sewing scissors as shown in Fig. 1 with the still images.

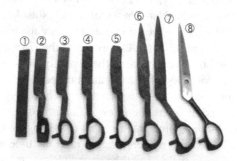

Fig. 1. Photo of the eight steps for manufacturing sewing scissors.

4 Process of Manufacturing Scissors

We observed the entire process by a video camera and classified into large steps and into small steps. The large steps include 4 process of works, the large steps 1 contains 8 small steps, the large steps 2 contains 3 small steps, the large steps 3 contains 1 small steps, the large steps 4contains 10 small steps. Process of manufacturing scissors is shown in Figs. 3, 4 and 5.

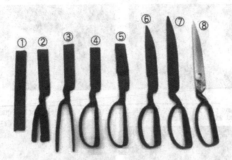

Fig. 2. Photo of the shape in the middle of manufacturing scissors (Photo credit; Cutlery Shop Furukawa).

5 Secret of Scissors with Good Sharpness

Figure 6 is the cross section when light is shined on the scissors when closing the scissors from opening position. Regardless of closing angle, it can been seen that the two blades touch at very limited range. Figure 7 shows the location where the two blades contact. The shape shown in the width was measured by the three-dimensional measuring device. The results are shown in Fig. 8.

In either case, the blade is shaped in a radiating line, which means the surface of the scissor blade is indented from the edge inward. This shape allows the edges to touch. This structure enables both blades to contact only at a point, not by a large contact surface (6). The process shown in Fig. 3 contributes to produce this mechanism.

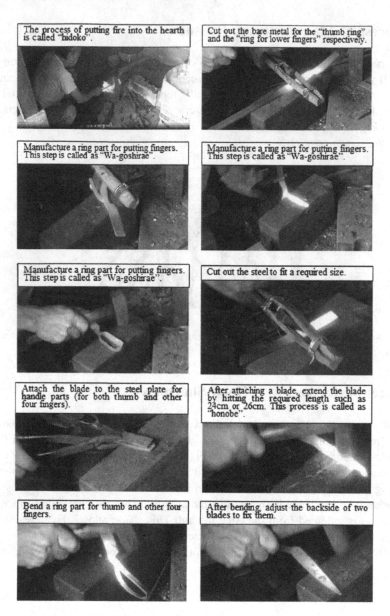

Fig. 3. Process of manufacturing scissors.

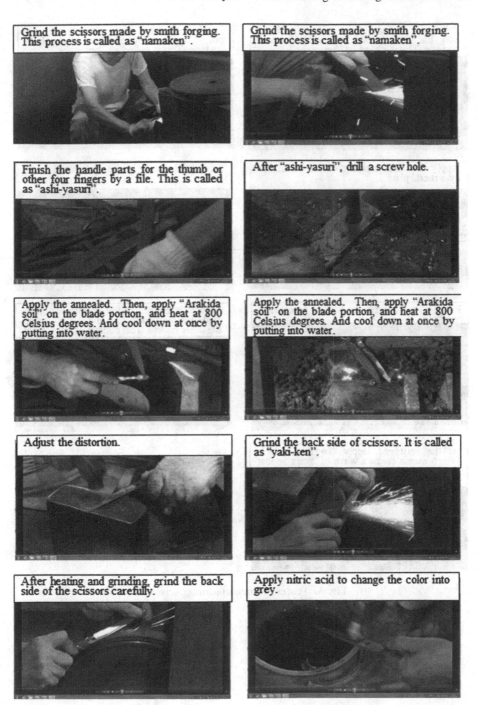

Grind the scissors made by smith forging. This process is called as "namaken".

Grind the scissors made by smith forging. This process is called as "namaken".

Finish the handle parts for the thumb or other four fingers by a file. This is called as "ashi-yasuri".

After "ashi-yasuri", drill a screw hole.

Apply the annealed. Then, apply "Arakida soil" on the blade portion, and heat at 800 Celsius degrees. And cool down at once by putting into water.

Apply the annealed. Then, apply "Arakida soil" on the blade portion, and heat at 800 Celsius degrees. And cool down at once by putting into water.

Adjust the distortion.

Grind the back side of scissors. It is called as "yaki-ken".

After heating and grinding, grind the back side of the scissors carefully.

Apply nitric acid to change the color into grey.

Fig. 4. Process of manufacturing scissors.

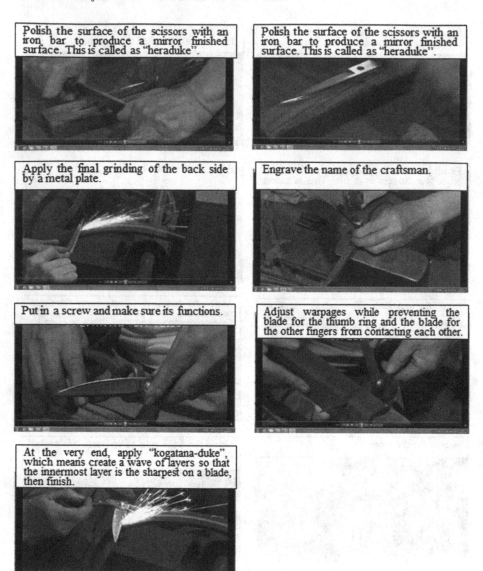

Fig. 5. Process of manufacturing scissors.

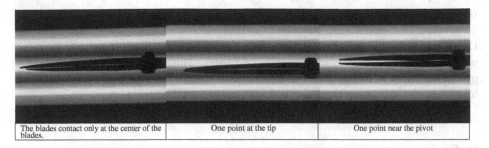

| The blades contact only at the center of the blades. | One point at the tip | One point near the pivot |

Fig. 6. Blades contact only at the center of the blades.

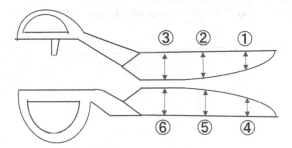

Fig. 7. Scheme of measuring locations.

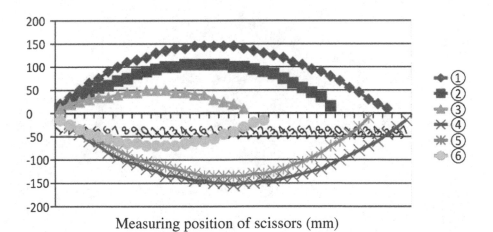

Measuring position of scissors (mm)

Fig. 8. Result of form measurement.

6 Conclusion

Using the method of forging Western scissors introduced to Japan in the late Edo era, we can record all processes of handmade craftsmen. This study enabled us to unveil a part of the secret of the sharpness of scissors, which tailors of high-class men's clothing love.

References

1. Okamoto, M.: Scissors, pp. 42–46. Ekuran-sha, Tokyo (1959)
2. Okamoto, M.: Scissors, pp. 233–255. Ekuran-sha, Tokyo (1959)

Expert vs. Elementary Skill Comparison and Process Analysis in VaRTM-Manufactured Carbon Fiber Reinforced Composites

Yasunari Kuratani[1(✉)], Kentaro Hase[2], Takahiro Hosomi[2],
Tomoe Kawazu[2], Tadashi Uozumi[3], Akihiko Goto[4],
and Hiroyuki Hamada[1]

[1] Kyoto Institute of Technology, Kyoto, Japan
kuratani@kado-corporation.com, hhamada@kit.ac.jp
[2] KADO Corporation, Tatsuno, Japan
{hase,hosomi,kawazu}@kado-corporation.com
[3] Gifu University, Gifu, Japan
uozumi@gifu-u.ac.jp
[4] Osaka Sangyo University, Daito, Japan
gotoh@ise.osaka-sandai.ac.jp

Abstract. VaRTM requires a preform to be manufactured before molding. However, it is often said that the accuracy of the preform affects the mechanical properties of the mold. Despite the progression of investigations into the automization of this process in recent years, preforms manufactured by hand still make up the majority, and the accuracy of these preforms lies in the ability of the worker. In this study, we have instructed three subjects with varying amount of years of experience working with composite materials, and manufactured VaRTM moldings. By analyzing the time taken, attitude and posture, and use of tools within the work process when layering, and by conducting an interlaminar shear strength test, we have acquired good results within the product quality of the mold, working time, and interlaminar shear strength in order of the number of years of experience. In the future, we will continue to research this subject so that we can focus on the creating a setup that has the same, consistent accuracy, regardless of the worker manufacturing the preform.

Keywords: CFRP · Vartm · Process analysis · Year of experience · Working posture

1 Introduction

Within the carbon fiber reinforced plastic industry (CFRP), the VaRTM molding method (Vacuum assisted Resin Transfer Molding) and the high-cycle RTM method (Resin Transfer Molding) are used for large molds. Research for the next generation of molding manufacturing technology is being actively pursued and used widely. With the VaRTM method, because there is no need to install equipment which will apply high temperatures and pressure, and because it can be used for complex shapes, it is

© Springer International Publishing Switzerland 2015
V.G. Duffy (Ed.): DHM 2015, Part I, LNCS 9184, pp. 133–142, 2015.
DOI: 10.1007/978-3-319-21073-5_14

considered a cost efficient and high-quality molding method. However, it requires that a fiber base-material preform is manufactured before molding. Manufacturing the preform takes a lot of time, and the accuracy of the preform affects the mechanical properties of the mold. In recent years, research into the automatic manufacturing of this preform have continued to progress; however, the majority are manufactured by hand.

Research of CFRP molding focusing on the flow and hardening of resins is currently underway, but the effect of the worker's manual labor is also considered to be an important factor. For example, in conjunction with analyzing the movements and work process of workers in hand lay-up molding and spray-up molding [1–3], Kikuchi et al. have begun tests that aim to scientifically explain the manual labor of workers in molding, such as investigating the subtly different effects that each worker had on their molding [4].

This research focused on VaRTM molding. However, this form of molding also has manual labor involved in its process, which is considered to have a large effect on the finished molding. Thus, we investigated the difference in the time it took the subjects, all of whom have varying years of experience working with composite materials, to manufacture the preform, and the mechanical properties of the test panel produced by the VaRTM molding, and how these factors affect the accuracy of the mold.

2   Experimental Method

2.1   Experimental Materials

We used a fiber base-material produced by SAERTEX, a carbon fiber NCF (Non-Crimp Fabric). The fixing agent was powder. (see Table 1) And we used a matrix resin produced by Axon Inc., EPOLAM5015 (main agent) and EPLOAM5015 (curing agent).

2.2   Molding Method

In order to stack the layers in the shape shown in Fig. 1 we manufactured the preform by layering the carbon fiber NCF, setting the silicon mold to produce a hat-shaped mold in the center, and then layering the same fiber, based on the layer structure chart shown in Table 1. The preform manufacturing process is comprised of three sections.

Table 1. Stacking sequence

Skin section			Hat-shaped section		
ply #	Fiber orientation (angular degree)	Thickness (mm)	ply #	Fiber orientation (angular degree)	Thickness (mm)
1	[+/−45]	0.25	1	[+/−45]	0.25
2	[0 /90]	0.25	2	[0 /90]	0.25
3	[90 /0]	0.25	3	[90 /0]	0.25
4	[−/+45]	0.25	4	[−/+ 45]	0.25
Total		1.00	Total		1.00

Sections 1 and 3 are the stacking sequence of the skin section and the stacking sequence of the hat-shaped mold, and Sect. 2 is setting the mold in order to create the hat shape (Table 2 shows the preform manufacturing process). After manufacturing the preform, resin is infused into the preform using the VaRTM method. After infusion, the preform is hardened at 25°C for 12 h, 40°C for 2 h, and then 80°C for another 2 h.

We informed the three subjects of the work process order and how to conduct the work beforehand, and provided them all with exactly the same tools. We also made them use a fiber base-material that had been cut the same size as the mold as well as auxiliary materials for the molding, all of which had been cut the same sizes. However,

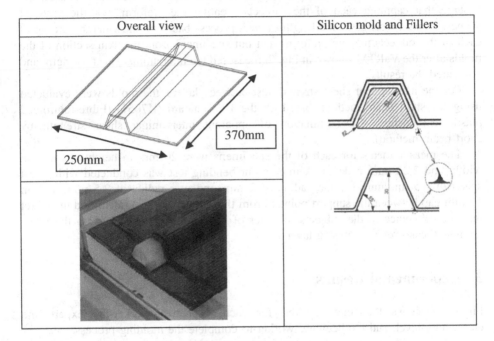

Fig. 1. CFRP perform

Table 2. Process flow of manufacturing preform

I	**the Skin Section (n=1~4)**
	n ply Fiber orientation confirmation
	n ply Stacking sequence
II	**Installation Section**
	setting the Silicon mold
	Fillers installation
III	**the Hat-Shaped Mold Section (n=1~4)**
	n ply Fiber orientation confirmation
	n ply Stacking sequence

despite specifying the tape used as an auxiliary material, we left the length to cut it and where to stick it up to the judgment of the subjects. The years of experience of the three subjects (how many years they have been working with composite materials) in order of most years of experience to least is Expert, Elementary and Beginner, with 8 years, 1.5 years, and 0 years of experience (first time) respectively.

2.3 Evaluation Method

For the subject's working posture and how they used the tools (iron), we divided up the time they spent on each of the processes and compared their actions based on the footage that captured each of the subjects creating the preform. For the physical properties, we investigated the length of each process based on the video recording of each of the subjects making preforms, cut out specimens from the skin section of the molds after the VaRTM, shown in Fig. 2, measured the interlaminar shear strength, and compared the results.

For the interlaminar shear strength test between layers, the molds were evaluated using the short beam method, based on the JIS standard (K7057) (Fibre-reinforced plastic composites – Determination of apparent interlaminar shear strength by short-beam method).

The measurements for each of the specimens were 20 mm in height, 18 mm in width, and 2.22 mm in depth. A three-point bending test was conducted with a test speed of 0.5 mm/min, support radius of 2 mm, indenter radius of 2.5 mm, and an 11 mm gap between the support points. From these tests, we have identified the effect that the difference in the subjects' number of years of experience had on the inter-laminar shear strength between layers.

3 Experimental Results

Figure 3 shows the time required for each respective worker-the expert, the elementary-level, and the beginner worker-to complete the molding process.

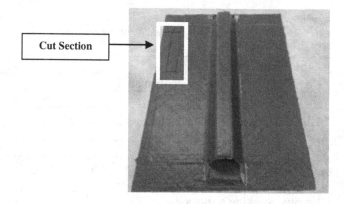

Fig. 2. Specimen cutoff

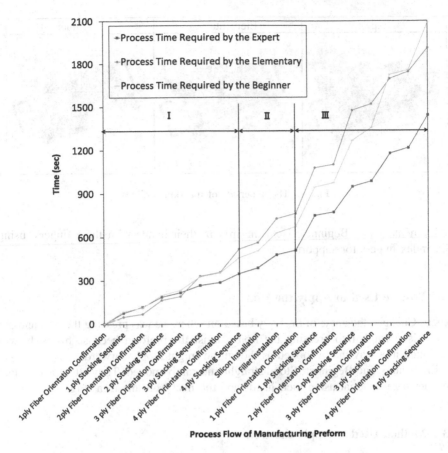

Fig. 3. Time required for each worker and process

The underside of the skin surface after the VaRTM showed the largest difference in the workers' level of experience (shown in Fig. 4). The experimental procedures for this research consisted of the subjects placing the silicon mold in order to create the hat shape, and then proceeding with the layering. However, if the worker does not make the fiber base-material fit and stack the layers while pressing an iron against the edges of the silicon mold, the edge line will rise up after the VaRTM, as is shown in Fig. 4, causing a difference in product accuracy. The preform's level of accuracy affects the mechanical properties of the mold. However, even in this experiment, the preform made by the subjects with little experience had visible edge lines in their specimens on the underside of the skin layer. Thus, this time, we analyzed the working posture and approach to applying the iron, which was used to join the fiber base-material.

3.1 Grip Used on the Iron

Expert: Held the iron in his hand with four fingers, gripping it tightly.

Expert	Elementary	Beginner
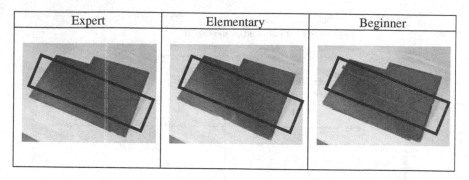		

Fig. 4. The underside of the skin surface

Elementary and Beginner: Held the iron in their hands with three fingers, using their index fingers for support.

3.2   Posture Used to Apply the Iron

Expert: Changed the angle of his body based on where he was pressing the iron and put all of his strength into pressing the iron against the preform because his body was positioned in a way that it looked as though he might topple forwards.

Elementary and Beginner: Stood straight and rarely moved. They attempted to join the fiber base-material using their hands and the heat from the iron (Fig. 5).

3.3   Method Used to Apply the Iron

We informed the subjects of the work procedures beforehand. However, aside from using the iron, we left how the fiber base-material is fitted into the mold up to each of the subjects. The reason for this is because that the purpose of this research was to increase preform accuracy through the worker by establishing the Beginner's way of learning, so we did not delve into explaining the finer points of molding.

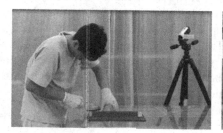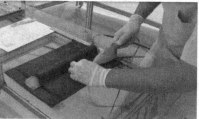

Fig. 5. Posture of expert

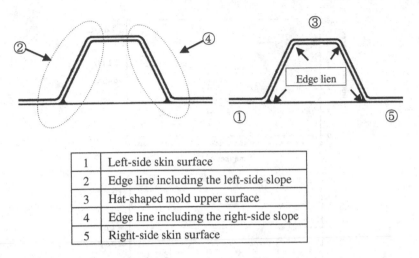

1	Left-side skin surface
2	Edge line including the left-side slope
3	Hat-shaped mold upper surface
4	Edge line including the right-side slope
5	Right-side skin surface

Fig. 6. Places the Iron was Pressed

Various differences arose in the order, places and angles in which each of the subjects applied the iron.

Thus, we divided the places on the molding that the iron was pressed against into five different places (see Fig. 6). We compared how long each of the subjects pressed the iron against the molding in the first ply layers and fourth ply layers for the hat-shaped mold (see Fig. 7).

Expert: Spent time on the edges and applied the iron while paying attention to the angle it was on because he understood the importance of fitting the fiber base-material into the edges of the silicon mold.

Elementary and Beginner: Spent a lot of time applying the iron to the skin surface rather than fitting it into the mold, attempting to secure the fiber base-material and quickly continue onto the next step.

Throughout the entire process, before applying the iron, the expert fitted the fiber base-material into the mold, pressed down the fiber base-material and mold with the hand that was not holding the iron so they would not move, and adjusted the iron's angle and the strength he was holding it down with, causing the fiber base-material to fill in excellently. For his posture when applying the iron, he stacked the layers while applying the iron, with his entire body pressing against the fiber base-material, preventing looseness between the layers. After the VaRTM, the resin flowed evenly into the fiber base-material, achieving a finish so clean that it is unclear where the mold is positioned just by inspecting it. However, the Elementary and Beginner subjects with little experience did not pay attention to the edges of the silicon mold (Fig. 6) when stacking the layers, but instead focused on securing the skin surface with the iron so that the fiber base material would not move. Thus, the fiber base-material was not properly stacked onto the edge line, resulting in the mold fitting being loose for the entire layering process, and sharp edge lines forming on the silicon mold on the underside of the skin surface after the VaRTM.

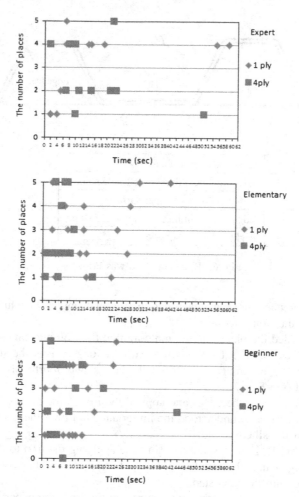

Fig. 7. Length of time and places each of the subjects pressed the iron

It was clear that because the last step in the process is vacuuming that, while that no major problems occur in the skin surface if the angle and other aspects of the fiber orientation have been properly layered, if you do not apply strength and use the iron evenly on when layering, the mold edge lines show on the underside of the product. Because we were able to check the differences in product quality just by looking at them, this time, we cut specimens out from skin sections which did not have edge lines showing and were also predicted to have few dispersions and twists in the fiber orientation (at the very least, they appeared exactly the same just by looking at them), and measured the interlaminar shear strength. However, as is shown in Fig. 8, differences were observed in the interlaminar shear strength among specimens in order of how many years' experience they had (Expert, Elementary and Beginner).

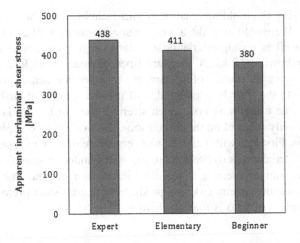

Fig. 8. Differences in the apparent interlaminar shear strength in each of the subjects

4 Discussion

From the testing the interlaminar shear strength, it was clear that even on the skin surface, which was believed to be unaffected by the number of years' experience that each of the subjects possessed, there was a difference in shearing strength due to the number of years' experience the subjects had, making it clear that the strength is proportionate to how many years' experience the worker has. Thus, we predict that, by taking cutoffs from various places on the hat-shaped layering surfaces and slanted sections, conducting an interlaminar shear strength test, pull test, and compression test, there will be a difference in strength, making further investigation necessary. In this research, we informed the subjects of the work procedure. However, because we did not inform them of the angle, posture, how to fit the fiber base-material, and the key places to apply the iron's heat on the fiber base-material when applying the iron, we predict that instructing the Elementary and Beginner subjects would cause a difference not just in their hand movements, but also in their posture and in their eye movements. We predict that there will be differences in the accuracy of future moldings.

5 Conclusion

In the future, we will need to research the effect that manufacturing preforms has on the mechanical properties of molds by investigating what the differences are in the strength, caused by the dispersion that the subjects create, through means such as recording the fiber orientation of each of the plies etc., subdividing the differences in strength caused by fiber orientation and dispersion in the fiber orientation, and clarifying the effects, such as strength caused by differences in the resin content. Therefore, because there was a lot of dispersion in the fiber density of the NCF we used this time, in the future, we will use a UD fiber base-material, which has a stable fiber density, focus on identifying the molding conditions and techniques of the workers, and continue to analyze. We would also like to cut out specimens from places besides the skin section, and as well as testing interlaminar shear strength, we would also like to use pull tests and industrial CT scans, measure fiber orientation angle and resin rate of impregnation, inspect the inside of specimens, measure the actual pressure that the workers apply onto the fiber base-material, and use the results for analysis.

We were unable to measure how much strength each of the workers applied this time because we only focused on the time it took the workers to complete the task for the work analysis. First, we will make the workers aware of how to appropriately setup the fiber base-material properly, and then we will conduct research that takes into consideration the aim of creating a molding instruction manual that includes vital points and an education system, enabling products with consistent preform accuracy to be created, regardless of who is making them.

References

1. Kikuchi, T., Koyanagi, T., Hamada, H., Nakai, A., Takai, Y., Goto, A., Fujii, Y., Narita, C., Endo, A., Koshino, T.: Biomechanics investigation of skillful technician in hand lay up fabrication method. In: Proceedings of the ASME 2012 International Mechanical Engineering Congress & Exposition, IMECE2012-86270, pp. 533–539 (2012)
2. Kikuchi, T., Hamada, H., Nakai, A., Ohtani, A., Goto, A., Takai, Y., Endo, A., Narita, C., Koshino, T., Fudauchi, A.: Relationships between degree of skill, dimension stability and mechanical properties of composites structure in hand lay-up method. In: Proceedings of the 19th International Conference on Composite Materials, pp. 8034–8042 (2013)
3. Kikuchi, T., Tani, Y., Takai, Y., Goto, A., Hamada, H.: Biomechanics investigation of skillful technician in spray-up fabrication method converting tacit knowledge to explicit knowledge in the fiber reinforced plastics molding. In: Duffy, V.G. (ed.) DHM 2014. LNCS, vol. 8529, pp. 24–34. Springer, Heidelberg (2014)
4. Kikuchi, T., Hamada, H., Nakai, A., Ohtani, A., Goto, A., Takai, Y., Endo, A., Narita, C., Koshino, T., Fudauchi, A.: Process analysis of hand lay up method by various experience persons. In: Proceedings of the 19th International Conference on Composite Materials, pp. 8113–8120 (2012)

The Relationship Between Mechanical Properties and the Method Technique of GFRP Plate by Hand Lay-up Method: Effect of the Workers Experience

Masakazu Migaki$^{(\boxtimes)}$, Keisuke Ono, Ryo Takematsu,
Yusaku Mochizuki, Eijutsu Ko, Daiki Ichikawa,
and Hiroyuki Hamada

Advanced Fibro-Science, Kyoto Institute of Technology,
Sakyō-ku, Kyoto, Japan
{iloveseta,ekusiek0223,mczk0520,i.athena.d5.mcg,
hhamada10294}@gmail.com, takematsu4@yahoo.co.jp,
hubo0400@163.com

Abstract. The aim of this research was focused on the relationship between the skill of an operator in the hand lay-up molding method and the mechanical properties of the molding composites. Glass fiber reinforced plastic (GFRP) plates were prepared using the hand lay-up method by five inexperience operators. The materials of GFRP included unsaturated polyester resin and chopped glass fiber mat. The working procedure of all operators was recorded by a video camera. Mechanical properties of the GFRP plates were carried out by tensile testing. The load-displacement curve was illustrated, which was used for characterizing the molding technique of various operators. The relationship of working times and mechanical strength of the GFRP was characterized, which impacted on the mechanical properties of the specimens. From the results, the relationship was considered separately in the first half and the second half of the working times. From the results, the step of degassing squeeze out air was significantly influenced the mechanical strength of the GFRP products. Therefore, the degassing step with the iron bar was the most affected on the mechanical properties of the GFRP plate making by the inexperience operator. It can be noted that the fully degassing out of the molding product strongly suggested for the hand lay-up method in order to maintain the high strength of the GFRP products.

Keywords: Hand lay-up · Glass cloth · Polyester · Impregnation · Composite

1 Introduction

FRP is referred to Fiber Reinforced Plastics by using resin and reinforcing fiber in order to improve the strength of the product. The important characteristics of the FRP are good thermal insulation, resistance to heat, weather and chemical, electrical insulating and radio wave transmitting. FRP can be manufactured to various shapes, free color decorating, light weight and excellent strength. Therefore, it is widely used in variety

V.G. Duffy (Ed.): DHM 2015, Part I, LNCS 9184, pp. 143–153, 2015.
DOI: 10.1007/978-3-319-21073-5_15

applications such as aerospace industry, railway, automobile, construction industry sports and some medical fields [1].

The fabrication methods of the FRP are including hand lay-up method, spray-up method and press method. The most common and traditional method is the hand lay-up method [2]. A general process of this method is pre-placed reinforced fiber in a mold and then impregnated resin to the fiber using a brash or a roller by a hand. The hand lay-up method is used for preparing the high or low volume productions, which is presented an advantage on method of complex shape products. However, a disadvantage of this process is also found. That is the quality of the products will be affected by the skill of operators [3]. In our series of study, glass fiber reinforced plastic (GFRP) plate was created by the hand lay-up method. We examined the difference in skills of individual operators in this method [4].

In this study, we focused on preparing the GFRP plate by the hand lay-up method from the difference of an individual workmanship. The targets of this research are five of inexperience operators of hand lay-up molding [5]. The working procedure and the working time of each operator from the hand lay-up method were recorded using a video camera. Mechanical properties of GFRP plates were carried out by tensile testing. The relationships of the total working times and other parametents of fabrication and the strength of each specimen from each operator were elucidated.

2 Experimental Methodology

2.1 Subject

The targets of this research are five of inexperience operators of hand lay-up molding. One operator made three GFRP plates, which each specimen was made by duration of three days.

2.2 Hand Lay-up Method

The procedures for creating the GFRP plate are listed in the following.

Step 1. Place reinforced fiber (glass fiber) in the mold plate.
Step 2. Pour the resin into the mold plate.
Step 3. Natural impregnated between the resin and the fiber.
Step 4. Use a roller for impregnated of the resin and the fiber.
Step 5. Degassing by using the iron bar.
Step 6. Free the mold plate by putting the weight.
Step 7. Wait for complete cure.

Figure 1 shows the hand lay-up mold plated used in this study. The hand lay-up method was used a roller in order to fabricated the resin on the smooth metal molded plate of 300 mm × 300 mm. After that 40 kg of the weight was applied in order to adjust the thickness and then the molded was left to cure for 24 h. In addition, the molded was put for 2 h in an oven at temperature of 100°C for completely curing of the resin.

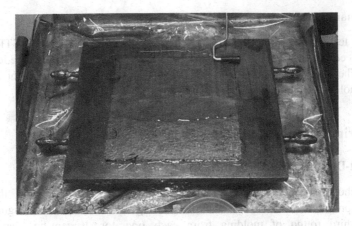

Fig. 1. Photograph of the hand lay-up mold plate

The targets of this research are five of inexperience operators of hand lay-up molding. One operator made three of GFRP plates, which each specimen was made by duration of three days. It measured the working time during the molding of each operator.

2.3 Measurements of Working Time

A video camera was used for recording the working of each operator. The camera was taken for the entire of making the GFRP plate until the laminating process was finished. The working time of the molding in each step was also recorded.

We focused on the impregnation of the resin and the fiber from the procedure of steps 3–5, which would impact on the properties of the molding. The working process significantly influenced on the properties of the GFRP molded article. The observations were included as the following.

1. Natural impregnation (sheet1).
2. Use the roller of the resin impregnation (sheet1).
3. Natural impregnation (sheet2).
4. Use the roller of the resin impregnation (sheet1).
5. Extrusion of resin.

2.4 Test Materials and Test Pieces

The resin was unsaturated polyester resin (RIGOLAC150HRBQTNW). The chopped glass fiber strand mat (M137, Owens Corning® Inc.) was used as the reinforced fiber. Kayamec M was used as curing agent. It was mixed at a ratio of 0.07 phr of the mass of the resin. The amount of resin was designated as 300 ml.

The size of the GFRP plate was 200 mm in length and 20 mm in width. Test pieces were prepared for three specimens.

2.5 Mechanical Properties

The tensile test was carried out by Intsron universal testing machine (INSTRON type 4206) at speed of 1 mm/min. The load cell was used at 10 tons. The gauge length was 100 mm. The load-displacement curve was illustrated, which was used for characterizing the molding technique of various operators. *1.

3 Experimental Results

3.1 Load-Displacement Diagrams

Figure 2 shows the load-displacement diagram of the tensile test of the GFRP specimens prepared at the first round of molding by each operator. Figure 3 presents the third round of molding from each operator. It can be seen that the load-displacement diagram of the first round molding showed the variation of each sample and the graphs were different from each operator as shown in Fig. 2. On the other hand, the load displacement curves from the third molding round by each operator presented some of an evenness of the displacement curves as illustrated in Fig. 3. These results would be used for indicating an experience and a skill of each operator in the hand lay-up method. Thus, the experience in the hand lay-up molding of the inexperienced person would be focused, especially on the technique for impregnating the resin. It can be said that it is difficult to improve their molding skill within three times of the molding.

3.2 Tensile Properties

The tensile strength of the GFRP as a function of the total working times is shown in Fig. 4. The total working times were focused on the step of natural impregnation, roller impregnation and degassing by the iron bar (extrude of resin). The working time of

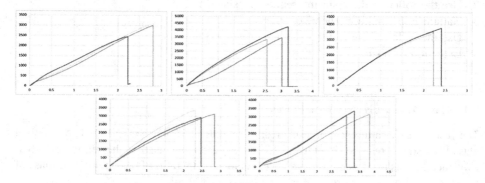

Fig. 2. The load displacement curve from tensile testing of the GFRP at the first round of molding by each operator.

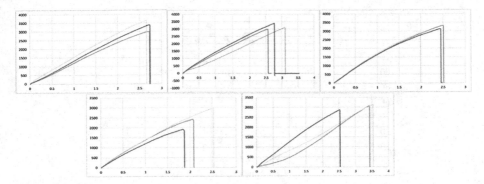

Fig. 3. The load displacement curve from tensile testing of the GFRP at the third round of molding by each operator.

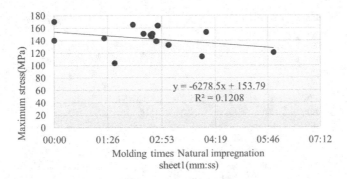

Fig. 4. The tensile strength as a function of the working time for natural impregnation (sheet1)

each research step obtained the variation of the tensile strength of the GFRP plates. From Fig. 4, we considered separately in the first half and the second half from the middle of the molding as illustrated in Figs. 5, 6, 7, 8, 9 and 10. Figure 5 shows the relationship of the tensile strength as a function of the degassing step. From this figure, the first half study (red line) showed a positive correlation while the second half study (blue line) showed a negative correlation between the tensile strength and the molding (working) time of the degassing step. It can be seen that the correlation coefficient of the second half was low. It might be attributed to unevenness of the molding from the operator.

Figures 6 and 7 show the results from the step of natural impregnation in the sheet 1 (first layer) and the sheet 2 (second layer), respectively. On the contrary, the results from the step of roller impregnation of the sheet 1 and sheet 2 are presented in Figs. 8 and 9. In addition, we illustrated the relationship of the total working times and the tensile strength is presented in Fig. 10. From these results, it could be observed the irregularity of the tensile strength at various molding times of the natural as well as the roller impregnation and the total working times from the inexperience operators (Figs. 11, 12, 13, 14 and 15).

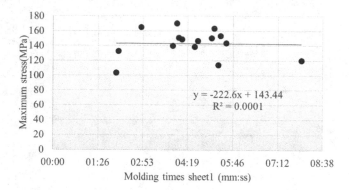

Fig. 5. The tensile strength as a function of the working time for impregnation with roller (sheet1).

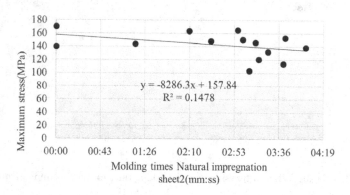

Fig. 6. The tensile strength as a function of the working time for natural impregnation (sheet2)

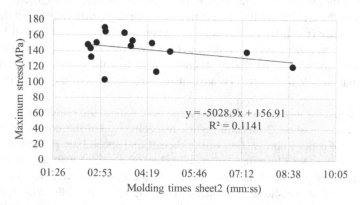

Fig. 7. The tensile strength as a function of the working time for impregnation with roller (sheet2).

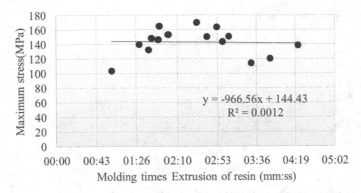

Fig. 8. The tensile strength as a function of the working time for the degassing by iron bar

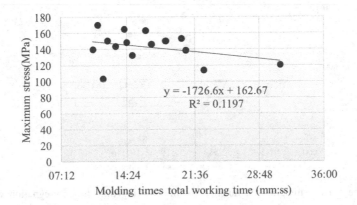

Fig. 9. The tensile strength as a function of the total working time

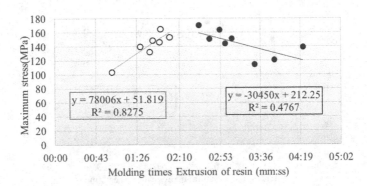

Fig. 10. The tensile strength as a function of the working time for the degassing by iron bar

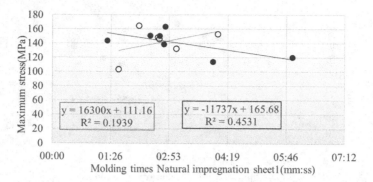

Fig. 11. The tensile strength as a function of the working time for natural impregnation (sheet1).

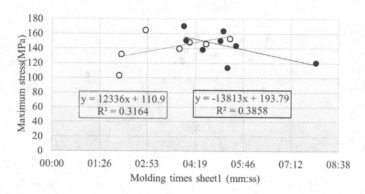

Fig. 12. The tensile strength as a function of the working time for impregnation with roller (sheet1).

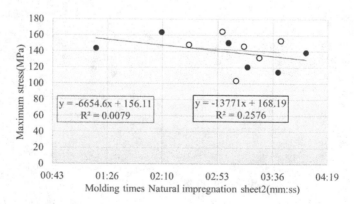

Fig. 13. The tensile strength as a function of the working time for natural impregnation (sheet2)

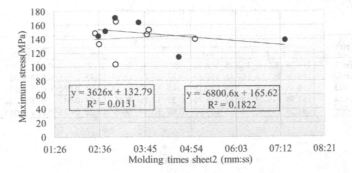

Fig. 14. The tensile strength as a function of the working time for impregnation with roller (sheet2).

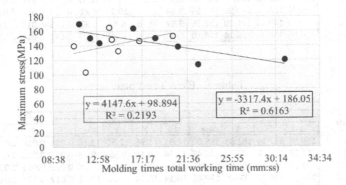

Fig. 15. The tensile strength as a function of the total working time

3.3   Correlation Table of the Working Time and the Tensile Strength

Table 1 summarizes the correlation coefficient from the results of the working time (time of each process, the first half and the second half) and the tensile strength of each analysis step. The correlation coefficient of the natural impregnation and the roller impregnation was low. On the other hand, the step of the degassing process showed the higher values of the correlation coefficient. From the results in Table 1, it can be considered that the experience of the operator is important to obtain the regularity of the strength of the GFRP plate specimens. It can be noted that the evenness of the tensile strength was found from the step of the degassing, especially at the first half of the molding process. This degassing step was significantly influenced the mechanical strength of the GFRP molding products. It can be considered that air bubble would remain in the plate when the degassing time was low, which effected on the declination of the mechanical properties of the GFRP plate. Therefore, the degassing step with the iron bar was the most affected on the mechanical properties of the GFRP plate making by the inexperience operator. It can be noted that the fully degassing out of the molding product strongly suggested for the hand lay-up method in order to maintain the high strength of the GFRP products (Tables 2, 3 and 4).

Table 1. E,σ,δ First plate

First plate	E				σ				δ			
	1	2	3	Ave.	1	2	3	Ave.	1	2	3	Ave.
subject1	114.95	82.48	113.25	103.56	7.82	7.70	9.11	8.21	0.017	0.012	0.015	0.015
subject2	148.06	143.88	160.43	150.79	10.57	10.23	10.57	10.45	0.018	0.027	0.023	0.023
subject3	159.45	157.64	193.38	170.16	11.46	11.32	10.14	10.97	0.030	0.025	0.032	0.029
subject4	152.98	149.27	129.12	143.79	10.91	12.89	8.20	10.67	0.017	0.013	0.026	0.019
subject5	131.24	139.00	149.53	139.92	10.90	10.44	9.40	10.24	0.026	0.015	0.033	0.025

Table 2. E,σ,δ Second plate

Second plate	E				σ				δ			
	1	2	3	Ave.	1	2	3	Ave.	1	2	3	Ave.
subject1	120.29	125.00	97.03	114.11	8.86	9.85	8.09	8.93	0.026	0.026	0.014	0.022
subject2	163.73	161.92	134.47	153.38	10.20	11.23	9.98	10.47	0.016	0.026	0.017	0.020
subject3	149.74	160.14	180.86	163.58	8.54	8.89	10.19	9.21	0.027	0.031	0.031	0.030
subject4	138.76	149.31	128.20	138.76	9.92	9.96	9.88	9.92	0.025	0.019	0.015	0.020
subject5	136.90	150.46	158.14	148.50	13.02	12.17	10.49	11.89	0.012	0.015	0.022	0.016

Table 3. E,σ,δ Third plate

Third plate	E				σ				δ			
	1	2	3	Ave.	1	2	3	Ave.	1	2	3	Ave.
subject1	150.08	182.29	162.63	165.00	12.01	11.96	12.50	12.16	0.016	0.016	0.018	0.016
subject2	155.09	135.58	148.76	146.47	11.14	12.14	9.65	10.98	0.018	0.014	0.027	0.019
subject3	142.97	145.80	162.56	150.44	11.32	11.85	11.57	11.58	0.025	0.031	0.016	0.024
subject4	118.36	149.15	93.92	120.48	10.14	10.94	9.58	10.22	0.012	0.025	0.011	0.016
subject5	134.39	136.86	126.16	132.47	10.59	10.86	10.89	10.78	0.016	0.011	0.013	0.013

Table 4. The correlation coefficient of the relationship between the tensile strength and the Conclusion.

Correlation table	Time of each process	First harf (White)	Second harf (Black)
Natural impregnation (sheet1)	0.25	0.44	0.67
sheet1	0.01	0.56	0.62
Natural Impregnation (sheet2)	0.33	0.09	0.51
sheet2	0.34	0.11	0.61
Extrusion of resin	0.03	0.91 *	0.7*
Total working	0.35	0.75 *	0.79 *

4   Conclusion

The relationship between mechanical properties and the working time in the hand lay-up method was presented in this study. The inexperience operators in the GFRP plate by the hand lay-up method were selected. The tensile strength as the function of the working time of the GFRP plate molding was different in each analysis step of the natural impregnation, the roller impregnation and the degassing process. The correlation coefficient from the relationship between the tensile strength and the working time of each analysis step indicated that the degassing process was significantly influenced on the mechanical strength of the GFRP molding products. Therefore, the degassing step with the iron bar was the most affected on the mechanical properties of the GFRP plate making by the inexperience operator. It can be noted that the fully degassing out of the molding product strongly suggested for the hand lay-up method in order to maintain the high strength of the GFRP products.

References

1. Japanese Standards Association JIS handbook nomber.26 Plastic
2. Tani, Y., Kikuchi, T., Otani, A., Nakai, A.: Molding operation and physical properties in hand lay-up molding. In: 57th Science Council of Japan Materials Engineering Union Lecture Papers, 25 November 2013, pp. 161–162 (2013)
3. Shimizu, T., Masaki, N., Murakami, S., Kanagawa, Y.: Stochastic simulation of tensile damage process of glass mat reinforced plastics
4. Unsaturated polyester resin, Showa Denko K.K. http://www.sdk.co.jp/products/44/63.html
5. Hand lay-up, spray-up molding (History of FRP60 years)

Researching Sounds Generated During the Second Lining Pounding Process

Yasuhiro Oka[1(✉)], Yuka Takai[2], Akihiko Goto[2],
Keisuke Ono[1], and Kozo Oka[1]

[1] Kyoto Institute of Technology, Kyoto, Japan
okayas@mac.com, oka@bokkodo.co.jp
[2] Osaka Sangyo University, Osaka, Japan
{takai,gotoh}@ise.osaka-sandai.ac.jp

Abstract. Japanese calligraphy and works of art, which are written and painted on paper and silk, are often lined with Japanese *washi* paper and strengthened from the reverse side. They are then treated with various binding methods based on the purpose of the item and how it is intended to be viewed. The hanging scroll, which is a perfect example of a binding format, is only displayed when it is meant to be viewed and is hung on an alcove or beam. When it is finished being used, it is rolled up tightly from the bottom and stored in a box. In order to repeatedly roll up and open a hanging scroll smoothly, the hanging scroll is lined with several layers of Japanese *washi* paper, which are pasted onto the reverse side of the scroll. A paste with a low adhesive strength which has been further diluted is used to prevent the adhesive from hardening after it has dried. The joined surfaces are then pounded with a brush to enhance the adhesion. The level of expertise of this technique is determined by the sound that is generated when pounded using the traditional method. This research measures the sound generated when the joined surfaces are pounded by an expert and a non-expert with the purpose of evaluating the specific features of both sets of sounds.

Keywords: Amplitude · Hanging scroll · Pounding brush

1 Introduction

In the 6th Century, around the time when Buddhism was introduced from the continent of Asia, various cultural works were brought to Japan. New cultures were introduced from overseas and Japan's own cultures gradually continued to flourish. Works of art from various fields depicted religious subjects, sceneries and genres, and calligraphy that depicted genuine records, sublimated to express beautifully, are known to be among those cultures. These works of art and calligraphies were prepared on paper and silk. Needless to say, paper and silk, which are organic materials, deteriorate and are easily deformed when exposed to air and light for long periods of time. Nevertheless, many works of art and calligraphies which are believed to have been created in Japan after the turn of the 8th Century are still being handed down to this very day. The strong determination that many people have to pass on these valuable works of art and calligraphies to the next generation is considered an achievement. However, at the

© Springer International Publishing Switzerland 2015
V.G. Duffy (Ed.): DHM 2015, Part I, LNCS 9184, pp. 154–164, 2015.
DOI: 10.1007/978-3-319-21073-5_16

same time, it is also believed that the method for binding works of art and calligraphy developed by Japan is the reason that many of these cultural works have been able to be passed on. The hanging scroll is a perfect example of this. Figure 1 shows an arrangement consisting of a hanging scroll which has been hung on an alcove with flowers placed in front of it to welcome guests. This hanging scroll is bound in a way so that it is only hung on an alcove or beam when it is meant to be viewed. Once it has finished being used, the hanging scroll is rolled up tightly from the bottom with the side that contains the work of art or calligraphy rolled up on the inside. It is then stored in a box. Figure 2 shows a hanging scroll being rolled up. In other words, the work of art or calligraphy which has been bound to the hanging scroll can be exposed to air and light, causes of deterioration, for a minimal duration, making it an excellent binding method.

They are unfurled and hung up on a wall for viewing but rolled up and stored in a box. The scroll needs to hang straight without causing any warps or undulations during display, but it also has to be able to be rolled up smoothly without creasing for storage. It is lined with Japanese *washi* paper in order to make these two functions possible. About four layers of Japanese *washi* paper is attached using starch paste for the purpose of lining. The adhesion needs to be supplied sufficiently when attaching the Japanese *washi* paper to withstand being rolled and unrolled, but if a starch paste with a high

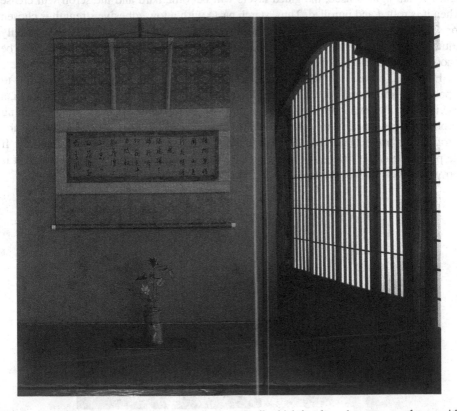

Fig. 1. An arrangement consisting of a hanging scroll which has been hung on an alcove with flowers placed in front of it

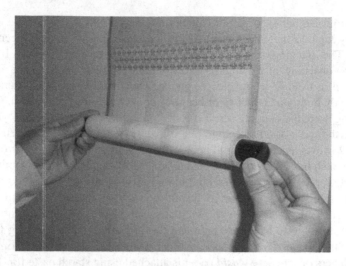

Fig. 2. Rolling up a hanging scroll

adhesive strength is used, the glued layers will become hard and the scroll will crease when it is rolled and unrolled. Thus, starch paste with a low adhesive strength is chosen for the lining adhesion from the second layer in particular. The paste is then heavily diluted with water so that it does not become hard after drying, allowing the scroll to be smoothly rolled and unrolled.

However, a paste with low adhesive strength is not able to sufficiently stick to Japanese washi paper. For this reason, the joined surfaces are pounded with a brush, a special skill that enhances the adhesion and has been handed down through hanging scroll craftsmen for several hundred years. In this research, this action of striking the scroll with a brush is referred to as "pounding". Figure 3 shows someone pounding. If the pounding is too strong, the lining paper can be damaged. On the other hand, if it is too weak, then the adhesion cannot be properly facilitated.

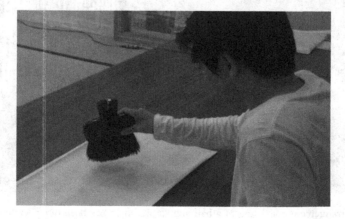

Fig. 3. Pounding

Similar to Japan's many traditional crafts which have a high degree of difficulty, watching and learning the skills of an expert is the primary method in which this skill has been passed down, making pounding difficult for non-experts to learn.

The level of expertise in this skill is sometimes measured in hanging scroll crafting workshops where this skill is put into practice every day primarily when experts use a brush on the joined surfaces, or more specifically, through the sound that is generated when the joined surfaces are pounded.

The subjects used in this research were an expert and a non-expert. This research analyzes the sounds generated by pounding, which has never been quantified until now. We expect this information to be of large assistance in learning how to pound.

2 Materials and Structure Used to Craft Hanging Scrolls

Usually, four layers of Japanese *washi* paper are stuck onto the back of where the work of art or calligraphy have been written or painted. Japanese *washi* paper called "*usu-mino* paper" is used for the first lining and glued directly to the back of the work of art or calligraphy. This Japanese *washi* paper, made from the plant fiber of a mulberry tree, is sturdy despite being so thin, and is resistant to water and other liquids. This properly supports the work of art or calligraphy from the reverse side and exists as what would be the "foundation" if using a building as a metaphorical example. It is manufactured in the Mino area in Gifu Prefecture. A wheat starch paste is used for the first lining adhesive. The wheat starch is gelatinized by stirring it in water for approximately one hour while applying heat to it, then it is left to gradually cool overnight before it is used. The starch paste has high adhesive strength.

For the second lining and all subsequent linings, this sturdy usu-mino paper and adhesively strong wheat starch paste cannot be used, and the lining cannot be layered. This is because using any more of these materials than is necessary causes the lining to harden after drying, preventing the scroll from being able to be neatly rolled and unrolled. Thus, misu paper, a Japanese washi paper which is even thinner and softer than usu-mino paper, is used for the second and third linings, and a Japanese washi paper called uda is used for the final lining. Misu paper and uda paper are made from mulberry tree, the same material used in usu-mino paper. Aged paste is added to misu paper, and white clay is added to uda paper.

A paste with a low adhesive strength called "aged paste" is used for the Japanese *washi* adhesive in the second lining and all subsequent linings. Aged paste is acquired by heating and gelatinizing wheat starch paste, sealing it in a pot and storing it in a cold, dark place for approximately ten years where it is left to mature. The starch is aged by storing it for a long period of time, and the molecular weight is considerably reduced due to enzymes which regenerate the microbes, giving aged paste a lower adhesive strength than normal starch pastes. Aged paste is normally diluted to about 3 % before it is used. It does not harden when it dries and does not crease, making it an essential material in allowing hanging scrolls to be repeatedly rolled and unrolled smoothly. Figure 4 shows Japanese *washi* paper and paste which have been layered and glued on the back of works of art and calligraphy.

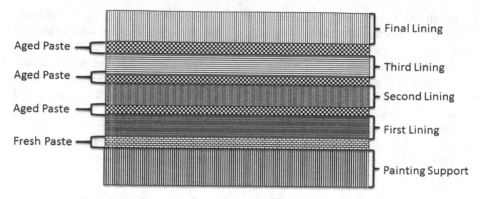

Fig. 4. A cross-section view of a hanging scroll with pasted layers of Japanese *Washi* paper

3   Adhesion Technique

The diluted aged paste, which is used for the second and all subsequent linings, hardly feels viscous when touched with a finger. As was previously mentioned, it has the advantage of not hardening after it dries, but on the other hand, it is not able to achieve adequate adhesive strength. Thus, the joined surfaces are pounded with a large brush called a pounding brush to facilitate adhesion. A worker continuously pounds with the pounding brush, starting from the front right and pounding in a forwards motion. Once the worker has reached the edge of the side furthest away from himself, he moves the pounding brush slightly to the left while continuing to pound. He then brings the pounding brush back towards himself. He pounds the joined surfaces which need to have their adhesion facilitated while repeating this forwards and backwards action. Figure 5 shows a diagram of the pounding brush's movements.

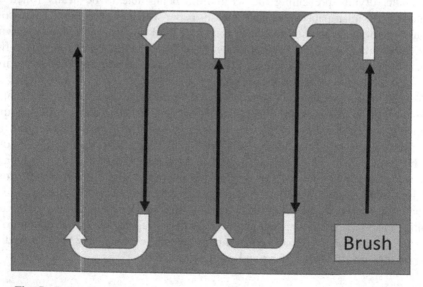

Fig. 5. Path of a pounding brush used to facilitate adhesion viewed from above

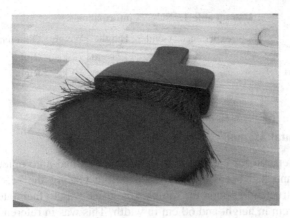

Fig. 6. Underside of the pounding brush which comes into direct contact with the joined surfaces

By repeatedly pounding as wide an area as possible on the joined surfaces with the underside of the pounding brush, shown in Fig. 6, adhesion can be facilitated without any unevenness. A non-expert, who needs to master the skill, is made aware that primarily, the wide area on the underside of the brush is supposed to strike the joined surfaces evenly. With each forwards and backwards action, the worker also changes which hand is holding the brush in order to prevent his arm from tiring and to allow continuous and stable pounding. The worker needs to be able to expertly use the underside of the brush the same way in both hands and pound the joined surfaces without any unevenness.

4 Measuring the Sounds Generated When Pounding

4.1 Purpose of Measuring

The level of expertise of the pounding technique is often determined by the sound that is generated when pounding. We instructed both an expert and a non-expert in the usual way of pounding. The sounds that were generated when they pounded were recorded by contact microphones, which were installed on the workbench. The difference in the level of expertise in performing this skill was investigated by measuring the amplitude of the sounds.

4.2 Test Subjects

The test subjects were an expert who has 22 years of experience in pounding, and a non-expert who only has 9 years of experience in pounding. The non-expert, with only 9 years of experience, is still learning the pounding technique, and is deemed to not yet be at a level where he is able to perform the task properly because he has not finished acquiring the skill. The details of each of the subjects are shown in Table 1.

Table 1. Subject information

Subject	Years of experience	Gender	Height	Weight	Dominant hand
Expert	22	Male	171 cm	72 kg	Right
Non-expert	9	Male	181 cm	60 kg	Right

4.3 Experimental Method

A sample was prepared for each of the subjects, which had a completed even-weave silk first lining and had been properly dried before placing the second lining. The subjects were instructed to pound the samples the usual way to facilitate adhesion. The samples were 35 cm in height and 60 cm in width. This was in reference to the size of the cloth lining which is selected when crafting hanging scrolls used in general events such as tea ceremonies.

In order to make the subjects work the same way they would when usually pounding, they were instructed to continue pounding until it was clear that the adhesion had been successfully facilitated.

Four contact microphones were installed on the workbench in order to measure the amplitude of the sounds that were generated when pounding. Figure 7 shows a diagram of the method used to measure the sounds. The sampling frequency was 48 kHz.

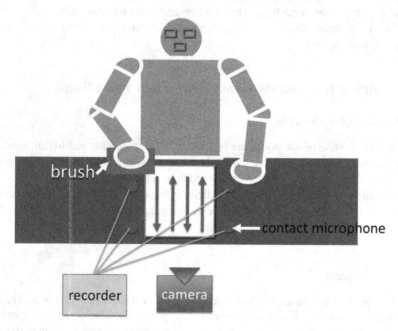

Fig. 7. Diagram of measuring method

5 Experimental Results

The number of times and the speed that the two subjects pounded were different. Both of the subjects began pounding from in front of themselves and proceeded to pound while switching the hand that was holding the brush each time it returned to the edge closest to them.

As is shown in the diagram in Fig. 8, both subjects started pounding just in front of themselves on the right hand side, continued pounding until they reached the left edge of the sample, and then returned while pounding from the left, all the way back to where they started in front of themselves on the right hand side. Once the brush had returned back in front of them on the right hand side, they then pounded until they reached the left edge, just like the first time. In other words, the brush moves 1.5 circuits around the surface when pounding. The expert pounded at total of 650 times, and the non-expert pounded a total of 591 times.

First, we compared the waveforms of the sounds recorded by the contact microphones that were generated when pounding. Some of the waveforms from the sounds collected from the expert's pounding are shown in Fig. 9, and some of the waveforms from the sounds collected from the non-expert's pounding are shown in Fig. 10.

When comparing both of the subjects' waveforms, it is evident that the amplitude of the sounds generated by the expert's pounding are larger than those of the non-expert's pounding, and that the amplitude of the expert's sounds were repeated with near-perfect consistency. We believe that, in contrast to the non-expert, the expert was able to use the pounding brush on a wide surface and pound effectively every time, achieving repeatedly large amplitude.

The amplitude of the non-expert's sounds were extremely low numerous times, sometimes achieving a waveform similar to that of the expert and sometimes not. This means that the non-expert was not always able to facilitate adhesion evenly and without irregularities on the joined surfaces, and indicates that the non-expert has not sufficiently mastered the pounding technique.

Figure 11 shows two smoothed waveforms – one from the expert's pounding that displayed consistent amplitude, and one which was observed numerous times in the

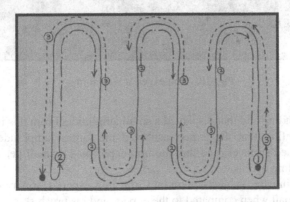

Fig. 8. Diagram showing the brush moving 1.5 circuits around the surface

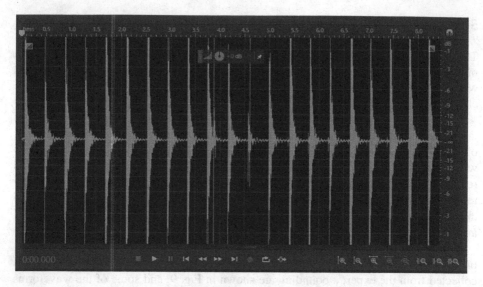

Fig. 9. Expert's waveforms

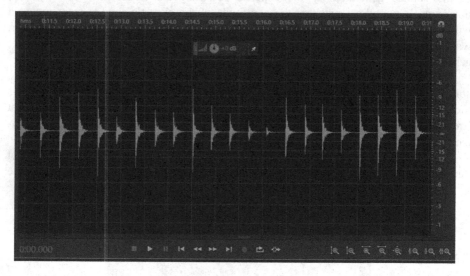

Fig. 10. Non-expert's waveforms

non-expert's pounding and that displayed a small amplitude. From this information, we were able to confirm that the expert achieved the largest amplitude directly after pounding the joined surfaces, and that the non-expert had a small peak in the second half of the pounding action.

When observing the subjects pounding, the non-expert's arm movements when pounding were small when compared to the expert, and his brush showed a tendency to

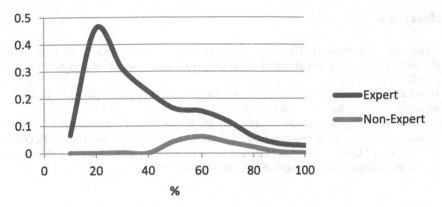

Fig. 11. Comparison of an expert and non-expert's waveforms

not pull back quickly from the joined surfaces directly after pounding. This is believed to be a factor that indicates that his waveforms were extremely small and different to those of the expert.

6   Conclusion

As stated earlier, the proficiency level of pounding with a pounding brush is often checked in workshops by the sound generated when pounding. Through this research, we have confirmed that the amplitude of the sounds generated by an expert's pounding are larger than those of a non-expert's pounding. We also confirmed that the sounds generated by a non-expert's pounding in one complete procedure of facilitating adhesion are not consistent and are both large and small in comparison to an expert. Within pounding, the ability to facilitate adhesion evenly over a wide area is strongly sought after. However, these results indicate that a non-expert's facilitation of adhesion is uneven when compared to an expert. This information is in agreement with the experimental results in the action analysis used to analyze similar pounding, which indicated that the expert's pounding action was able to be consistently reproduced in contrast to the non-expert's pounding action. Furthermore, this information is also in agreement with the peeling load results of samples that had actually been pounded in the peeling test. In the peeling test, by calculating the standard deviation of the peeling load from samples created by an expert and non-expert, it was revealed that the expert's sample had less dispersion than the non-expert's sample.

From this experiment, we have been able to quantify proficiency level in pounding for the first time by measuring the difference in sounds generated when pounding, indicating the accuracy of the method for evaluating proficiency level currently used in workshops.

Acknowledgements. This research was the recipient of JSPS Grant-in-Aid for Scientific Research #25350327.

References

1. Hayakawa, N., Kigawa, R., Kawanobe, W., Higuchi, H., Oka, Y., Oka, I.: Basic research of the physical properties and chemical compositions of aged paste. Conserv. Sci. **41**, 15–28 (2002)
2. Hayakawa, N., Kimijima, T., Kusunoki, K., Oka, Y.: Effects of the pounding brush as an adhesive. Conserv. Sci. **43**, 9–16 (2004)
3. Nishiura, T.: Adhesive effects of pounding by brush. Sci. Picture Framing 99–107 (1997)
4. Hayakawa, N., Kigawa, R., Nishimoto, T., Sakamoto, K., Fukuda, S., Kimishima, T., Oka, Y., Kawanobe, W.: Characterization of Furunori (aged paste) and preparation of a polysaccharide similar to Furunori. Stud. Conserv. **52**(3), 221–232 (2007)

EMG Activity Analysis of Expert Skills on Handheld Grinding Work for Metallographic Sample

Takuya Sugimoto[1(✉)], Hisanori Yuminaga[2], Hiroyuki Nishimoto[3], and Akihiko Goto[4]

[1] Kyoto Institute of Technology, Kyoto, Japan
t-sugi@koyo-kinzoku.com
[2] Kansai Vocational College of Medicine, Osaka, Japan
yuminaga@kansai.ac.jp
[3] Takeda Pharmaceutical Company Limited, Tokyo, Japan
hiroyuki.nishimoto@outlook.com
[4] Osaka Sangyo University, Osaka, Japan
gotoh@ise.osaka-sandai.ac.jp

Abstract. Carburizing is the most common heat treatment process for hardening ferrous alloy. The quality assurance of carburizing process requires metallographic analysis of case depth, retained austenite, intergranular oxidation, and carbide network by means of metallographic sample. Metallographic preparation consists of sectioning, mounting, plane grinding, polishing to mirror surface. It is difficult for non-expert to prepare metallographic sample with global mirror surface because preparation skill needs long time experience in this field. In this study, the difference of EMG activity during handheld grinding motion for metallographic specimen between expert and nonexpert execution was analyzed. The expert's abductor pollicis brevis, extensor carpi radialis brevis, and triceps brachii were working activity than the other muscles. We considered that these muscle activity balance by the expert contribute to the stable grinding conditions and good surface finish.

Keywords: Grinding · Expert · Metallographic preparation · EMG

1 Introduction

Carburizing is one of the most common case hardening techniques used for ferrous gear part. In addition to a surface hardness measurement by Rockwell hardness tester or Micro Vickers hardness tester, the quality of test specimens was evaluated by effective case depth measurement and a metallurgical examination. The metallurgical examination includes retained austenite; network carbide, inter-granular oxidation depth; and grain size measurements [1]. A near surface microstructure is required to accurately examine test specimens acquired from a heat treatment lot. The preparation process of the test specimen consists of sectioning, hot-mounting with epoxy resin, and grounding by SiC papers and alumina suspension. After the grinding, the test specimen is inspected with microscope ×100–1000.

© Springer International Publishing Switzerland 2015
V.G. Duffy (Ed.): DHM 2015, Part I, LNCS 9184, pp. 165–173, 2015.
DOI: 10.1007/978-3-319-21073-5_17

During the preparation process, if the test specimen is altered, or edge rounded, accurate metallographic information cannot be obtained. Resin or core perlite is softer than the case martensite, and therefore can be ground quicker. If this occurs, the surface of the specimen becomes rounded which prevents a microscopic, near surface microstructure analysis. Difficulty arises when pin-pointing the exact cause of process failure, especially when evaluating the quality of the heat-treatment process. The preparation process of this specimen is standardized by ASTM E3 [2]. LE Samuels established the foundation for the theory of preparation of a specimen [3]. And Smith MF compared the outcome of thermal sprayed specimens created by different abrasives [4]. However, a study was not conducted on how skills are acquired when handling a specimen, which experts obtain through long-term experience. In fact, the obtained near surface microstructure may differ dependent on the skill of an expert, or non-expert. The hardness and shape characteristics of the specimens vary depending on their components. Experts change their grinding and polishing processes according to the specimen's respective components. For the efficient transfer of the skills from expert to non-expert, it is necessary to compare and clarify the difference between the expert and non-expert execution. In this study aim to analyze the difference in muscle activity during the grinding motion of metallographic samples between expert and non-expert.

2   Experimental Method

2.1   Subjects

Four males were joined in the experiment. 20 years of experience in grinding was called as an expert. 5 years of experience in grinding process was called as a non-expert 1. 2 years of experience in grinding process was called as a non-expert 2. 0 year of experience in grinding process was called as a beginner.

2.2   Motion Analysis Method

Gear shape made of 9310 Steel NiCr–Mo alloy (AMS6265) were used as the sample to be ground. One grinding machine (Refine Tec Ltd, STO-228B) was used for the experiment. This machine has one rotating table. The grit P120 SiC abrasive which was usually used for plane grinding process was used for the experiment. To analyze each technician's technique, each subject grasped a specimen for metallographic examination and pressed it down on a rotating disk (300 rpm) to grind the surface of the specimen. The activity of the upper limb on the subject's dominant side, which operated the grinder, was recorded from a side view using a digital video camera (HC-V520 M, Panasonic) for analysis. In order to measure actual motions and muscle activities during the grinding process, we carried out the recording in synchronization with the EMG and behavior measurements.

2.3   Electromyographic Measurement System

Electromyography analysis was conducted using an EMG multi-channel telemeter system WEB-1000 (NIHON KOHDEN CORPORATION). It is a machine to capture and measure the electrical activity for change of muscle electric potential and the marks possible an investigation of muscle synergies, as well as muscle predominance in specific patterns of movement.

The sampling frequency rate was fixed at 1000 Hz and the data loaded into computer via A/D converter for analysis. In order to evaluate the relationship between hand and upper limb while holding a metallographic sample, we attached EMG markers at eight positions: on the middle fibers of the deltoid (D), the pectoralis major (PM), the biceps brachii (BB), the triceps brachii (T), the extensor carpi radialis brevis (ECRB), the flexor carpi radialis (FCR), the abductor pollicis brevis (APB), and the 1st dorsales interossei muscles (1/D) as shown in Fig. 1. The grinding motion, conducted in 5 s for three times, was subject to EMG waveform analysis.

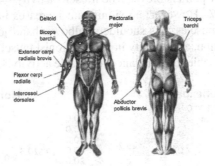

Fig. 1. The measured muscle

2.4   Data Analysis

Average Rectified Value of EMG (mVsec) during the three plane grinding motions for 5 s was calculated. The above mean value (mVsec) was divided by the maximal voluntary capacity corresponding to each muscle.

2.5   Surface Roughness

The final surface roughness and profile were examined with a surface profile measuring device (Taylor-Hobson, Talysurf PGI +; Taylor Hobson; x-direction resolution: 0.25 μm, and, y-direction resolution:0.8 nm). The measuring speed was 0.5 mm/s. We performed seven measurements respectively. Four measurements were from the epoxy on each gear tip to the other side of the epoxy. Three measurements were from the epoxy on each gear root to the other side of the gear. After the measurement, Rmax, was calculated by the software in accordance with the profile data.

2.6   %MVC Mean EMG of the Subjects

The %MVC Mean for each of the subjects is shown in Fig. 2.

The maximum overall muscle activity of the beginner was about 20 %, and even in his triceps brachii muscle and the flexor carpi radialis muscle, the muscle activity percentage remained in the 30 s, which is considered quite low.

The non-expert 1 exhibited a maximum muscle activity of 100 % in his triceps brachii muscle, and showed 66.2 % muscle activity in his flexor carpi radialis, which is quite high. As for his other muscles, the values for his 1/D and APB were slightly high, but all other muscles were only up to 20 % and hardly exhibited any muscle activity.

The non-expert 2 exhibited over 50 % muscle activity in his triceps brachii. However, he only exhibited just under 40 % muscle activity in his flexor carpi radialis, and less than 20 % in all other muscles, not exhibiting any significant muscle activity.

The expert exhibited just under 50 % muscle activity in both his triceps brachii and flexor carpi radialis, and an increase in muscle activity of approximately 70 % was observed in his abductor pollicis brevis. The muscle activity in his interossei dorsales was approximately 30 %. However, no significant increases in muscle activity were observed in any other muscles. His shoulders, elbows, hand joints and thumbs were effectively fixed in position, and activity in the antagonist muscle decreased effectively in reciprocation to this, achieving a balance in muscle activity.

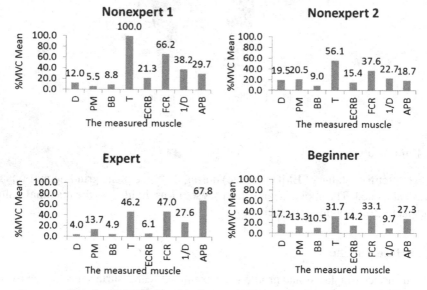

Fig. 2.   %MVC Mean EMG for each muscle on each subject

2.7   Comparing MVC Percentages Per Muscles Among the Subjects

The %MVC Mean per muscles among the subjects is shown in Fig. 3.

Deltoid. Beginner - 17.2 %; non-expert 1–12 %; non-expert 2 - 19.5 %: 4 %; expert - 4 %.

Excluding the expert, the subjects showed just over 10 % of muscle activity, making it clear that very little muscle activity was occurring. In comparing these values to the 4 % muscle activity observed in the expert, it was clear that no notable muscle activity occurred in the deltoid. The deltoid is the muscle that is used when the shoulder joint is turned outwards, and in comparing the expert to the other subjects, it was clear that he hardly used his.

Pectoralis Major. Beginner - 13.3 %; non-expert 1–5.5 %; non-expert 2–20.5 %; expert - 13.7 %.

The expert had slight muscle activity with a value of 13.7 %, a value that was considered significantly different to the other subjects. This indicates that the expert used the pectoralis major to hold the shoulder joint in position when the rotational force from the rotating grinder's disc acted upon the specimen.

Biceps Brachii. Beginner - 10.5 %; non-expert 1–8.8 %; non-expert 2–9 %; expert - 4.9 %.

The non-experts showed less than 10 % muscle activity while the expert showed slight muscle activity with 4.9 %.

This muscle is the muscle that bends the elbow, but it was clear that each of the subjects did not actively bend their elbows to press the specimen against the grinder disc. Furthermore, the expert showed less than 5 % muscle activity, a value that was still significantly lower than the other subjects, making it clear that he hardly used it.

Triceps Brachii. Beginner - 31.7 %: non-expert 1–100 %; non-expert 2–56.1 %; expert - 46.2 %.

The expert's muscle activity in the triceps brachii was 46.2 % and no significant difference was observed to both the beginner and the non-expert 2. However, it was confirmed that the non-expert 1 had significantly high muscle activity with a value of 100 %. This indicates that the non-expert 1 was over-extending his elbow when pressing the specimen against the grinder disc. All of the other subjects extended their elbows with about 30 % to 50 % muscle activity.

Extensor Carpi Radialis Brevis (ECRB). Beginner - 21.3 %; non-expert 1–15.4 %; non-expert 2–6.1 %; expert - 14.2 %.

The maximum muscle activity for all the subjects was less than approximately 20 %. The expert was observed to have 14.2 % muscle activity, which was not significantly different to the other subjects. The ECRB is the muscle that flexes the hand joint, but it was clear that less than approximately 20 % of muscle activity occurs when pressing the specimen against the grinder disc.

Flexor Carpi Radialis (FCR) Beginner - 33.1 %; non-expert 1–66.2 %; non-expert 2–37.6 %; expert - 47 %.

The FCR is the muscle that operates the hand joints and fingers. It is a muscle that is necessary when grasping the specimen. It was clear that the expert had 47 % muscle activity (approx. 50 %) when grasping the specimen while holding it against the grinder

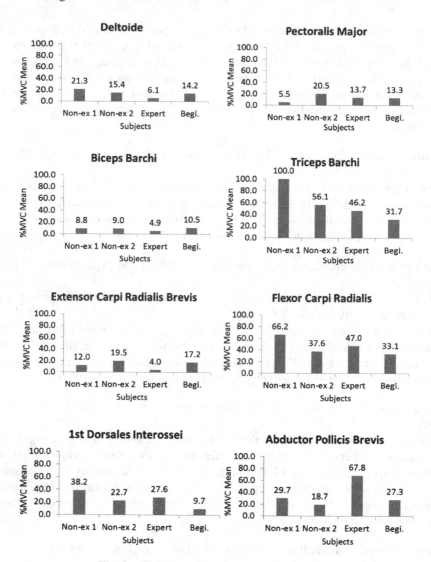

Fig. 3. %MVC per Muscles among the Subjects

disc. For the other subjects, the beginner and the non-expert 2 both gripped the specimen with a muscle activity percentage in the 30 s, which was roughly the same as the expert. However, it was clear that the non-expert 1 had just under 70 % muscle activity when grasping the specimen.

Interossei Dorsales (1/D) Beginner - 9.7 %; non-expert 1–66.2 %; non-expert 2–22.7 %; expert - 27.6 %.

The 1/D is one of the muscles that stabilizes the thumb when grasping an object. However, it was clear that the expert only showed 27.6 % muscle activity (approx. 30 %)

in his 1/D. Both the non-experts also used between approximately 20 % and 40 %. And the beginner hardly used his, with only 9.7 % activity.

Abductor Pollicis Brevis (APB) Beginner - 27.3 %; non-expert 1–29.7 %; non-expert 2–18.7 %; expert - 67.8 %.

The APB is one of the muscles that stabilizes the thumb when grasping an object. However, the beginner and the non-experts only used between 20 % and 30 % muscle activity in their APBs, while the expert had 67.8 % muscle activity in his APB, making it clear that he used his much more in comparison to the other subjects. It is clear that the muscle activity that occurred in the expert's APB was entirely different to the other subjects.

2.8   The Final Surface Roughness of the Sample Ground by Each Subject

Figure 4 shows the final surface roughness mean of the sample ground by each subject. Rt is Sum of height of the largest profile peak height Rp and the largest profile valley Rv within an evaluation length. The variability of the surface roughness by the expert was significantly smaller than that by the other subjects (P < 0.05).

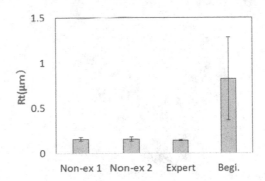

Fig. 4. The final surface roughness of the sample ground by each subject

3   Discussion

The expert's decreased muscle activity in his deltoid and biceps brachii, and his significantly increased muscle activity in his abductor pollicis brevis distinguish him from the other subjects. In comparison to the other subjects, the expert showed hardly any use of their deltoid and abductor pollicis brevis while grinding.

The deltoid is the muscle that turns the shoulder joint outwards, and the biceps brachii is the muscle that bends the elbow. When all of the subjects in this experiment pressed the specimen against the grinding disc using the positioning of their arms, they hardly used their deltoid and biceps brachii. However, the expert showed exceptionally low muscle activity in these two muscles.

The expert also showed the most activity in the abductor pollicis brevis in comparison to the other subjects. Figure 4 shows the schematic diagram of the expert's grasping hand. The abductor pollicis brevis is the muscle that acts when the thumb is in the palmar abduction position, and it is imperative when grasping objects. The position in which this muscle acts is called the "intrinsic plus position". The intrinsic plus position flexes only the MP joint. The PIP and DIP joints flex in the extension position. This is a position that is typically observed in experts of all occupations. However, holding an object in this position and maintaining the position is extremely difficult. This is because this position is significantly different to the regular position in which a person holds an object using their fingers. The display of significantly increased muscle activity in the expert's abductor pollicis brevis meant that this muscle was being actively used when grasping the specimen. The fact that this activity was not observed in the other test subjects indicates that they were not grasping the specimen in this position. Having a steady thumb is also extremely important in maintaining this position, and keeping the thumb in a fixed position requires use of the abductor pollicis brevis. The abductor pollicis brevis has Type 1 characteristics and is typically highly resistant to fatigue. It is clear that the expert was able to continue to press the grinding specimen against the grinding disc effectively because of this (Fig. 5).

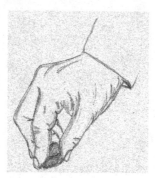

Fig. 5. The schematic diagram of the expert's grasping hand

4   Conclusion

The following results were obtained in this experiment by comparing the difference in muscle activity of an expert when grinding to subjects who were not experts:

1. The expert had low muscle activity in his deltoid and biceps brachii compared to the other subjects.
2. The expert had significantly high muscle activity in his abductor pollicis brevis and grinded in the intrinsic plus position.
3. An increase in muscle activity was observed in the expert's abductor pollicis brevis, extensor carpi radialis brevis, and triceps brachii compared to his other muscles. Activity in the antagonist muscle also decreased effectively in reciprocation to this, achieving a balance in muscle activity.

References

1. Vander, G.F.: Metallography: Principles and Practices. McGraw-Hill, ASM international (1984)
2. ASTM International. Standard Guide for Preparation of Metallographic Specimensof, E3-11 (2011)
3. Samuels, L.E.: Metallographic Polishing by Mechanical Methods. ASM International, USA (2003)
4. Smith, M.F.: A comparison of techniques for the metallographic preparation of thermal sprayed samples. J. Therm. Spray Tech. **2**, 287–294 (1993)

Difference in Polishing Process of FRP Between Expert and Non-expert

Takuya Sugimoto[1(✉)], Daiki Ichikawa[1], Hiroyuki Nishimoto[2],
Yoshiaki Yamato[3], and Akihiko Goto[4]

[1] Kyoto Institute of Technology, Kyoto, Japan
t-sugi@koyo-kinzoku.com, daikiichikawa0113@yahoo.co.jp
[2] Takeda Pharmaceutical Company Limited, Tokyo, Japan
hiroyuki.nishimoto@outlook.com
[3] Kure National Collage of Technology, Hiroshima, Japan
yamato@kure-nct.ac.jp
[4] Osaka Sangyo University, Osaka, Japan
gotoh@ise.osaka-sandai.ac.jp

Abstract. One of the quality assurance methods for steel and composite materials is to verify material constitutes and structures of polished specimens by microscope. We prepared a sample used for microscope analysis in the following method: first, cut a sample from the cross-section, and mount with the epoxy resin, and then grind it. This process requires long craftsmen's experience to grind a sample properly for microscope test. In this research, we comparably evaluated the differences in grinding sound and comprehension skills between the expert and the non-expert. As a result, we found that the expert was more sensitive to the difference in the sounds generated during grinding process. He comprehended the state of a grinding sample by the sound generated during grinding and adjusted his grinding force in a wider range.

Keywords: Polish · CFRP · Expert · Microscopic analysis

1 Introduction

The steel and composite materials are essential in the production of automobiles, construction machinery, transport equipment such as airplanes, and construction structures [1–9]. These materials are selectively used according to necessary strength and application purpose. However, the strength and mechanical properties of steel and composite materials can't be determined by appearance. In addition to the tensile and strength tests, it is necessary to verify the metallographic and laminate structures for making sure if material constitutes and structures are suitable for desired applications. And when verifying the metallographic and laminated structures, ground specimens are used for microscope tests [10]. This method enables us to comprehend the phase states of metal structures, the depth of grain boundary oxidations, austenite residue amount measurements, and the dispersion states of cementite [11–12]. Moreover, the microscope test of composite materials can verify the resin impregnation states, the existence of voids, and fiber bundle states [13].

© Springer International Publishing Switzerland 2015
V.G. Duffy (Ed.): DHM 2015, Part I, LNCS 9184, pp. 174–181, 2015.
DOI: 10.1007/978-3-319-21073-5_18

As for the preparation method of a sample used for microscope analysis, first cut a sample from the cross-section, mount with the epoxy resin, and then grind it. The sample preparation method is specified by ASTM E3 [14]. Based on the fundamental theory for specimen preparation designed by Samuels et al. [15], Smith et al. suggested the comparative evaluation method of finishing qualities of thermal sprayed specimen made from different grinding materials [16]. However, there is no research about the necessary skills for the sample preparation. It required the high skills obtained through long years experiences for creating samples accurately for test use. The strengths and sizes of samples vary depending on characteristics of components, so that only skilled workers can comprehend the components' properties and adjust the grinding conditions properly. In this study, we analyzed the grinding process on the subjects with different proficiency. We also presume that the important information to grasp a grinding state properly is the sounds generated during grinding. We evaluated the sensitivity to the sounds generated during grinding works on the subjects. And also measured that the pressing forces of the subject's figures during grinding process. And then discussed how the difference in pressing forces of the figures and sensitiveness to grinding sounds affect the grinding process and finishing quality.

2   Measurement Method

We adopted two craftsmen as the subjects for this study; one has 25 years grinding experience, who is referred as "expert." The other has only 2.5 years grinding experience and is referred to as "non-expert." The CFRP is laminated with a seven-layer made by a hand-lay-up method and was used as grinding samples. After cutting the CFRP specimen, it was heat mounted by epoxy resin with 31.7 mm thickness in the outer diameter (Durofast, Struers,).

2.1   Grinding Process Analysis

Using a grinding machine (by Refinetec, STO-228B) which the subjects daily used, the motion of a subject pressing a specimen on the grinding sheet was analyzed. The grinding was done by P120, P400, P800, and P1200 SiC grinding sheet and 5μ, 0.3μm of alumina suspension.

Test Method. The motions that a subject gripped a specimen and pressed on a rotating grinding plate were recorded by a video camera for analysis. The test conditions such as the rotating speed of the grinding plate and water supply were the same for the both subjects. After the grinding process, we interviewed the subjects regarding the grinding process when necessary. The finished surfaces were evaluated by microscope (Eclipse MA-100, Nikon).

Results. The Total Grinding Time: Figure 1 shows the total grinding time of the subjects. The expert took 525 s and the non-expert took 637 s in the total grinding time respectively. The time that the expert spent for grinding was 112 s shorter. As for the total grinding time per each grinding particle size, the expert spent shorter time for all particle sizes, except the 0.3 μm.

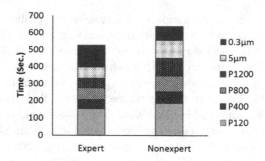

Fig. 1. The total grinding time of the subjects

The Average Grinding Time: During the grinding process, both subjects pressed the samples on the rotating grinding plate and they repeated this motion. Figure 2 shows the average time that the subject pressed the sample against the rotating plate. As the results shows, for all particle sizes of SiC and alumina grinding sheets, the expert showed greater variation in average time of pressing samples on the grinding sheets. When we interviewed the expert regarding this result, he remarked that he was doing this unconsciously. But he adjusted the pressing forces and time based on the feedback from the grinding sounds and the sense transmitted from the grinding sample.

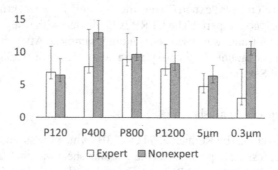

Fig. 2. The average time that the subject pressed the sample against the rotating plate between subjects.

Final Finished Surface: Figure 3 shows the final finished surface of the ground specimens done by the subjects respectively. Comparing the finished surface done by the non-expert, we found that warp and weft clearly appeared on the finished surface of the expert's sample. This suggested that the expert ground the warp and weft, and resin in the uniform manner.

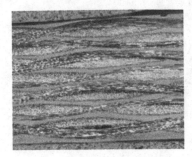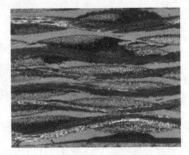

Fig. 3. The final finished surface of the ground specimens by each subject

2.2 Susceptibility Test of Grinding Sound

As the results of process analysis, we found that the expert comprehended the grinding conditions using the sound generated during grinding work. Thus, we tested the susceptibility of each subject to the sound generated by grinding. The grinding sounds were recorded beforehand and used for this test.

Test Method. We recording the grinding sound using a digital recorder, PCM (Pulse Code Modulation) recorder (R-26, Roland). The microphone was in-built in a linear PCM recorder. The sampling frequency was 44,100 Hz and the number of quantization bits was 16 bits. The grinding sound was recorded using an automatic grinding machine (IMT, Rana-3) with P120 grinding sheet, which both subjects had in daily use. The pressure range was 10–20 according to the usual levels to both subjects. While increasing the pressure with every 1, we recorded the grinding sound for 5 s on each pressure level, respectively. The Fig. 3 shows the location of the grinding machine and the recorder. Recording was conducted under the same environment where the subjects are usually working. Before the test, both subjects had time to make sure of the difference in the sound generated on each pressure level. We varied the pressure levels from 10–20. In the test, the subjects heard the standard grinding sound (10 N) once again. And then we increased the pressure level gradually from 10 N. The subjects answered the grinding sound corresponding to each pressure level from 10 N to 20 N, only with sound recognition.

Results. We examined the subjects' comprehension levels to the grinding sound with varying pressure levels by every 1 N from the standard grind sound (10 N) to 20 N. Figure 4 shows the results of each subject and the actual pressure levels. Regarding the difference between the actual pressure levels and the results, while the deviation range of the expert were within ± 1 N for all pressure levels, the non-expert selected the sound on the same pressure level (16 N) three times. This results suggested that the non-expert was less susceptible to the grinding sound compared to the expert. And the non-expert said that he sometimes judged sounds only with the volume. Also during the experiment, he no longer determined the standard grinding sound.

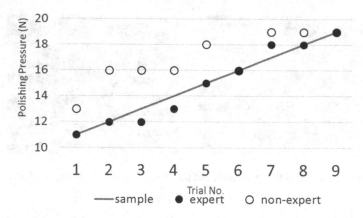

Fig. 4. The results of each subject and the actual pressure levels

2.3 Griping Force During Grinding Process

According to the results of process analysis, the expert varied the force to press a sample on the grinding machine. We thus measured the gripping force of the specimen during the grinding process using a pressure sensor (Pressure Profile Systems Inc., Finger TPSII). The sensor thickness was at 2 mm and the sensitivity was 0.045 kg. We attached sensors on the thumb, index finger, middle figure and ring finger which the subjects usually use during grinding process. The data acquisition frequency was set at 40 Hz. Since the wet grinding was carried out with water, to avoid any effect to the sensors, the subjects wore very thin finger stalls during the experiment.

Test Method. Using a grinding machine (by Refinetec, STO-228B) which the subjects daily used, we analyzed the motions when the subjects pressed the gripped specimen on the grinding sheet. First, we asked the subjects to perform grinding with usual force for three times. Then, perform another three times with maximum pressure. Other grinding conditions such as rotating speed of grinding plate and water supply were in the same manner as usual.

Results. Figure 5 shows the average force that the each subject gripped a sample. The total amount of the average grip force of the expert was 7.15 kg, while the non-expert showed 3.18 kg. The result of the expert was more than two-fold of that of the non-expert. Moreover, regarding the total amount of the average grip force at the maximum pressure, the expert showed 186 %, which was much greater than 152 % of the non-expert.

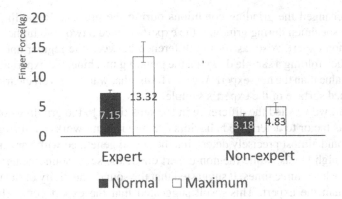

Fig. 5. The total amount of the average grip force between subjects

3 Discussion

As shown in Fig. 2, the standard deviation of the time while the expert pressed the specimen on the grinding sheet was greater than that of the non-expert. This suggested that the expert varied the grinding conditions more than the non-expert. In the interview with the expert, he perceived the grinding efficiency based on grinding sound. In order to verify the correlation between the grinding pressure and sound, we examined if the subject could identify the grinding sound corresponding to each pressure level. With this experiment, we found that the expert could identify the grinding sound within ±1 N error range. This suggested that the expert could comprehend the grinding pressure level based on the skills cultivated through his long-term experience. Moreover, at the time of maximum pressure, the force gripping a sample of the expert increased with 86 % more than that in normal procedure. We assumed that the broad experience of the expert allowed him to relax, so that he could perform grinding works without overstrain. He therefore, was not overwhelmed by the disturbance occurred on the rotation plate by rotation force, and maintained stability in pressing the sample down on the rotating plate. On the other hand, the non-expert overstrained and couldn't perform well. Thus, the difference in the values between the normal and maximum rates was not as great as the expert. Furthermore, the expert enhanced the grinding pressure by utilizing the differences between the normal and maximum pressures levels. This enabled the grinding work efficiently, so that the total grinding time of the expert was shorter than that of the non-expert.

4 Conclusion

In this study, we compared the differences of the grinding process done by the expert and non-expert in the preparation of the specimens for CFRP microscope analysis. As the result, the standard deviation of the time when the expert had pressed the non-abrasive sample on the grinder was greater than that of the non-expert. It suggested that the expert had changed the grinding conditions during the process. Regarding the force gripping the specimen during grinding, the expert showed a two-fold higher value than that of the non-expert. Also, as for the difference between the regular and maximum pressures when folding a sample down on the grinding machine, the expert also showed the greater value than the non-expert. We also found that warp and weft clearly appeared on the finished surface of the expert's sample.

Moreover, we verified the difference in the sensitivity to the grinding sound that is considered as factor to determine behaviors during grinding works. In the experiment, the expert could almost precisely determine the sound generated with varying pressure from low to high levels, while the non-expert chose the same sound generated by the same pressure level three times. It suggested that the sound sensitivity of the non-expert was lower than the expert. This result suggested that the expert comprehended the grinding states with the sound generated during grinding. He re-created the optimal grinding conditions with a wide range of pressure adjustments, which induced the finished surface with high-uniformity.

References

1. Nakayama, Y.: Trend of composite material and process for aircraft structure. vol. 26, no. 2, pp. 35–38. Materials Integration, T.I.C (2013)
2. Hoshi, H.: Repair and recycle of aircraft composite structure. J. N.D.I **60**(9), 541–545, 01 September 2011. Non-destructive inspection, The Japanese Society for Non-destructive inspection
3. Hasegawa, R.: Cutting tool for aircraft and applications. Precis. Eng. **75**(8), P953–P957 (2009)
4. Nakamura, M.: Manufacturing technology of aircraft airframe structure. Precis. Eng. **75**(8), P941–P944 (2009)
5. Izui, H.: New materials and manufacturing technologies required for next-generation aircraft. Precis. Eng. **75**(8), P937–P940 (2009)
6. Yonemoto, K., Yamamoto, Y., Okuyama, K., Ebina, T.: Application of CFRP with high hydrogen gas barrier characteristics to fuel tanks of space transportation system. Jpn. Soc. Aeronaut. Space Sci. **7**(26), P13–P18 (2009)
7. Jinno, M.: Fabrication process of composite materials for aircraft structure. Soc. Polym. Sci. **57**(9), 770 (2008)
8. Trends in aircraft usage. Nikkei Monozukuri, vol. 643, P61–P65, April 2008
9. Sasajima, M., Yamaguchi, Y., Ishikawa, T.: Outline of national project on advanced materials and process development for next generation aircraft structure. J. Jpn. Soc. Aeronaut. Space Sci. **54**(631), P228–P234 (2006)
10. Netsushorigijutsunyuumon. Jpn. Soc. Heat Treat. **3** (2001)
11. Sugioka, N., Kitada, M., Nishijima, M.: Metallurgical microstructure of the spear blade manufactured from the end of muromachi period to the Edo period. Jpn. Inst. Metal Mater. **75**(5), 185–191 (2013)
12. Tanaka, M., Kitada, M., Nishijima, M.: Microstructure and nonmetallic inclusion in Japanese percussion lock gun fabricated in the late Edo period. Jpn. Inst. Metal Mater. **74**(12), 779–787 (2010)
13. Hayes, B.S., Gammon, L.M.: Optical microscopy of fiber-reinforced composites. First printing, ASM International (2010)

14. Standard guide for preparation of metallographic specimen, ASTM E3–01. ASTM International (2007)
15. Samuel, L.E.: Metallographic polishing by mechanical methods. ASM International (2003)
16. Smith, M.F.: A comparison of techniques for the metallographic preparation of thermal sprayed samples. J. Therm. Spray Technol. **2**(3), 287–294 (1993)

An Investigation on Skillful Gel-Coat Techniques and its Application to Beginner's Application

Erika Suzuki[1], Tetsuo Kikuchi[1,2(✉)], Yuka Takai[3], Akihiko Goto[3], and Hiroyuki Hamada[2]

[1] Toyugiken Co., Ltd., Minamiashigara-shi, Kanagwa, Japan
{erika-suzuki,tetuo-kikuchi}@toyugiken.co.jp
[2] Department of Advanced Fibro-Science, Kyoto Institute of Technology, Kyoto, Japan
hhamada@kit.ac.jp
[3] Osaka Sangyo University, Osaka, Japan
{takai,gotoh}@ise.osaka-sandai.ac.jp

Abstract. Gel Coating has been used for forming composite structures since ancient times. On the other hand, gel coating work itself relies on human skills, which means that the finish differs according to the operator carrying out the work, the quality of the product differs among parts depending on the ease of forming. Hence highly specialized control technique and the tradition of skill are required to ensure the consistent stability of product quality. Therefore, in this study, motion analysis experiment of gel coating experts by MAC 3D System was conducted to obtain objective data on an expert applier's skills (the default value) with compared to the non-expert one. Furthermore, dimensional stability measurements were made, and an investigation of the correlation to an expert's application techniques was conducted in order to pass the suitable training and communicating technical skills to advanced management engineering and inexperienced appliers.

Keywords: Dimension stability · Motion analysis · Explicit knowledge

1 Introduction

Gel Coating relies on the skill of the person doing the applying. Gel Coating is an important process which determines the appearance of product. This NG of operation is related to product NG straightly. Moreover, controlling the thickness of Gel Coating is very difficult because of it may become thin and the color may become transparent. However, when the thickness is thick, especially before the Gelling coat gel, it will drop at the vertical plane. The dropped vestige will make bad appearance on product surface. As a result of its difference from common Gel Coating, it isn't able to judge the quality of Gel Coating, the gel coat failure would generate a large loss. For this reason, motion analysis of the spray up method process was conducted to obtain objective data on an expert applier's skills (the default value). Furthermore, dimensional stability measurements were made, and an investigation of the correlation to an expert's

V.G. Duffy (Ed.): DHM 2015, Part I, LNCS 9184, pp. 182–191, 2015.
DOI: 10.1007/978-3-319-21073-5_19

application techniques was conducted. In this way, suitable training and communicating technical skills can be passed on to advanced management engineering and inexperienced appliers. Also, the degree of master craftsmanship (called *takumi* in Japanese) needs to be quantified, so that more advanced technology will become manageable.

2 Methodology

2.1 Subjects

In this study, two people were tested: an expert gel coating craftsman (male, 54 years old, 32-year work career) and a non-expert (male, 25 years old, 1-year work career). The biological data of the subjects is shown in Table 1. One was left handed, and another was right handed. They didn't have physical handicaps or a disease that restricted their work. The purpose and method of this study were explained in advance to the subjects. Their consent to participate was obtained.

Table 1. Biological data of subjects

Subject	Age	Years experience	Height (cm)	Weight (kg)	Dominant-hand
Expert	54	32	169	66	left
Non-expert	25	1	168	62	right

2.2 Analysis Objective

The object of the analysis was to evaluate the work done for making gel-coated plate. The size of the mold was 1820 mm high and 910 mm wide. A blue rectangle (1250 mm × 800 mm) was drawn on the 1 m^2 spray region (Fig. 1).

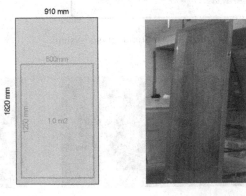

Fig. 1. Mold used in this study (1820 mm high, 910 mm wide)

2.3 Gel Coating

The gel coating machine that was used was made in Japan. As a base material, the vinyl ester resin was used.

2.4 Dimensional Stability

To compare the dimensional stability of the expert and non-expert, the surface coarseness of the plane of the acquired molded product was measured. A micrometer was used for measuring thickness.

All samples (1250 mm × 800 mm) obtained in the experiment were cut and divided into 16 sections. Moreover, the thickness of the cross section of each area was measured every 10 mm. About 1,110 data points were obtained per subject.

2.5 Measurement Techniques of Operator's Skill Level

Motion analysis (Figs. 2, 3) and eye movement measuring (Fig. 4) were done from start to finish for the entire work process. The experiment was performed under the same circumstances as their usual workplace so that the subjects could work as normal. Moreover, instructions—except restrictions for measurement—were omitted so that the subjects could work at their own pace. In addition, three-dimensional motion and eye movements were measured separately.

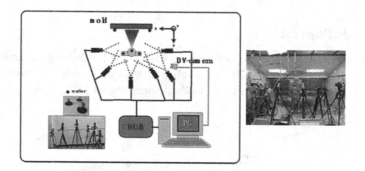

Fig. 2. Motion analysis system

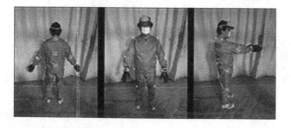 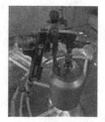

Fig. 3. 19 markers were attached to the subject's body (infrared reflective markers were reflected as white).

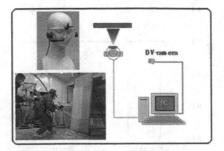

Fig. 4. Eye movement measurement system

3 Results and Considerations

3.1 Dimensional Stability

The dimensional stability (thickness distribution) of the expert and non-expert are shown in Fig. 5. The classification by color in the figure is every 0.2 mm.

The expert's average thickness was 0.27 mm and the coefficient of variation (C.V.) value was 13.2 %. On the other hand, the average thickness for the non-expert was 0.19 mm and the C.V. value was 29.4 %. As the theoretical thickness of this study was 0.3 mm, the non-expert's thickness distribution was thin and the C.V. value was also large (Fig. 6). In particular, there are very thick regions in the bottom of product done by non-expert. This dimensional stability shows that the expert had precise thickness control. In other words, the expert's loss of gel coating also decreased. Improving the gel coating technology would substantially contribute to dimensional stability and reduced waste.

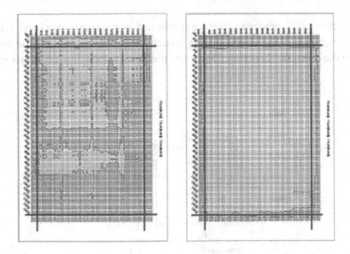

Fig. 5. Comparison of thickness distribution (left: non-expert, right: expert) (Color figure online)

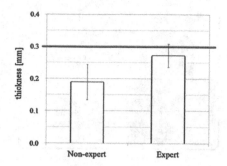

Fig. 6. Comparison of thickness distribution

3.2   Process Analysis

First, each motion under work was defined, and could be divided into two motions: first the "horizontal stroke" and second the "vertical stroke". The "stroke" was defined as the one-way movement of the gel coating in the horizontal and vertical direction of the mold (Fig. 7).

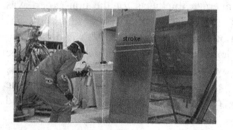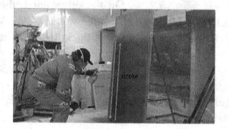

Fig. 7. Definition of "horizontal stroke" and "vertical stroke"

There are great differences between experts and non-experts workers, especially in operation time (Fig. 8). The daub done by experts was even no matter the longitudinal direction and the constant direction. However, the non-experts don't conduct in this way.

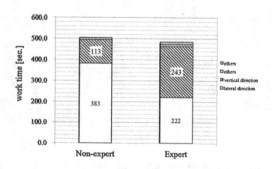

Fig. 8. Comparison of work time

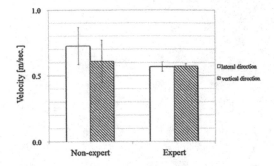

Fig. 9. The mean work time per stroke for each process

Next, the mean velocity of the stroke in each process was compared (Fig. 9). The experts daubed in same speed both in the longitudinal direction and in the content direction, thus less deviation can be concluded.

3.3 Motion Analysis

The operations at the time of the gel coating by the expert and non-expert were compared. Attention was paid to the motion of the gun of gel coating. The difference in motion was especially noted (Fig. 10). Here, the x axis is defined as the direction perpendicular to the spray. The y axis is defined as the spray direction. And the z axis is defined as the height direction.

To better understand the series of motions, the "crookedness expansion movements" of the expert and non-expert were compared. The angle variations between the knee, greater trochanter and shoulder (right side) are shown in Figs. 11 and 12. The expert had a wide angle variation (wide arc) and it turns out that this is the stable angle variation. Moreover, it is clear that the expert is further "crooked" by about 50 degrees, and it turns out that the "crookedness expansion movement" for each stroke by the expert was performed smoothly. That is, the expert is performing the "crookedness expansion movement" efficiently while on tiptoes.

The difference in the angle variation can be clearly seen from this figure. Moreover, because of the efficient body movement of experts, spray guy is always perpendicular

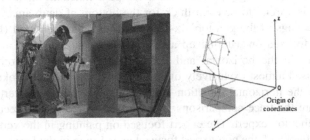

Fig. 10. Motion analysis

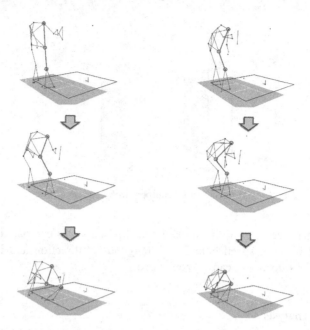

Fig. 11. The comparison of the angle variations (right side) between the knee, greater trochanter and shoulder (left: non-expert, right: expert).

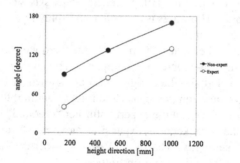

Fig. 12. Angle between the knee, greater trochanter and shoulder (right side)

to the lower part of daub area. Thus, daub loss declined and stable size of product can be gained. However, the angle of spray gun is not perpendicular, the loss may increase and then, there is a trend to be even thick for the bottom of daub area.

Next, the tracings of the gun top's x-z coordinates were measured (Fig. 13).

The expert focused on painting up and down first, but also paid attention to the alternate coating in the horizontal and vertical directions. On the other hand, the non-expert focused almost exclusively on painting with horizontal strokes (Fig. 14).

In addition, the horizontal direction coating is thicker than the vertical direction coating. Here are the trace comparisons in horizontal and vertical directions between the expert and the non-expert. The expert focused on painting in the vertical direction paint. On the other hand, the non-expert focused on painting in the horizontal direction.

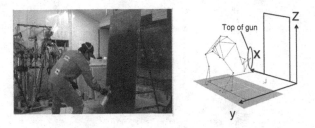

Fig. 13. Tracing of the gun top

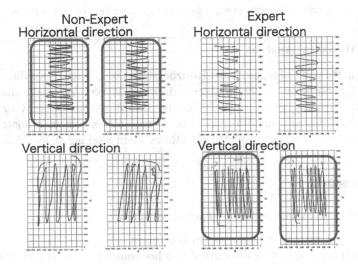

Fig. 14. The comparison of the tracings of the gun top's x-z coordinates (left: non-expert, right: expert).

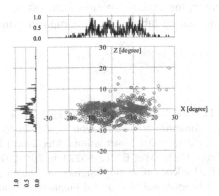

Fig. 15. Comparison of points of view for expert (in case of horizontal direction)

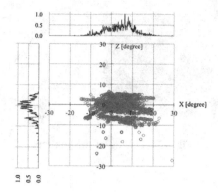

Fig. 16. Comparison of points of view for non-expert (in case of horizontal direction)

3.4   Eye Movement Analysis

By observing the point-of-regard track, Horizontal axis is x, longitudinal direction is z, learn that the movement in the transverse direction is very even and smooth, the vertical direction was always stable. That is, skilled workers were very intently watching the daub area, rather than the obviously unstable movement of non-experts in different directions and absent-minded sometimes when working (Figs. 15 and 16).

4   Conclusions

The results for the expert can be summarized as follows:

1. The thickness of coating by the expert is uniform.
2. The expert sprayed in both the vertical and horizontal sections at a similar pace.
3. The expert's main focus was on the vertical coating.
4. The expert's eyes covered a wider range than the specified area

Furthermore, it was found that the above four points can be incorporated into the educational tools of non-experts and intermediates, sharply reducing the skill acquirement time. Moreover, the expert's motion data was fed to a gel coating robot, resulting in minimal errors during fabrication of composite panels.

References

1. Kikuchi, T., Koyanagi, T., Hamada, H., Nakai, A., Takai, Y., Goto, A., Fujii, Y., Narita, C., Endo, A., Koshino, T.: Biomechanics investigation of skillful technician in hand lay up fabrication method. In: The ASME 2012 International Mechanical Engineering Congress & Exposition, Houston, Texas, USA, IMECE2012-86270, p. 288 (2012)
2. Karimi, A., Manteufel, R.: Understanding why engineering students take too long to garaduate. In: The ASME 2013 International Mechanical Engineering Congress & Exposition, San Diego, California, USA, IMECE2013-65367 (2013)

3. Miller, A., Samples, J.: Building a community – how to enrich an engineering technology program with identity, presence and pride. In: The ASME 2013 International Mechanical Engineering Congress & Exposition, San Diego, California, USA, IMECE2013-65034 (2013)
4. Kobus, C.J.: Storytelling – a most powerful tool in shaping lesson plans in engineering education. In: The ASME 2013 International Mechanical Engineering Congress & Exposition, San Diego, California, USA, IMECE2013-65604 (2013)
5. Zhang, Z., Yang, Y. Hamada, H.: Mechanical property of glass mat composite with open hole. In: The ASME 2012 International Mechanical Engineering Congress & Exposition, Houston, Texas, USA, IMECE2012-87270, p.79 (2012)
6. Shirato, M., Kume, M., Ohnishi, A., Nakai, A., Sato, H., Maki, M., Yoshida, T.: Analysis of daubing motion in the clay wall craftsman: influence on several kinds of clay with different fermentation period on the daubing motion properties. In: Symposium on Sports Engineering: Symposium on Human Dynamics 2007, Japan, pp. 254–257 (2007)
7. Kikuchi, T., Fudauchi, A., Koshino, T., Narita, C., Endo, A., Hamada, H.: Mechanical property of CFRP by carbon spray up method. In: The ASME 2013 International Mechanical Engineering Congress & Exposition, San Diego, California, USA, IMECE2013-64144, p. 63 (2013)
8. Kikuchi, T., Hamada, H., Nakai, A., Ohtani, A., Goto, A., Takai, Y., Endo, A., Narita, C., Koshino, T., Fudauchi, A.: Relationships between degree of skill, dimension stability and mechanical properties of composites structure in hand lay-up method. In: The 19th International Conference on Composite Materials, Montreal, Canada, pp. 8034–8042 (2013)

Numerical Analysis on "Kana-Ami" Structure Between Expert and Non-expert

Zelong Wang[1(✉)], Ken-ichi Tsuji[2], Toru Tsuji[2], Koji Ishizaki[1(✉)],
Yuka Takai[3], Akihiko Goto[3], and Hiroyuki Hamada[1]

[1] Advanced Fibro-Science, Kyoto Institute of Technology, Kyoto, Japan
simon.zelongwang@gmail.com
[2] Kana-Ami Tsuji, Kyoto, Japan
tsujiken@kanaamitsuji.com
[3] Department of Information Systems Engineering, Osaka Sangyo University,
Osaka, Japan
gotoh@ise.osaka-sandai.ac.jp

Abstract. "Kana-ami" is a kind of metal wire network in Japan, which was once prevailed many years ago in the old Japan and has been decreased in the development of social industrialization. In previous research, the characteristics of the "Kana-ami" hexagonal structure were clarified, the metal wire net of "Kana-ami" made by expert presented the convex shape in vertical direction so that helps buffer the fall. The results confirmed the superiority of the product made by expert. In this research, the actual structure of "Kana-ami" was clarified by X-Ray. And the advantage of the expert's product was confirmed. The three-dimensional analysis method was applied to present the different actual structure.

Keywords: Kana-ami · Three-dimensional scanning · X-Ray · Expert · Non-expert

1 Introduction

"Kana-ami" is a kind of metal wire network in Japan as shown in Fig. 1. It's employed as one kitchen instrument (Bread grill) or fence knitting for cultural relic, which was once prevailed many years ago in the old Japan and has been decreased in the development of social industrialization. Additionally, traditional handcrafts are handed down mainly through oral teaching and extempore creation, making proceed of teacher-student relations, family relations and art education.

However, it is very difficult for learner to copy the weaving motion from master. Usually, the master only can pass the every essential to the prentice but the rest were on your own. Therefore, the technique of tradition handcrafts is reliant on apperceiving heavily as "Kana-ami". Without apperception, it cannot be learnt no matter how hard you study, which was considered as the special tacit knowledge. And quantified the correct apperception of master is the main target in this study.

In previous research, the expert's motion of the "Kana-ami" weaving process was clarified, which was "brief, frequent, fast" during the twisted cross [1–3]. As the same time, the different "Kana-ami" hexagonal structure in vertical direction between expert

© Springer International Publishing Switzerland 2015
V.G. Duffy (Ed.): DHM 2015, Part I, LNCS 9184, pp. 192–200, 2015.
DOI: 10.1007/978-3-319-21073-5_20

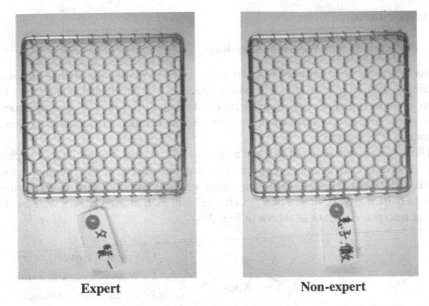

| Expert | Non-expert |

Fig. 1. The Japanese traditional handicraft of "Kana-ami"

and non-expert also was explained in the free fall experiment by high-speed camera [4, 5]. The metal wire net of "Kana-ami" made by expert presented the convex shape in vertical direction so that helps buffer the fall. The results confirmed the superiority of the product made by expert.

Therefore, the accurate identification and effective expression of the hexagonal structure of "Kana-ami" were focused in this study. The Industrial CT (X-Ray) system was applied, through scanning the whole metal wire network products made by expert and non-expert, The "Kana-ami" structure was orientated and recorded base on X-Ray there-dimensional scanning.

The velocity, acceleration, and jerk were also calculated as the same time, in order to further analysis the feature of motion between expert and non-expert. As well know, the hardest part about movement for a learner is the motion changing moment, which the velocity and direction of movement generated uncertain changing. However, the structure difference caused by different weaving motion was very difficult to explore, which was directly affect the "Kana-ami" product performance.

In additionally, the precise three-dimensional structure was observed and analyzed. The characteristics of hexagonal structure for expert and non-expert were compared. It was confirmed previous conclusion that the expert's structure was presented a curve shape and reasonable orientation. It is means that expert' motion was able to weaving a curve hexagon of "Kana-ami" mental wire network.

The purpose of this paper was through three-dimensional orientation scanning by X-Ray to clarify the "Kana-ami" structure features between expert and non-expert's motion in order to demonstrate expert's motion can generate excellent "Kana-ami" product, which was considered as a current movement technique of "Kana-ami" weaving method.

2 Experiment

2.1 Participants and Weaving Procedure

In this study, the two masters with 46 years and 10 years wire netting technique experience were employed as participants, which called expert and non-expert. The expert and non-expert not only have parent child relationships but also have mentoring relationship. And both of them would be committed to heritage this Japanese handicraft technique of "Kana-ami".

The subjects were required to make a "Kana-ami" product. Figure 1 shows a photo of one of completed samples. As same with previous research, two twisted crossed were called "Twisted cross" during the whole weaving process. "First twisted cross", "Second twisted cross", "Right-line", "Left-line" and each inside vertexes were used to call the hexagon elements as shown in Fig. 2.

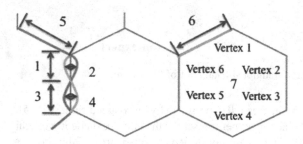

1	Length of First twisted cross
2	Width of First twisted cross
3	Length of Second twisted cross
4	Width of Second twisted cross
5	Length of "Right-line"
6	Length of "Left-line"
7	6 Vertex angle

Fig. 2. The industrial CT system of "Toscaner"

2.2 Experimental Process

The three-dimensional orientation structure of "Kana-ami" was measured by industrial CT. (High resolution miniature CT TOSCANER - 32300 mu FD/32300 mu hd; Toshiba Co. Ltd.), which X-ray tube voltage generator was 230 kv, and the focus size was 4 microns (without wire). The spatial resolution was 5 microns.

The expert and non-expert's "Kana-ami" products were scanned by industrial CT system through X-Ray as shown in Fig. 3. The three-dimensional data of expert and non-expert's "Kana-ami" products were analyzed by the software of "Solidworks".

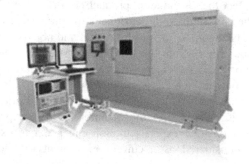

Fig. 3. The industrial CT system of "Toscaner"

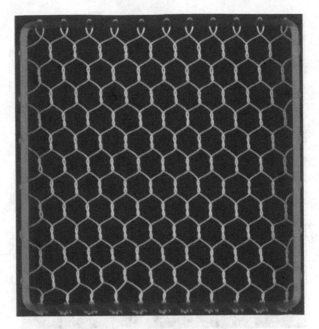

Fig. 4. The perspective drawing of expert's "Kana-ami"

3   Result and Discussion

3.1   Interval-Timing Analysis

The image results of three-dimensional scanning were shown in Figs. 4 and 5 (Expert and Non-expert). The whole final "Kana-ami" products of expert and non-expert were presented by X-Ray technology. Threshold value was adjusted into the most clear level.

3.2   Interval-Timing Analysis

The numerical models of the whole product made by expert and non-expert were illustrated in Figs. 6 and 7 respectively. The hexagons features of expert and non-expert created by three-dimensional scanning were demonstrated as the same with previous research, which was proceeded by digital image processing technology.

In the overall view, as shown in Figs. 6 and 7, both vertex 1 and 4's average angle value of 5 knitted samples by expert showed nearly 100°, which were approached 95° at the same location of non-expert. Expert and non-expert's angle values of vertex 2 and 5 were almost higher than vertex 3 and 6. The expert s vertex angle of 1 and 4 were bigger than non-expert. On the contrary, compared with non-expert, expert's vertex 2 and 6 were smaller then non-expert. 3rd hexagon on 3rd line at the same location made by expert and non-expert were focused on Fig. 8(a) and (b).

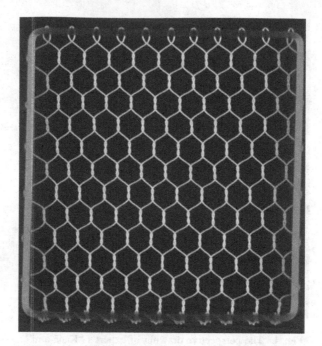

Fig. 5. The perspective drawing of non-expert's "Kana-ami"

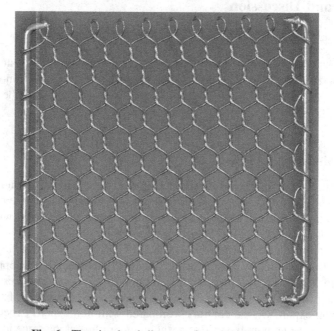

Fig. 6. The simulated diagram of expert's "Kana-ami"

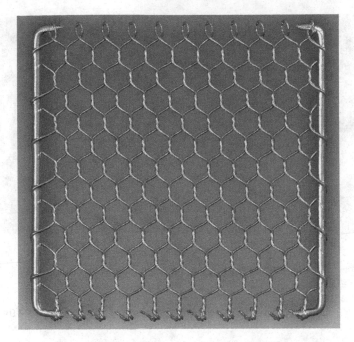

Fig. 7. The simulated diagram of non-expert's "Kana-ami"

The bulge direction of 'Right-line' at the same location made by expert and non-expert were focused in frontal side as shown in Fig. 8(a) and (b).

Compared with non-expert, the bulge direction of 'Right-line' by expert was upper ward as red arrow in Fig. 8(a), which was considered that higher than non-expert more than 0.05 mm in previous research. The bulge direction of the 'Right-line' by non-expert was down ward as red arrow in Fig. 8(b).

The bulge direction of 'Right-line' at the same location made by expert and non-expert also were focused in axial side as shown in Figs. 9(a) and 10(a). And the expert and non-expert's outline of schematic diagram located at the hexagon were shown in Figs. 9(b) and 10(b).

As same with above result, the bulge direction of 'Right-line' by expert was upper ward as red arrow in Fig. 9. The bulge direction of 'Right-line' by non-expert was left upper ward as red arrow in Fig. 10. It was confirmed the result of previous research that different making motion technique was deemed to the main reason for the differences in structure of final products between expert and non-expert, which was directly affected the hexagonal shape, which was deemed that expert's shape of "Right-line" was made under suitable rotation angle.

According to this result, the curve shape of "Right-line" was similar between expert and non-expert. However, the bulge direction was different. The expert bulge direction was upper ward, which was showed more significant radian and more convex to the frontal side. The non-expert bulge direction was convex to left upper side.

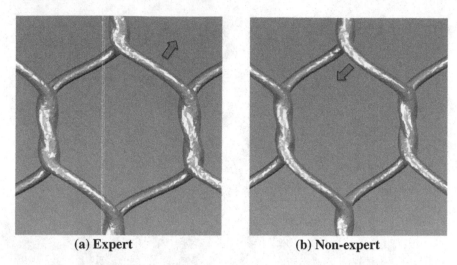

(a) Expert   (b) Non-expert

Fig. 8. The 3rd hexagon on 3rd line in frontal side

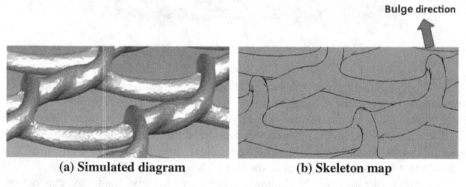

(a) Simulated diagram   (b) Skeleton map

Fig. 9. The expert's 3rd hexagon on 3rd line in axial side

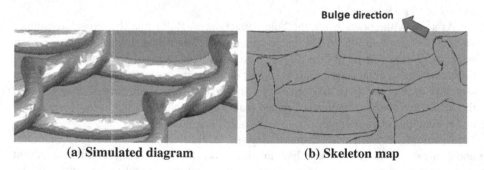

(a) Simulated diagram   (b) Skeleton map

Fig. 10. The non-expert's 3rd hexagon on 3rd line in axial side

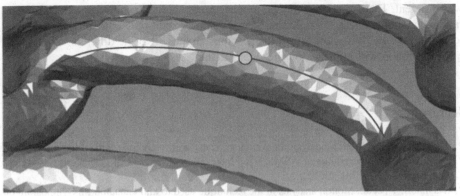

(a) Expert

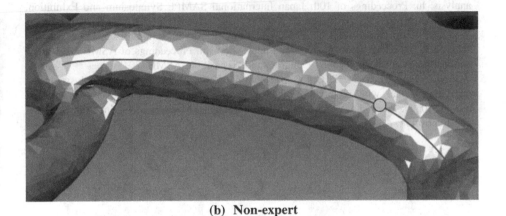

(b) Non-expert

Fig. 11. The curve shape of "Right-line" for expert and non-expert in inclined side

The peak of curve shape for "Right-line" and "Left-line" was illustrate on Fig. 11, which the expert and non-expert were shown in Fig. 11(a) and (b) respectively. As shown in Fig. 11, the peak of the 'Right-line' made by expert was located in the central as shown in yellow color. However, the peak of the 'Right-line' made by non-expert was located in the down side as shown in yellow color, which was closed with next "First twisted cross". And the length of the "Right-line" made by expert was shorter than non-expert's. It was second main reason that the expert's "Right-line" was more convex to frontal side than "Non-expert".

4 Conclusions

As a conclusion, the three-dimensional structure of expert and non-expert's "Kana-ami" product was accurate scanning. The result of "Right-line" shape was shown the similar curve between expert and non-expert. However, the bulge direction was different. The expert bulge direction was upper ward, and showed more significant radian and more convex to the frontal side. The non-expert bulge direction was convex to left upper side. It was confirmed the previous suppose that the different "Kana-ami" making motion will influence on the final product.

References

1. K, Tusji., et al.: Motion analysis of weaving 'Kana-ami' technique with different years of experience. In: Proceedings of ASME 2012 International Mechanical Engineering Congress and Exposition, ASME (2012)
2. Tatsunori, T., et al.: Motion analysis of the technique used to knit kanaami. In: Symposium on Sports Engineering: Symposium on Human Dynamics, pp. 258–261 (2007)
3. Tatsunori, T., et al.: Human motion of weaving 'Kana-ami' technique by biomechanical analysis. In: Proceedings of 10th Japan International SAMPE Symposium and Exhibition, TC-1-3 (2007)
4. Wang, Z. Endo, A. Koshino, T. Tsuji, T. Tsuji, K.: Evaluation of metal wire network "Kana-ami" structure between expert and non-expert. In: Proceedings of ASME 2013 International Mechanical Engineering Congress and Exposition, ASME (2013)
5. Wang, Z. Tsuji, K. Tsuji, T. Goto, A. Takai, Y. Yang, Y. Hamada, H.: Analysis on the three-dimensional wire orientation of "Kana-ami" metal network between expert and non-expert. In: Proceedings of ASME 2014 International Mechanical Engineering Congress and Exposition, ASME (2014)

Motion Analysis of Interval Time During "Kana-ami" Making Process

Zelong Wang[1]([✉]), Ken-ichi Tsuji[2], Toru Tsuji[2], Yuka Takai[3],
Akihiko Goto[3], and Hiroyuki Hamada[1]

[1] Advanced Fibro-Science, Kyoto Institute of Technology, Kyoto, Japan
simon.zelongwang@gmail.com
[2] Kana-ami Tsuji, Kyoto, Japan
tsujiken@kanaamitsuji.com
[3] Department of Information systems Engineering, Osaka Sangyo University,
Osaka, Japan
gotoh@ise.osaka-sandai.ac.jp

Abstract. In this paper, the motion making technique of Japanese traditional handicraft was analyzed by motion analysis system. Two experts were employed as expert and non-expert for comparison. The feature of interval time for each main work process was paid attention. The subjects' interval timing during the weaving process was clarified to investigate the proficiency of weaving technique quantitatively. It is found that expert was able to go into working state easily.

Keywords: Kana-ami · Interval timing · Motion analysis · Expert · Non-expert

1 Introduction

"Kana-ami" is a classical traditional handicraft product of metal wire network in Japan as shown in Fig. 1. It's employed as one kitchen instrument (tofu scooping) or fence knitting for cultural relic, which was once prevailed many years ago in the old Japan and has been decreased in the development of social industrialization. Additionally, traditional handcrafts are handed down mainly through oral teaching and extempore creation, making proceed of teacher-student relations, family relations and art education.

However, it is very difficult for learner to copy the weaving motion from master. Usually, the master only can pass the every essential to the prentice but the rest were on your own. Therefore, the technique of tradition handcrafts is reliant on apperceiving heavily as "Kana-ami". Without apperception, it cannot be learnt no matter how hard you study, which was considered as the special tacit knowledge. And quantified the correct apperception of master is the main target in this study.

In previous research, the expert's motion of the "Kana-ami" weaving process was clarified, which was "brief, frequent, fast" during the twisted cross [1–3]. As the same time, the different "Kana-ami" hexagonal structure in vertical direction between expert and non-expert also was explained in the free fall experiment by high-speed camera [4, 5]. The metal wire net of "Kana-ami" made by expert presented the convex shape in vertical direction so that helps buffer the fall. The results confirmed the superiority of the product made by expert.

© Springer International Publishing Switzerland 2015
V.G. Duffy (Ed.): DHM 2015, Part I, LNCS 9184, pp. 201–211, 2015.
DOI: 10.1007/978-3-319-21073-5_21

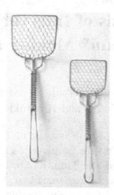

Fig. 1. The Japanese traditional handicraft of "Kana-ami"

Refer to the previous conclusions, the reasonable decoding and the effective expression of expert's motion were focused in this research. The motion analysis system was applied, through extracting each main work of twisted cross during the "Kana-ami" weaving process, both expert and non-expert's fingers trajectory of twisted cross was recorded and separated base on there-dimensional coordinate system. The velocity, acceleration, and jerk were also calculated as the same time, in order to further analysis the feature of motion between expert and non-expert.

As well know, the hardest part about movement for a learner is the motion changing moment, which the velocity and direction of movement generated uncertain changing. However, every movement changing has to experience a process of acceleration direction changing, which was jerk value around zero as called interval-timing moment in this research.

In additionally, the interval-timing of each twisted cross was found and summarized. The characteristics of interval timing for expert and non-expert were compared. It was discovered that the expert's interval timing of each weaving process was reduced gradually as the weaving progresses. It is means that expert was able to enter the working state quickly, and change every movement essential with short interval timing.

The purpose of this paper was through motion analysis to clarify the interval-timing between expert and non-expert's motion in order to find a current movement technique of "Kana-ami" weaving method.

"Kana-ami" was all made by hand work, so the processing motion technique makes a big effect on final products' quality and craftsman's long-term working efficiency.

2 Experiment

2.1 Participants

In this study, the two masters with 46 years and 10 years wire netting technique experience were employed as participants, which called expert and non-expert. The expert and non-expert not only have parent child relationships but also have mentoring relationship. And both of them would be committed to heritage this Japanese handicraft technique of 'Kana-ami'.

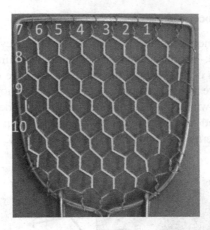

Fig. 2. Metal wire network pattern of 'Kana-ami' product

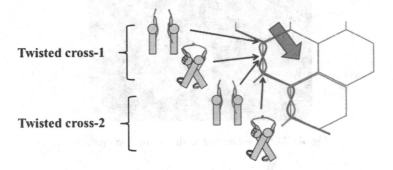

Fig. 3. The two main twisted crosses process of hexagonal pattern

2.2 Weaving Procedure

The subjects were required to make a "Kana-ami" product. Figure 2 shows a photo of one of completed samples. The hexagonal pattern was started and twisted from 1st oblique row to 10th oblique row according to weaving order. Figure 3 was illustrated a schematic detailing the making process of a hexagonal pattern of wire network. As shown in Figs. 2 and 3, the "Kana-ami" product was consisted by 48 hexagons, which were established by two twisted crosses on both sides. Therefore, the weaving process of two twisted crosses was the main work during the whole "Kana-ami" weaving process. As shown in Fig. 3, the first twisted cross was called as "Twisted cross-1" and the second twisted cross was called as "Twisted cross-2". The "Twisted cross-1" and "Twisted cross-2" were paid attention in this paper.

2.3   Experimental Process

The three-dimensional motion capture system was used for evaluating the motion of making wire nets. (Hawk-I; Motion Analysis Co. Ltd.) The infrared reflection markers were affixed at 21 points on the body of the subject to analyze motion during the wire netting as shown in figure. And six cameras captured the position of each marker in the X, Y and Z directions with 100 Hz sampling rate. All markers position data were synchronized and entered into a computer. All subjects (10 products) were recorded under the former predetermined condition as shown in Fig. 4.

Fig. 4. The measurement setting of motion analysis

2.4   Interval-Timing Analysis

The data of expert and non-expert's motion during the period of each twisted cross was extracted from the motion analysis system. The motions were categorized into 4 types according to the finger and twisted cross as shown in Fig. 5, which were called as

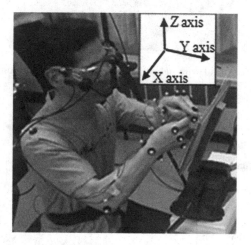

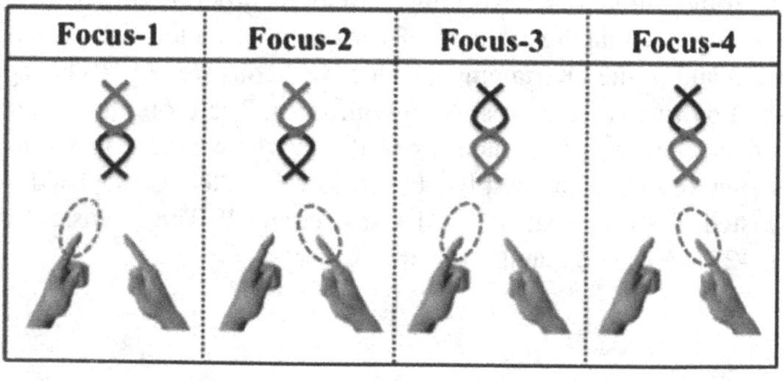

Fig. 5. Focus illustration of interval-timing process

"Focus-1", "Focus-2", "Focus-3", "Focus-4". As shown in Fig. 5, the "Focus-1" was focused on the left index finger during the process of "Twisted cross-1", the "Focus-2" was focused on the right index finger during the process of "Twisted cross-1". And the "Focus-3" and "Focus-4" were focused on the left and right index fingers during the process of "Twisted cross-2".

All the acceleration changing moment of four types data was found, which the jerk value around zero, which also was the acceleration direction of transient variation. The interval-timing was defined as a period in the range of the average acceleration changing when the jerk was around zero. One "Kana-ami" product has 48 hexagons consisted of 70 times trials of two twisted crosses. The motion of "Focus-1" at the first hexagon on 2nd oblique row by non-expert was presented as an example, whose velocity, acceleration and jerk were shown in Figs. 6, 7 and 8. The interval timing

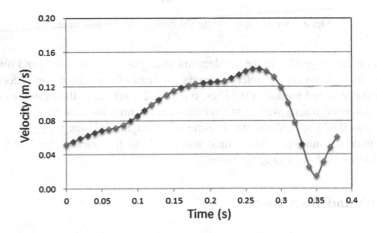

Fig. 6. An example of interval-timing plot on velocity figure

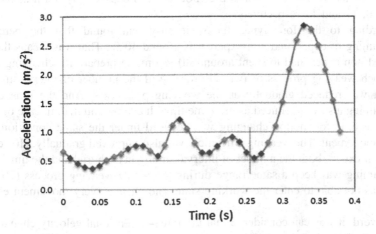

Fig. 7. An example of interval-timing plot on acceleration figure

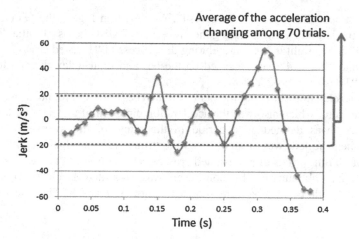

Fig. 8. An example of interval-timing plot on jerk figure

moments on the range of average acceleration changing moment was found out as red marks in Fig. 8. Accordingly, interval-timing moment of the velocity and acceleration were illustrated as red marks on the Figs. 6 and 7. Therefore, in the example case, the number of interval timing was eight, and the average time for each interval-timing for this trial was 0.026 s. And the whole time of example trial was 0.39 s, the percent between interval-timing and whole time was 53.85 %. It is means that 53.85 % time was used to prepare for changing motion.

3 Result and Discussion

The number of interval-timing, average time of interval-timing, and the percent between interval-timing and whole time for 70 trails were summarized according to the four types focus ("Focus-1", "Focus-2", "Focus-3", "Focus-4"), which illustrated into Figs. 9, 10, 11 and 12 respectively.

According to the four types focus, it easy can found that the percent of interval-timing of expert and non-expert was around 40 %. That was means that both expert and non-expert had to spent around 40 % time to prepare for changing motion during each weaving process of twisted cross. And the number of interval-timing in each trial was reduced gradually as the weaving progresses. And the time of each interval-timing also was reduced as the same time. It can be said that, in case of expert, the prepare time for motion changing was reduced under the same condition of the effective movement. The weaving efficiency was also improved gradually. However, in case of non-expert, both the number of interval-timing in each trial and the time of each interval-timing was keep a same range during the whole weaving process (70 trials). Expert was not able to enter the working state, and change every movement essential quickly.

In a word, it was can considered that the three-dimensional velocity changes need successively through the process of vector acceleration and deceleration. It is has to

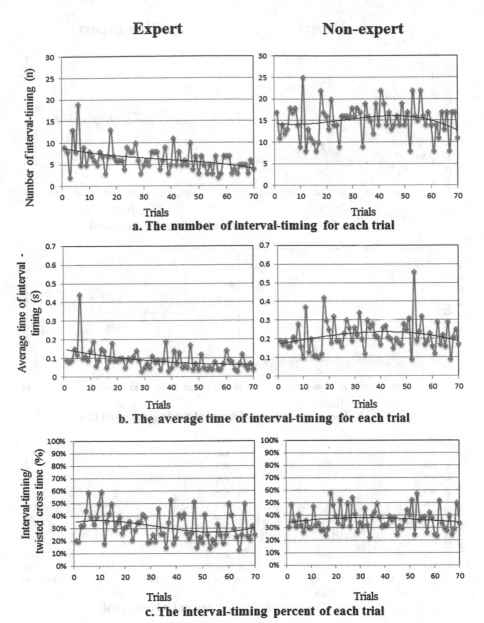

a. The number of interval-timing for each trial

b. The average time of interval-timing for each trial

c. The interval-timing percent of each trial

Fig. 9. "Focus-1" comparison between expert and non-expert

take a short process of uniform acceleration when the acceleration direction was changing, because the behavior motion completely controlled by the brain and requires action time. Therefore, the interval-timing was an important feature of motional proficiency.

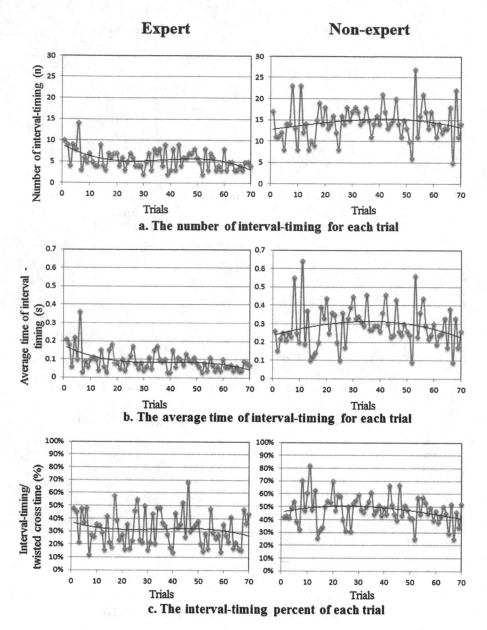

a. The number of interval-timing for each trial

b. The average time of interval-timing for each trial

c. The interval-timing percent of each trial

Fig. 10. "Focus-2" comparison between expert and non-expert

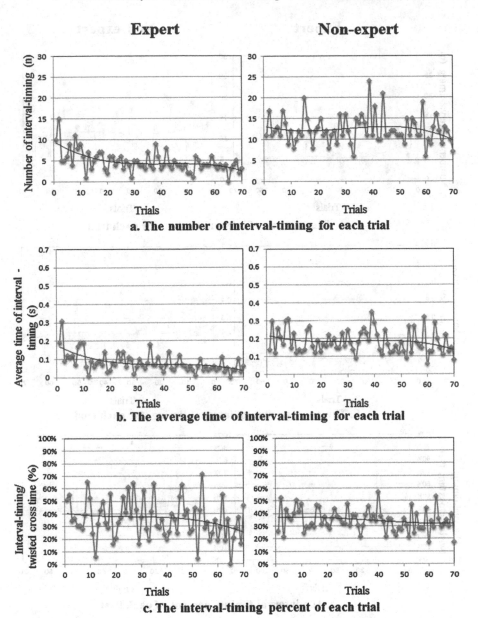

Expert   **Non-expert**

a. The number of interval-timing for each trial

b. The average time of interval-timing for each trial

c. The interval-timing percent of each trial

Fig. 11. "Focus-3" comparison between expert and non-expert

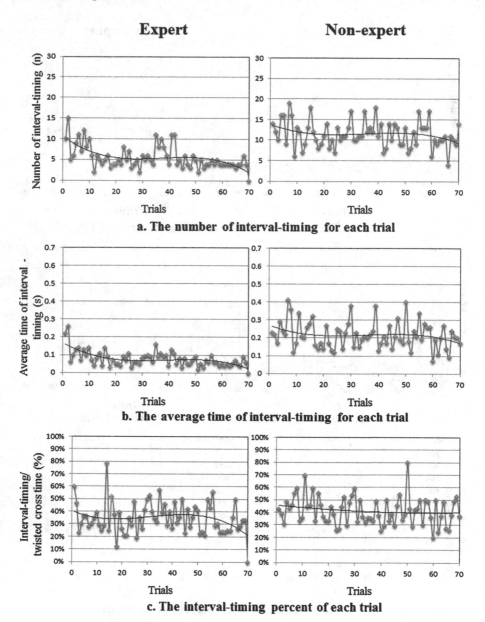

a. The number of interval-timing for each trial

b. The average time of interval-timing for each trial

c. The interval-timing percent of each trial

Fig. 12. "Focus-4" comparison between expert and non-expert

4   Conclusions

As a conclusion, both expert and non-expert spent round 40 % time to make interval timing movement for each trial. Because the number and time of "Interval-timing" was reduced gradually in case of expert, the completion time of each weaving trail was shown significant reduction. It is can considered that expert can change motion state skillfully, and easier to enter a right working state smoothly.

References

1. Tusji, K., et al.: Motion analysis of weaving 'Kana-ami' technique with different years of experience. In: Proceedings of ASME 2012 International Mechanical Engineering Congress & Exposition, ASME (2012)
2. Tatsunori, T., et al.: Motion Analysis of the Technique Used to Knit Kanaami. In: symposium on sports engineering: symposium on human dynamics, pp. 258–261 (2007)
3. Tatsunori, T., et al.: Human motion of weaving 'Kana-ami' technique by biomechanical analysis. In: Proceedings of 10th Japan International SAMPE Symposium & Exhibition, TC-1-3 (2007)
4. Wang, Z., Endo, A., Koshino, T., Tsuji, T., Tsuji, K.: Evaluation of metal wire network "Kana-ami" structure between expert and non-expert. In: Proceedings of ASME 2013 International Mechanical Engineering Congress & Exposition, ASME (2013)
5. Wang, Z., Tsuji, K., Tsuji, T., Goto, A., Takai, Y., Yang, Y., Hamada, H.: Analysis on the three-dimensional wire orientation of "Kana-ami" metal network between expert and non-expert. In: Proceedings of ASME 2014 International Mechanical Engineering Congress and Exposition, ASME (2014)

Brain Activity Analysis on "Kana-Ami" Making Process

Zelong Wang[1(⊠)], Ken-ichi Tsuji[2], Toru Tsuji[2], Yuka Takai[3], Akihiko Goto[3], and Hiroyuki Hamada[1]

[1] Advanced Fibro-Science, Kyoto Institute of Technology, Kyoto, Japan
simon.zelongwang@gmail.com
[2] Kana-Ami Tsuji, Kyoto, Japan
tsujiken@kanaamitsuji.com
[3] Department of Information Systems Engineering, Osaka Sangyo University,
Osaka, Japan
gotoh@ise.osaka-sandai.ac.jp

Abstract. In this paper, the brain wave activity and saliva α-armylase for expert and non-expert was measured during five test of "Kana-ami" fatigue. Two experts were employed as expert and non-expert for comparison. The feature of subjects' working state and physical condition for each trial test was paid attention. It is found that expert was able to keep charging and concentrate working state even the body under the fatigue condition.

Keywords: Kana-ami · Brain wave · Saliva α-armylase · Expert · Non-expert

1 Introduction

"Kana-ami" is a classical traditional handicraft product of metal wire network in Japan as shown in Fig. 1. The history of Japanese "Kana-ami", the wire netting ware in Kyoto, goes back more than ten centuries. Used as kitchen utensils in Kyoto cuisine, these tools have been cherished by chefs in the city through the ages. However, "Kana-ami" handicraft technique has been declined in the development of social industrialization.

Additionally, on the one hand, traditional handcrafts are handed down mainly through oral teaching and extempore creation, making proceed of teacher-student relations, family relations and art education. On the other hand, a lot of traditional craftsman consider their work is monotonous and tedious even if very meaningful. It is very important to overcome the obstacles of focus on proceeding one thing for a long time.

However, it is very difficult for learner to keep concentrate the working state from master. Usually, the master only can pass the every essential to the prentice but the rest were on your own even with a long-term practice. Similarly, "Kana-ami" making process is a long and boring period. In order to make a good quality "Kana-ami" product, craftsman always keep the high concentration during the making process. However, long-term concentration is easier to make craftsman tired and affect the overall product beauty finally.

© Springer International Publishing Switzerland 2015
V.G. Duffy (Ed.): DHM 2015, Part I, LNCS 9184, pp. 212–219, 2015.
DOI: 10.1007/978-3-319-21073-5_22

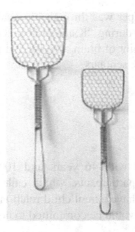

Fig. 1. Japanese traditional handicraft of "Kana-ami"

In previous research, the expert's motion of the "Kana-ami" weaving process was clarified [1–3]. As the same time, the different "Kana-ami" hexagonal structure in vertical direction between expert and non-expert also was explained in the free fall experiment by high-speed camera [4, 5]. The results confirmed the superiority of the product made by expert. It was considered that expert could keep a reasonable tempo and interval-timing during long-term proceeding. Referred to previous study, the results of five continuous "Kana-ami" product making fatigue tests clarified that non-expert with 10 years experience is difficult to keep continuous a good working mental status with long-time making process.

In this study, cooperating with "Kanaami Tsuji" workshop, it is one of the few workshops to focus only on the "Kana-ami" production in Japan. Two craftsmen were employed as experts, called expert and non-expert, which have parent-child and Master-apprentice relationships. Expert is the excellent metal wire net designer of Kyoto in 2009 and 2010 with 46 years experience. Non-expert would be determining to continue the Japanese traditional handicraft technique, which has 10 years weaving experience.

The brain activity analysis was employed to evaluate subject's brain concentration condition during "Kana-ami" product making process. The brain wave analysis system was applied, the subjects was required to make five "Kana-ami" continuously. Both expert and non-expert's brain wave activity was recorded one by one. The five trials of expert and non-expert's α and β brain wave ratio were calculated to present the working state. The saliva α-armylase activities for each trial of expert and non-expert were measured and used for assessing their physical recovery and levels of fatigue.

In additionally, the result of expert's α and β brain wave were shown a steady ratio during the whole process of five trials "Kana-ami" making. However, the expert shown the large saliva α-armylase changing, which was considered that expert was physical fatigue easily because older characteristic. Therefore, expert can keep a good working condition under fatigue state.

And the purpose of this paper was through the evaluation and analysis of crafts-man's brain activity difference during "Kana-ami" making process to found the rela-tionship between expert key point of brain activity and their working state and finally provide a reference for the new scholars.

2 Experiment

2.1 Participants

In this study, the two masters with 46 years and 10 years wire netting technique experience were employed as participants, which called expert and non-expert. The expert and non-expert not only have parent child relationships but also have mentoring relationship. And both of them would be committed to heritage this Japanese handicraft technique of 'Kana-ami'.

2.2 Experimental Process

The subjects were required to make five "Kana-ami" products continuously. The brain wave activities of expert and non-expert were recorded by EEG system (electroen-cephalogram, MindSet; NeuroSky) as shown in Fig. 2. The saliva α-armylase activity also was measured by saliva α-armylase system (NIPRO) before the experiment and after the production for each product each as shown in Fig. 3.

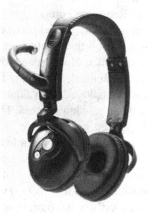

Fig. 2. Brain wave activity system

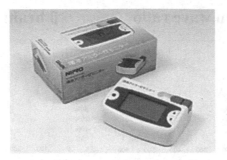

Fig. 3. Saliva α-armylase activity

3 Results and Discussions

3.1 Analysis Result of α and β Brain Wave

Figures 4 and 5 showed brain wave α and β occupation ratio comparison between expert and non-expert during fiver continuous trial tests. It is worthwhile to find that expert's α and β ratio kept constant and similar value at the level of 30 % and 70 % respectively during five continuous trial tests. However, non-expert displayed irregular α and β ratio trial through all the trials with rise-fall trend from trial to trial. In order to investigate the change of brain wave activity of expert and non-expert along with increasing trial test number, average value of α wave for each trial were also calculated and plotted in Fig. 6. It demonstrated that expert could keep a stable mental condition with low relaxation (α) and high concentration (β) balance during continuous 5 trial weaving process. By contrast, non-expert's brain wave behavior was not stable, sometimes concentrated in work and sometimes relaxed without limit by significant increasing of α ratio, which was considered to be a key factor affected stability of final product's quality.

3.2 Saliva α-Armylase Activity Discussion

As well know that saliva α-armylase could be a kind of effective indicator of fatigue and stress condition Here, in Fig. 7 Saliva α-armylase of both expert and non-expert subjects were measured just after each product weaving trial, and five times of continuous saliva test data was plotted. In general, both expert and non-expert subjects showed increasing fatigue symptom change after continuous five trial tests.

It is obvious to note that expert's saliva value increased significantly along with increasing test trial with larger value than non-expert. And non-expert also displayed a linear increasing trend with prolonged trial test time. Due to expert's longer occupation experience, it was confused to find that expert's big fatigue change than non-expert. However, when we considered the factor of both two subjects' characteristic ages, expert was elder than non-expert with nearly 30 years. Referred to the research of relationship between saliva test and human characteristic, people with larger ages would easily generate a large amount of saliva α-armylase. Therefore, expert's physical

α brain wave ratio   β brain wave ratio

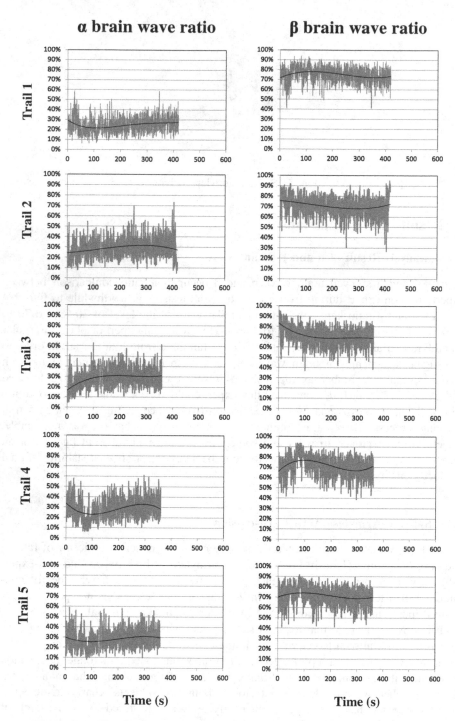

Time (s)   Time (s)

Fig. 4. Five trials α and β brain wave ratio of expert

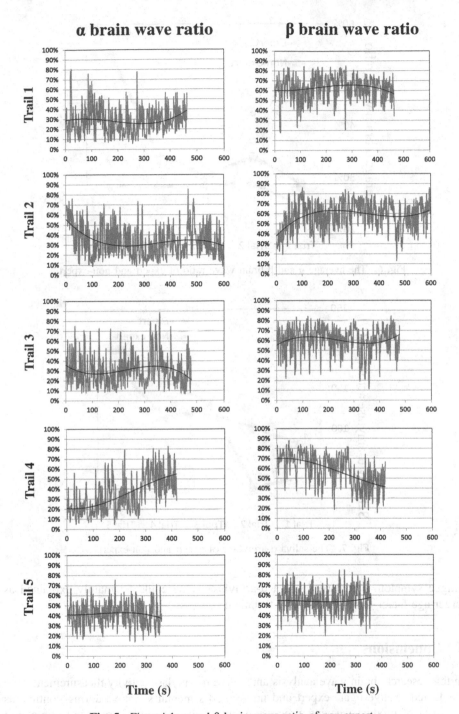

Fig. 5. Five trials α and β brain wave ratio of non-expert

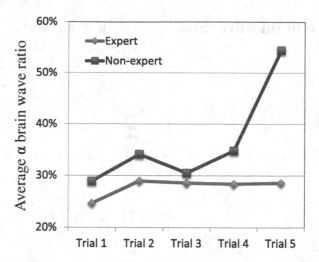

Fig. 6. The average α and β brain wave ratio of expert and non-expert

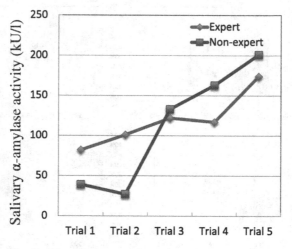

Fig. 7. The saliva α-armylase of expert and non-expert

fatigue symptom with larger saliva α-armylase value could be mainly explained as larger age factor but not caused by technical process.

4   Conclusions

In this research, brain wave analysis and saliva α-armylase activity measurement were conducted to investigate expert and non-expert's mental situation during continuous five trial of product weaving process. As a conclusion, both expert and non-expert presented the severer physical fatigue status during continuous test trial by trial.

Furthermore, expert's sharper increasing of saliva α-armylase in a wider range because of larger age factor was also clarified. However, the expert's brain wave showed a fairly steady ratio of α wave ratio and β wave ratio. Combined two tests results together, it could be demonstrate that expert was able to control his body fatigue and concentrate for long-term weaving process.

References

1. Tusji, K., et al.: Motion analysis of weaving 'Kana-Ami' technique with different years of experience. In: Proceedings of ASME 2012 International Mechanical Engineering Congress and Exposition, ASME (2012)
2. Tatsunori, T., et al.: Motion analysis of the technique used to knit kanaami. In: Symposium on Sports Engineering: Symposium on Human Dynamics, pp. 258–261 (2007)
3. Tatsunori, T., et al.: Human motion of weaving 'Kana-Ami' technique by biomechanical analysis. In: Proceedings of 10th Japan International Sampe Symposium and Exhibition, TC-1–3 (2007)
4. Wang, Z. Endo, A. Koshino, T. Tsuji, T. Tsuji, K.: Evaluation of metal wire network "kana-ami" structure between expert and non-expert. In: Proceedings of ASME 2013 International Mechanical Engineering Congress and Exposition, ASME (2013)
5. Wang, Z. Tsuji, K. Tsuji, T. Goto, A. Takai, Y. Yang, Y. Hamada, H.: Analysis on the three-dimensional wire orientation of "kana-ami" metal network between expert and non-expert. In: Proceedings of ASME 2014 International Mechanical Engineering Congress and Exposition, ASME (2014)

Modeling Human Work
and Activities

Human Performance Modeling for Dynamic Human Reliability Analysis

Ronald Laurids Boring[✉], Jeffrey Clark Joe, and Diego Mandelli

Idaho National Laboratory, Idaho Falls, ID, USA
{ronald.boring,jeffrey.joe,diego.mandelli}@inl.gov

Abstract. Part of the U.S. Department of Energy's (DOE's) Light Water Reactor Sustainability (LWRS) Program, the Risk-Informed Safety Margin Characterization (RISMC) Pathway develops approaches to estimating and managing safety margins. RISMC simulations pair deterministic plant physics models with probabilistic risk models. As human interactions are an essential element of plant risk, it is necessary to integrate human actions into the RISMC risk framework. In this paper, we review simulation based and non simulation based human reliability analysis (HRA) methods. This paper summarizes the foundational information needed to develop a feasible approach to modeling human interactions in RISMC simulations.

Keywords: Human reliability analysis · Probabilistic risk assessment · Simulation · Modeling

1 Introduction

1.1 Risk-Informed Safety Margin Characterization (RISMC)

The Risk-Informed Safety Margin Characterization (RISMC) Pathway within the United States (U.S.) Department of Energy's (DOE's) Light Water Reactor Sustainability (LWRS) Program develops and delivers approaches to manage safety margins for nuclear power plants [1, 2]. This important information supports the nuclear power plant owner/operator decision-making associated with near and long-term operation. The RISMC approach can optimize plant safety and performance by incorporating a novel interaction between probabilistic risk simulation and mechanistic codes for plant-level physics. The new functionality allows the risk simulation module to serve as a "scenario generator" that feeds information to the mechanistic codes.

When evaluating the safety margin, what we want to understand is not just the frequency of an event like core damage, but how close we are (or are not) to key safety-related events and how might we increase our safety margin. The RISMC Pathway uses a probabilistic margin approach to quantify impacts to reliability and safety. As part of the quantification, we use both probabilistic (via risk simulation) and mechanistic (via physics models) approaches. Safety margin and uncertainty quantification rely on plant

© Springer International Publishing Switzerland 2015
V.G. Duffy (Ed.): DHM 2015, Part I, LNCS 9184, pp. 223–234, 2015.
DOI: 10.1007/978-3-319-21073-5_23

physics (e.g., thermal-hydraulics and reactor kinetics) coupled with probabilistic risk simulation. The coupling takes place through the interchange of physical parameters (e.g., node pressure) and operational or accident scenarios.

In order to perform advanced safety analysis, the RISMC project has a toolkit that was developed internally at Idaho National Laboratory (INL) using the Multiphysics Object Oriented Simulation Environment (MOOSE) [3] as the underlying numerical solver framework. This toolkit consists of the several software tools, which include:

- Reactor Excursion and Leak Analysis Program (RELAP-7) [4]: the code responsible for simulating the thermal-hydraulic dynamics of the plant.
- Reactor Analysis and Virtual Control Environment (RAVEN) [5]: it has two main functions: (1) act as a controller of the RELAP-7 simulation and (2) generate multiple scenarios (i.e., a sampler) by stochastically changing the order and/or timing of events.

1.2   Human Reliability Modeling within RISMC

In past RISMC studies, human interactions have been modeled in a simplified manner. We used the method described in [6] to model human related actions, which are based on the Standardized Plant Analysis Risk-Human Reliability Analysis (SPAR-H) model [7] contained in Systems Analysis Programs for Hands-on Integrated Reliability Evaluations (SAPHIRE). The SPAR-H model characterizes each operator action through eight parameters called performance shaping factors (PSFs) that are used to compute the probability that an action will happen or not; the probability values are then inserted into the fault and event trees that contain such events.

However, from a simulation point of view we are not seeking to determine *if* an action is performed but rather *when* such an action is performed. Thus, we need a probability distribution function (pdf) that defines the probability that a human related action occurs as a function of time. Because most human reliability analysis (HRA) methods like SPAR-H do not provide a dynamic account of human actions or the PSFs, it is desirable to review modeling outside HRA such as human performance modeling.

1.3   Importance of HRA Simulation Approaches

Cacciabue [8] and others (e.g., [9]) have outlined the importance of simulation and modeling of human performance for the field of HRA. Specifically, simulation and modeling address the dynamic nature of human performance in a way that has not been found in most HRA methods. Concurrent to the emergence of simulation and modeling, several authors (e.g., [10, 11]) have posited the need for dynamic HRA and have begun developing new HRA methods or modifying existing HRA methods to account for the dynamic progression of human behavior leading up to and following human failure events. Currently, there is strong interest in the fusion of simulation and modeling with HRA (e.g., [12–16]).

2 Traditional Static HRA Methods

Swain [17], Hollnagel [18], and Boring [19] state that the practice of HRA started in the 1950s, with the first symposiums meeting in the 1960s, and that the development of formal HRA engineering methods started in the ensuing years when it was applied to modeling human performance in the construction of nuclear weapons and nuclear power reactors. The seminal HRA method for nuclear energy, a Technique for Human Error Rate Prediction (THERP) [20] was developed during this time, and its final version was developed partly as a response to the accident at Three Mile Island. Since the 1980s, there has been a proliferation of HRA methods, which have attempted to improve various aspects of early methods. Which aspects of the early methods were addressed depended greatly on the developers of the new method and the issue or issues they were trying to address.

Boring et al. [21] summarized past attempts to compare and categorize HRA methods, and noted that many of those attempts ended up with complex and non-orthogonal schemes due to the number and variety of published HRA methods. One example of a fairly complex summary is Chandler et al. [22], which compared many HRA methods across multiple dimensions, including the methods':

- Features and capabilities;
- Source (i.e., technical basis and/or data basis), approach, and treatment of dependencies and recovery;
- Error identification and human error probability (HEP) estimation approach;
- Resource requirements; and
- Cost and availability of method, tools, and data.

NUREG-1842 [23], and more recently NUREG-2127 [24] also provide comprehensive comparative summaries of HRA methods used by the nuclear industry. The reader is encouraged to review these categorization schemes to understand the various approaches to grouping and comparing HRA methods.

2.1 Shortcomings of Non-simulation Based HRA

As Hollnagel [18] has pointed out, non-simulation based HRA methods are essentially modeled after traditional probabilistic reliability assessment (PRA). That is, these methods use the same basic approach PRA uses to model equipment reliability, with two key exceptions. The first is that the modeling of equipment failures is replaced by modeling human failures at tasks and/or activities. The second exception is that wider uncertainty bands are used to account for the increased variability in human performance relative to equipment performance, which is often attributed to individual differences between people, the time-dependent nature of many human tasks, and the non-orthogonality of factors that influence human performance. Inherent to this approach, given the assumptions about how these HRA methods conceive of and model human performance, is the goal of calculating the probability of a human error or erroneous action.

One primary shortfall with non-simulation HRA methods is the assumption that PSFs do not influence one another when, in fact, there is clear psychological evidence that PSFs frequently interact. For example, a limited amount of time to perform the task (i.e., time pressure) affects the person's stress level when performing the task. Both time pressure and stress are commonly identified as separate PSFs in many HRA methods, which are used individually to directly modify the HEP in an additive fashion. Simply adding PSFs together simplifies the method, but it also eliminates any mathematical accounting for their potential interaction or influence upon one another. If these HRA methods are included in a simulation framework with this erroneous assumption that PSFs are independent and additive, the propagation of this error will lead to inaccurate HEP estimates.

This PSF example is just one of many issues with non-simulation based HRA methods. Others, including Swain [17] and Dougherty [25] have expounded on a range of issues with non-simulation based HRA methods that can greatly affect their ability to be effectively incorporated into simulation frameworks. Broadly speaking, issues include:

- The accuracy of HRA's HEP predictions has not been satisfactorily demonstrated, and
- The time-dependence of human actions (i.e., dependency) is not effectively modeled for purposes of quantifying HEPs.

These issues, among others, need to be addressed with simulation based HRA methods in order for them to be effectively included into simulation frameworks.

The weaknesses in existing HRA methods are likely to be challenges in developing an approach to dynamic HRA. Recent work (for example, [26] and [27]) has focused on improving the accuracy and validity of HRA methods. Most of this work emphasizes the use of data collected in full-scope nuclear control room simulators such as the Human Systems Simulation Laboratory (HSSL) at INL (see [28] and [29]). Simulator studies may be invaluable stepping stones for building models required for simulation based HRA.

3 Simulation Based HRA

3.1 Introduction

In the face of any unresolved debate over different HRA methods, what advantage can be had by positing yet another approach? There exist developments—namely in human performance modeling—that do not fit the classification of existing HRA methods. Human performance modeling utilizes virtual scenarios, virtual environments, and virtual humans to mimic the performance of humans in actual scenarios and environments. What sets this form of HRA apart is that it provides a dynamic basis for HRA modeling and quantification. Traditional HRA methods have featured largely static task analyses of operating events as the underlying basis of performance modeling. These methods have also relied on performance estimations mapped to similar previous performance derived through empirical data or expert opinion. Simulation based HRA differs from its antecedents in that it is a dynamic modeling system that reproduces human decisions and actions as the basis for its performance estimation.

Simulation based HRA may also augment previous HRA methods by dynamically computing PSF levels to arrive at HEPs for any given point in time. More importantly, simulation based HRA may present the decision points that operators make while engaging with the plant. These decision points are crucial anchors to plant performance, and no plant model can claim to model performance accurately without accounting for the nuances of human operations that determine the evolution of events.

3.2 Non-HRA Human Performance Modeling

Meister [30] suggests that HRA filled an important void early in the evolution of human factors by centering on prediction. Much of classic human factors has centered on the collection of data on the interaction of humans with designed systems. The purpose of such data is to improve the design of the system, ultimately to optimize human performance in terms of criteria such as usability, efficiency, or safety. HRA has instead attempted to predict human performance, specifically human errors, that can occur in such human-machine interactions. The purpose of HRA is therefore not typically to improve the design of the system so much as to determine what factors impact the safe human operation of that system. Over time, HRA has been joined by another predictive tool, namely human performance modeling.

Human performance modeling is an umbrella term used to describe systems that simulate human decision making and actions. Human performance modeling is largely synonymous with cognitive simulation and artificial intelligence, although it has in practice applied to unified systems that attempt to account for a broad range of human cognition. In contrast, variants of cognitive simulation or artificial intelligence may focus on modeling specific cognitive mechanisms instead of providing integrated models of multiple cognitive mechanisms. This distinction is analogous to the differences found in hardware component vs. system models, respectively. Young [31] suggests that human performance models vary on a number of dimensions, including:

- The psychological theories underpinning the modeling,
- The complexity of the human activity,
- Models vs. applied simulations, and
- The use of actual vs. conjectured human behavior.

There are numerous human performance modeling systems available. For example, [32] reviews human performance modeling systems that they have been applied to aerospace at the National Aeronautics and Space Administration (NASA), including the following systems:

- Adaptive Control of Thought-Rational (ACT-R 5.0),
- Air Man-machine Integration Design and Analysis System (Air MIDAS), which is a variant of MIDAS,
- Distributed Operator Model Architecture (D-OMAR), and
- Attention-Situation Awareness (A-SA) systems.

A recent review by Pew [33] for the golden anniversary issue of the journal Human Factors chronicles other human performance modeling systems, including:

- Various versions of the Micro Saint task modeling system,
- The General Problem Solver,
- The State, Operator, and Result (SOAR or Soar) system,
- The Goals, Operators, Methods, and Selection Rules (GOMS) approach,
- The Executive-Process Interactive Control (EPIC) system,
- ACT-R, and
- MIDAS.

Recalling a general distinction between models and simulations, all of these systems offer models of cognition, but only Micro Saint, Soar, ACT-R, MIDAS, and EPIC are fully implemented simulation systems.

As noted, a defining characteristic of human performance modeling systems is that they mimic human decision making. Russell and Norvig [34] identify two general types of decision making used in human performance modeling systems. The first, historically speaking, is the deductive artificial intelligence approach, which consists of software systems that make simple deductive conclusions given coded representations. Two famous implementations include systems to prove logical theorems such as the General Problem Solver and logical programming languages such as PROLOG. The second logical reasoning type is the inductive system. Such a system, commonly called a production system, is capable of inferring from given contextual representations to produce new representations. The human performance modeling systems already described in [32, 33] mostly fit within this latter type of decision making. The advantages of inductive over deductive systems are striking: inductive systems can learn given minimal information, whereas deductive systems must avail preprogrammed information. Both, nonetheless, have their uses: the deductive General Problem Solver, for example, is quite effective at solving mathematical theorems, a domain that is certainly cognitive yet often falls outside the capacity of human cognition. The inductive logic production systems such as ACT-R, Soar, and Micro Saint, are more humanlike in their approach, making them suitable for simulating human performance realistically.

3.3   HRA and Human Performance Modeling

Gore and Smith [35] point out that despite a common focus on human performance, HRA and human performance modeling have not been well integrated. Human performance modeling systems have not been used to model those human behavioral contexts that lead to human error, nor to predict the rates of unsuccessful human performance. Yet, such an extension of human performance modeling is a logical bridge to HRA. Infusing HRA concepts like human error and HEPs into human performance modeling increases the utility of such systems.

Importantly for the present purposes, human performance modeling takes HRA out of the static models that are the mainstay of current Level 1 PRA applications.[1] While

---

[1] A Level 1 PRA concerns potential core damage; Level 2 PRA concerns potential release of radioactivity (i.e., a severe accident); Level 3 PRA concerns potential consequences of a severe accident in terms of health and environment.

current HRA methods have proven robust in their application to Level 1 PRA, the methods are optimized for heavily proceduralized activities within the control room. Level 2 and 3 PRA require analyses of less proceduralized activities involving the dynamic interplay of control room and balance-of-plant and responder personnel. Current HRA methods are, with few exceptions, not validated for such applications. Human performance modeling affords the opportunity to extend current HRA approaches to novel domains by simulating Level 2 and 3 scenarios and the human activities within those scenarios.

There have been efforts to implement human performance modeling for HRA:

- A framework for using NASA's MIDAS system for HRA has been laid out [36] but has not been implemented to date.
- ACT-R has been extended to model errors in the Human Error Modeling Architecture (HEMA) [37] in research funded by the Office of Naval Research. While the conceptual design was published in 2005, an implementation of the system has not been made public to date.
- A production system inspired by ACT-R and Soar has been developed in conjunction with the University of Oldenburg to model errors by pilots and drivers [38]. This system helps identify sources of errors but does not predict their frequency.
- A demonstration model in Micro Saint has mapped workload from the NASA Taskload Index (TLX) to the ATHEANA and SPAR-H HRA methods [39]. This research stops short of using the methods' performance shaping factors to quantify human error. Its primary purpose in its current inception is to provide a mapping of existing workload simulation data to a format that is compatible with HRA methods.
- The Accident Dynamics Simulator-Information Decision and Action in Crew (ADS-IDAC) system [40] was developed specifically for HRA applications, tying together a cognitive model, a decision making engine, performance shaping factors, and a dynamic event simulator. This implementation was further extended in [41, 42] to include a crew response model for emergency operations and severe accidents in nuclear power plants.

3.4 HRA and Human Performance Modeling of Severe Accidents

While other human performance modeling systems have achieved an otherwise adequate level of maturation in their domains, only the ADS-IDAC system requires minimal extensions to be used for HRA. Extending other human performance modeling systems to include HRA would require costly and time-consuming extensions of those preliminary efforts in [36–39].

In fact, ADS-IDAC recently was integrated with Methods for Estimation of Leakages and Consequences of Releases (MELCOR) code to evaluate a station blackout (SBO) at a pressurized water reactor (PWR) [43]. The project encountered significant technical difficulties, including challenges in the integration of ADS-IDAC with MELCOR. Instead of fully integrating the two programs, the authors suggest using an external script to jointly execute the two programs and manage interfacing data. RISMC's toolkit is well-suited to this approach and might be a solution to the technical difficulties encountered previously.

However, coding ADS-IDAC scenarios requires significant resources. As with other HRA methods, ADS-IDAC was developed for Level 1 analysis. As such, the method is built around written procedures, with every procedure step and sub-step explicitly coded. Scenarios without written procedures are coded using "mental procedures" that can be activated when certain parameters or conditions are met. The level of detail in this model (and the associated resources required to implement it) may be too specific for the HRA modeling desired in the RISMC framework.

In any case, ADS-IDAC offers the most mature HRA-based human performance modeling currently developed. This model can be seen as the starting point for incorporating human actions into dynamic, simulation based risk assessment.

4 Conclusions

4.1 Selection of an HRA Approach for RISMC

For infrequent occurrences, including incidents at power plants, there is often inadequate operations experience to provide data-based quantification of human performance in HRA. Utilities, researchers, and regulators who wish to determine the risk significance of such past events retrospectively will utilize HRA estimation methods to the extent that they encompass the PSFs and scenarios at play in the event. However, because of the scarcity of available data, it is often necessary to utilize expert estimation techniques, which have historically been fraught with poor inter-analyst reliability [44].

Human performance modeling avoids the shortcomings of applying an HRA quantification method in a poorly suited domain or utilizing expert opinion to arrive at the human contribution to the risk of an event. Instead, by scripting a scenario that closely matches the past event, it is possible to generate simulation runs with virtual personnel to arrive at an estimate of the frequency with which human performance elevated the risk of the scenario. This approach increases the veracity of risk estimation.

Equally promising, so-called unexampled events, particularly severe accident scenarios, stand to benefit from human performance modeling by allowing virtual operators to engage in the evolution of events and provide a range of decisions and actions that might impact plant response. This form of simulation based HRA is a crucial evolution of risk analysis for the plant and one that can only be accomplished by coupling virtual operator models with advanced plant simulations. This problem set is the challenge of RISMC and presents an important opportunity to advance both HRA and the state of plant models.

4.2 Next Steps: Severe Accident Modeling and Need for Simulation Based HRA

In order to develop an approach for simulation based human reliability modeling, several questions need to be addressed:

- What level of detail should be modeled? Is it appropriate to model operator cognition and every operator action, as in ADS-IDAC, or is a more high-level model sufficient? Perhaps a hybrid approach (e.g. the course-grain and fine-grain model proposed in [20]) should be adopted. This question is particularly relevant in Level 2 and Level 3 analysis, as these events are much less familiar to operators and procedures are not available for many of these scenarios. As we move away from prescribed human interactions with the plant, step-by-step analysis of operator actions becomes more difficult and more speculative.

- What PSFs must be considered in simulation based HRA? PSFs are unlikely to remain constant throughout a scenario, and interactions between performance shaping factors must be addressed.
- If an existing HRA method (or methods) is used, which method best suits the RISMC toolkit? SPAR-H was selected for RISMC's first, simple HRA model [6]; perhaps this is a reasonable choice going forward. ADS-IDAC features nearly 60 PSFs [40]; yet development efforts may be best spent validating a subset of these PSFs like the eight found in SPAR-H [7].
- When and how can empirical data and simulator studies be used to support dynamic HRA? Existing sources such as previous simulator study data may be useful, and INL's HSSL provides a platform for collecting further data if desired.

Most of these questions are tied to the tension between a highly realistic but resource-intensive model and a model that is easy to implement and modify but perhaps too simplistic. The targeted balance between these two ends is complicated by the uncertainty surrounding human performance that has plagued HRA since its inception. In the next phase of this project, we will attempt to address these concerns and recommend an optimal approach for RISMC HRA.

5 Disclaimer

This work of authorship was prepared as an account of work sponsored by an agency of the United States Government. Neither the United States Government, nor any agency thereof, nor any of their employees makes any warranty, express or implied, or assumes any legal liability or responsibility for the accuracy, completeness, or usefulness of any information, apparatus, product, or process disclosed, or represents that its use would not infringe privately-owned rights. Idaho National Laboratory is a multi-program laboratory operated by Battelle Energy Alliance LLC, for the United States Department of Energy under Contract DE-AC07-05ID14517.

References

1. Smith, C., Rabiti, C., Martineau, R.: Risk Informed Safety Margin Characterization (RISMC) pathway technical program plan, Idaho National Laboratory, Idaho Falls (2011)
2. Madelli, D., Smith, C., Riley, T., Nielsen, J., Schroeder, J., Rabiti, C., Alonsi, A., Kinoshita, R., Malijovec, D., Wang, B., Pascucci, V.: Overview of new tools to perform safety analysis: BWR station black out test case. In: Proceedings of PSAM 12 Conference, Honolulu (2014)
3. Alfonsi, A., Rabiti, C., Mandelli, D., Cogliati, J., Kinoshita, R.: Raven as a tool for dynamic probabilistic risk assessment: software overview. In: Proceedings of M&C2013 International Topical Meeting on Mathematics and Computation, LaGrange Park, IL (2013)

4. David, R.B., Gaston, D., Martineau, R., Peterson, J., Zhang, H., Zhao, H., Zou, L.: RELAP-7 Level 2 Milestone report: demonstration of a steady state single phase PWR simulation with RELAP-7, Idaho Falls (2012)
5. Alfonsi, A., Rabiti, C., Mandelli, D., Cogliati, J., Kinoshita, R.: Raven as a tool for dynamic probabilistic risk assessment: software overview. In: Proceeding of M&C2013 International Topical Meeting on Mathematics and Computation, LaGrange Park, IL (2013)
6. Mandelli, C., Riley, T., Schroeder, J., Rabiti, C., Alfonsi, A., Nielsen, J., Maljovec, D., Wang, B., Pascucci, V.: Support and modeling for the boiling water reactor station black out case study using RELAP and RAVEN, Idaho Falls (2013)
7. Gertman, D.I., Blackman, H.S., Marble, J.L., Byers, J.C., Smith, C.L.: The SPAR-H human reliability analysis method. NUREG/CR-6883 (2005)
8. Cacciabue, P.C.: Modeling and simulation of human behavior for safety analysis and control of complex systems. Saf. Sci. **28**, 97–110 (1998)
9. Lüdke, A.: Kognitive Analyse formaler sicherheitskritischer Steuerungssysteme auf Basis eines integrierten Mensch-Maschine-Models. Akademische Verlagsgesellschaft, Berlin (2005)
10. Jae, M.S., Park, C.K.: A new dynamic HRA method and its application. J. Korean Nucl. Soc. **27**, 292–300 (1995)
11. Sträter, O.: Evaluation of human reliability on the basis of operational experience, GRS-170. Garching bei München, Gesellschaft für Anlagen- und Reaktorsicherheit (GRS) mbH (2000)
12. Mosleh, A., Chang, Y.H.: Model-based human reliability analysis: prospects and requirements. Reliab. Eng. Syst. Saf. **83**, 241–253 (2004)
13. Reer, B., Dang, V.N., Hirschberg, S.: The CESA method and its application in a plant-specific pilot study on errors of commission. Reliab. Eng. Syst. Saf. **83**, 187–205 (2004)
14. Sträter, O.: Cognition and Safety: An Integrated Approach to Systems Design and Performance Assessment. Ashgate, Aldershot (2005)
15. Boring, R.L.: Modeling human reliability analysis using MIDAS. In: Proceedings of the Fifth International Topical Meeting on Nuclear Plant Instrumentation, Controls, and Human Machine Interface Technology (NPIC-HMIT), pp. 1270–1274 (2006)
16. Trucco, P., Leva, M.C., Sträter, O.: Human error prediction in ATM via cognitive simulation: preliminary study. In: Proceedings of the 8th International Conference on Probabilistic Safety Assessment and Management (PSAM8), vol. Paper 0268, pp. 1–9 (2006)
17. Swain, A.: Human reliability analysis: need, status, trends and limitations. Reliab. Eng. Syst. Saf. **29**(3), 301–313 (1990)
18. Hollnagel, E.: Human reliability analysis. In: Karwowski, W. (ed.) International Encyclopedia of Ergonomics and Human Factors, 2nd edn. CRC Press, Boca Raton (2006)
19. Boring, R.: Fifty years of THERP and human reliability analysis. In: Probabilistic Safety Assessment and Management and European Safety and Reliability Conference, 16B-Th3-5, Helsinki, Finland (2012)
20. Swain, A., Guttmann, H.: Handbook of human reliability analysis with emphasis on nuclear power plant applications. Final report. NUREG/CR-1278, Washington, DC (1983)
21. Boring, R., Hendrickson, S., Forester, J., Tran, T., Lois, E.: Issues in benchmarking human reliability analysis methods: a literature review. Reliab. Anal. Syst. Saf. **95**, 591–605 (2010)
22. Chandler, F., Chang, Y.H., Mosleh, A., Marble, J., Boring, R., Gertman, D.: Human Reliability Analysis Methods: Selection Guidance for NASA, Washington, DC (2006)
23. U.S. nuclear regulatory commission: evaluation of human reliability analysis methods against good practices, NUREG-1842, Washington, DC (2006)

24. U.S. nuclear regulatory commission: the international hra empirical study: lessons learned from comparing HRA methods predictions to HAMMLAB simulator data, NUREG-2127, Washington, DC (2014)
25. Dougherty, E.: Human reliability analysis—where shouldst thou turn? Reliab. Eng. Syst. Saf. 29(3), 283–299 (1990)
26. Groth, K.M., Smith, C.L., Swiler, L.P.: A bayesian method for using simulator data to enhance human error probabilities assigned by existing HRA methods. Reliab. Eng. Syst. Saf. 128, 32–40 (2014)
27. Shirley, R.B., Smidts, C.S., Li, M., Gupta, A.: Validating THERP: assessing the scope of full-scale validation of the technique for human error rate prediction. Ann. Nucl. Energy 77, 194–211 (2015)
28. Boring, R.L., Agarwal, V., Joe, J.C., Persensky, J.J.: Digital full-scope mockup of a conventional nulcear power plant control room, phase 1: installation of a utility simulator at the Idaho National Laboratory, INL/EXT-12-26367, Idaho National Laboratory, Idaho Falls (2012)
29. Boring, R., Agarwal, V., Fitzgerald, K., Hugo, J., Hallbert, B.: Digital full-scope simulation of a conventional nuclear power plant control room, phase 2: installation of a reconfigurable simulator to support nuclear plant sustainability, INL/EXT-13-28432, Idaho National Laboratory, Idaho Falls (2013)
30. Meister, D.: The History of Human Factors and Ergonomics. Lawrence Erlbaum Associates, Mahwah (1999)
31. Young, M.J.: Human performance model validation: one size does not fit all. In: Proceedings of the Summer Simulation Conference, San Diego, CA, pp. 732–736 (2003)
32. Foyle, D.C. (ed.): Human Performance Modeling in Aviation. CRC Press, Boca Raton (2008)
33. Pew, R.W.: More than 50 years of history and accomplishments in human performance model development. Hum. Factors 50(2), 489–495 (2008)
34. Russell, S.J., Norvig, P.: Artificial Intelligence—A Modern Approach. Prentice-Hall, Englewood Cliffs (1995)
35. Gore, B.F., Smith, J.D.: Risk assessment and human performance modelling: the need for an integrated systems approach. Int. J. Hum. Factors Model. Simul. 1(1), 119–139 (2006)
36. Boring, R.L., Gertman, D.I., Tran, T.Q., Gore, B.F.: Framework and application for modeling control room crew performance at nuclear power plants. In: Proceedings of the Human Factors and Ergonomics Society 52nd Annual Meeting (2008)
37. Fotta, M.E., Byrne, M.D., Luther, M.S.: Developing a Human Error Modeling Architecture (HEMA). Found. Augment. Cogn. 11, 1025–1031 (2005)
38. Lüdtke, A., Weber, L., Osterloh, J.-P., Wortelen, B.: Modeling pilot and driver behavior for human error simulation. In: Duffy, V.G. (ed.) ICDHM 2009. LNCS, vol. 5620, pp. 403–412. Springer, Heidelberg (2009)
39. Laux, L., Plott, C.: Using operator workload data to inform human reliability analyses. In: Joint 8th IEEE HFPP/13th HPRCT Conference (2007)
40. Chang, Y.H.J., Mosleh, A.: Cognitive modeling and dynamic probabilistic simulation of operating crew response to complex system accidents, parts 1–5. Reliab. Eng. Syst. Saf. 92, 997–1101 (2007)
41. Coyne, K.A.: A predictive model of nuclear power plant crew decision-making and performance in a dynamic simulation environment. University of Maryland Ph.D. Dissertation, College Park (2009)
42. Li, Y.: Modeling and simulation of operator knowledge-based behavior. University of Maryland Ph.D. Disertation, College Park (2013)

43. LaChance, J., Cardoni, J., Li, Y., Mosleh, A., Aird, D., Helton, D., Coyne, K.: Discrete Dynamic Probabilistic Risk Assessment Model Development and Application, Albuquerque, NM (2012)
44. Boring, R., Gertman, D., Joe, J., Marble, J., Galyean, W., Blackwood, L., Blackman, H.: Simplified Expert Elicitation Guildeline for Risk Assessment of Operating Events, Idaho Falls (2005)

Improvement of Needle Bar in Textile Machine by Hitting Process

Kontawat Chottikampon[1(✉)], Suchalinee Mathurosemontri[1],
Hitoshi Marui[1], Ryo Marui[2], Hiroyuki Nishimoto[1],
and Hiroyuki Hamada[1]

[1] Kyoto Institute of Technology, Kyoto, Japan
{ruklongtime, zucha_k_t_89}@hotmail.com,
rugger.hitoshi@gmail.com,
hiroyuki.nishimoto@outlook.com, hhamada@kit.ac.jp
[2] Marui Textile Machinery Co. Ltd., Osaka, Japan
ryo@marusans.com

Abstract. The research conducted was to study the hitting process of a needle bar used within textile machinery and how to improve its efficiency and performance. A needle bar consists of a brass bar attached with a number of small pins. The primary focus was learning technique while straightening the needle bar. In order to join pins and brass bar together, the soldering is applied. The result from the heat transfer during soldering process can cause the brass pins to bend, which is undesirable for finished product. A soldering expertise uses hitting movement technique to modify and straighten the brass bar. Even though soldering process is the only step in making the brass bar; however, its method is considered very complicated and requires refinement and specialization from the maker.

Keywords: Needle bar · Hitting process · Linking machine

1 Introduction

The linking machine is using for joining knitted fabric pieces together to form a garment. Linking is a method of seaming/attaching pieces of a garment together after the pieces have been knitted on a flat-bed knitting machine. The linking process requires a skilled operator, and is used mainly for high-end knitted apparel. In the linking process, a slacker course of loops of yarn is created on the linking machine, which connects two pieces of fabric together.

For over thirty years of experience in soldering, a man who first started his own business became an expert in making a needle bar in textile industry. This specific part is the important component of a linking machine. The needle bar is very useful and faster for the seaming process of garments. The fabric has been set on the pins of needle bar that will guide a needle of a sewing machine. This specific part was produced by man-made technique, which strongly influenced by personal skill and experience. The most important process in producing a needle bar is to know how to place each pins onto the groove perfectly. Soldering pin to pin is necessarily in this process. The heat transfer during soldering process has an extensive effect to the pins row and the brass

© Springer International Publishing Switzerland 2015
V.G. Duffy (Ed.): DHM 2015, Part I, LNCS 9184, pp. 235–244, 2015.
DOI: 10.1007/978-3-319-21073-5_24

bar to bend in zigzag pattern. The straightening process or hitting process is required after soldering process in order to make a straight needle bar. For this reason, a skilled needle bar maker uses his own sensations and experience to re-shape the brass bar.

2 Experimental

The linking machine is using for joining knitted fabric pieces together to form a garment. Linking is a method of seaming/attaching pieces of a garment together after

2.1 Fabrication Process of Needle Bar

The straight brass bar (4.5 × 92.0 × 0.2 cm) is prepared as the basement of needle bar. Small slots that using as the channel for placing the needle pins are marked on the brass bar by using the groove cutter machine. The groove cutter machine and the slotted brass bar are shown in Figs. 1 and 2, respectively.

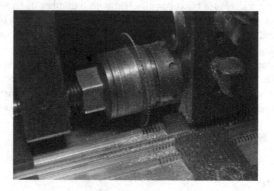

Fig. 1. The groove cutter machine

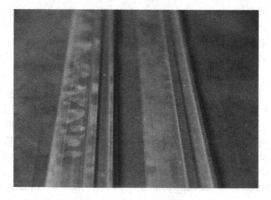

Fig. 2. The slotted brass bar

In this research, the needle bar number seventh is studied. The "number seventh" means the amount of pins placed onto grooves within an inch (seven pins per inch). In the middle of a brass bar, seven pins are placed onto the groove one by one and the metal plate is used to hold the pins with the brass bar as presented in Fig. 3.

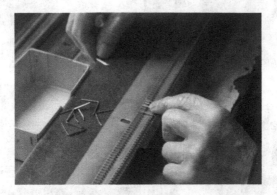

Fig. 3. Pin setting step

The pins are joined together with the slotted brass bar by the soldering process. Soldering is a process in which two or more metal items are joined together by melting and flowing a filler metal (solder) into the joint, the solder having a lower melting point than the adjoining metal [1].

The soldering process of needle pins and brass bar is shown in Fig. 4. In order to remove impurities that can obstacle the joint, the flux is applied prior the soldering process (Fig. 4a). The solder is applied on the heated soldering head (Fig. 4b) and consequently tapped on soldering area (Fig. 4c) to let the solder melting and covering the soldering area (Fig. 4d). Then the soldering process continues to the next part of the brass bar from the middle portion (Fig. 4e). After that the needle bar maker continues to place more pins at the end of each side of the brass bar (Fig. 4f) and repeat soldering (working from the side towards in the middle of the brass bar) until the pins are all placed and covered all length of the brass bar (Fig. 4g).

The post soldering processes consist of the scrap removal and the straightening of the needle bar. The needle bar maker uses the file to scrape an excess dust and smoothen the brass bar's surface after soldering process as shown in Fig. 5.

2.2 The Straightening of the Needle Bar

In general, the needle bar, which is attached with a number of pins, is supposed to straight in order to be able to insert into the linking machine. However the heat transfer during soldering process causes an extensive effect to the needle bar to bend in an arch shape as illustrated in Fig. 6 [2, 3]. Furthermore, the arch shape of the needle bar has caused the alignment of the pins to shift. The needle bar is not productive if the pins are not aligning in straight line.

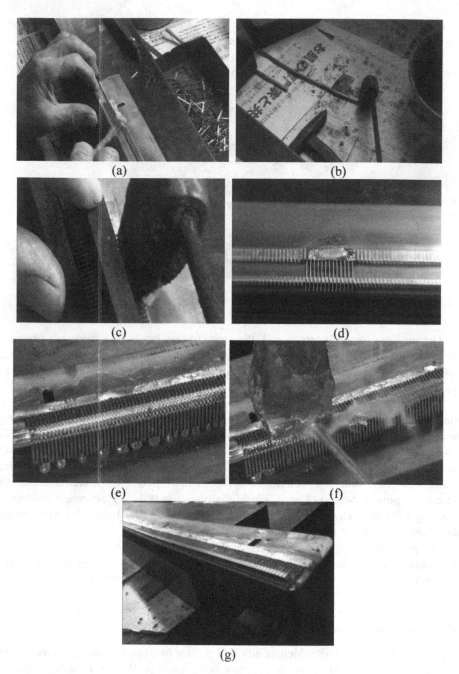

Fig. 4. Soldering process of the brass bar: (a) Apply flux, (b) Preparation of the solder and the heated soldering head, (c) Tap the soldering head on the soldering area, (d) Complete soldered area, (e) Extended soldering area, (f) Continue to solder on other area of brass bar and (g) The finished soldered brass bar.

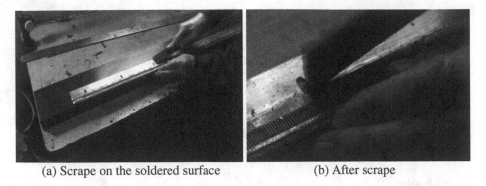

| (a) Scrape on the soldered surface | (b) After scrape |

Fig. 5. The scrap removal process: (a) Scrape on the soldered surface, (b) After scrape

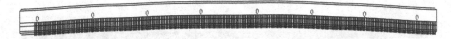

Fig. 6. The arch shape bending of the needle bar after soldering process

In order to modify the needle bar, the needle bar maker uses hitting technique. The needle bar was hit for several cycles with different hitting positions and frequency as shown in Fig. 7. The hitting positions start from the center of the needle bar from the first hitting cycle and gradually expand until covering the overall length of the needle bar.

3   Results and Discussion

3.1   Effect of Hitting Process on Gap Length Between Pins

In order to evaluate the effect of hitting process on the straightening of needle bar, the gap lengths between both pin's base and pin's tip are measured. The gap distance between base of needle pin and between tip of needle pin are plotted in Figs. 8 and 9, respectively. It can be seen that the gap distance between both base and tip of the needle pin gradually decrease with the increasing of hitting cycle especially at the hit positions. The effect of hitting process on the decreasing of the gap distance is more pronounce for the pin's tip than the pin's base. The average gap distance between the pin's tip decrease from 2.749 mm before hitting to 2.693 mm after the sixth hitting cycle. This indicates the hitting process straightened the needle bar.

The needle bar was placed on the flat table in order to measure the curvature of the needle bar. The curvature is determined by the gap length between the surfaces of the table to the surface of needle bar (h) as illustrated in Fig. 10. The higher gap length refers to the higher curvature of the needle bar.

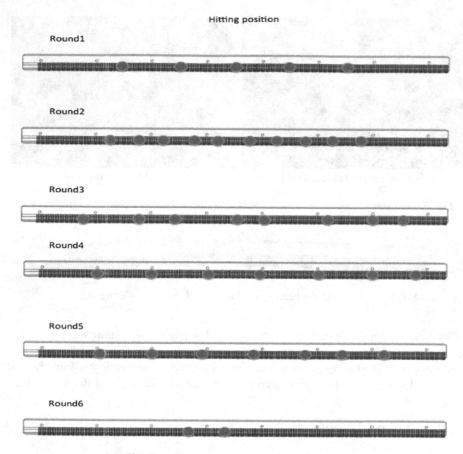

Fig. 7. The hitting process of the needle bar

The comparison of the gap distance under the needle bar between prior and after hitting process is shown in Fig. 11. The curvature of the needle bar after soldering process show highest value ($\sim$0.6 mm) at the center of needle bar due to the effect from the heat transfer during soldering process. By the application of hitting process, the curvature decreases by 30 percentage and shows highest value at 0.4 mm.

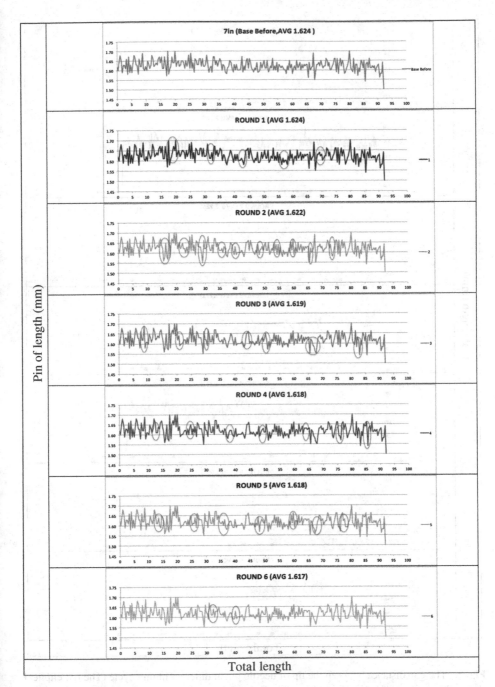

Fig. 8. The gap distance between the base of needle pin at different hitting cycle (The red eliptical shows the position of hitting in each cycle) (Color figure online).

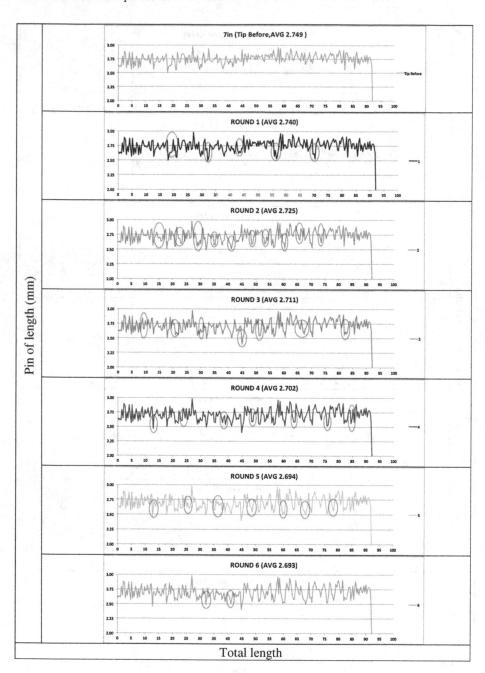

Fig. 9. The gap distance between the tip of needle pin at different hitting cycle (The red eliptical shows the position of hitting in each cycle) (Color figure online).

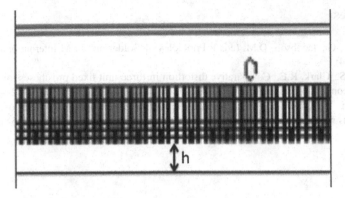

Fig. 10. The measurement of curvature of needle bar

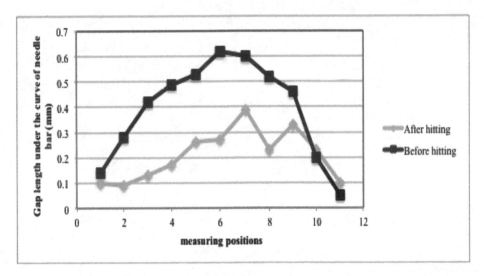

Fig. 11. The gap length under the curve of needle bar before and after hitting process

4   Conclusion

The preparation of the needle bar, which is an important part of the linking machine, was studied. The soldering process was used to joint the needle pins with the brass bar. Heat transfer while soldering has an extensive effect onto the brass bar to bend in an arch shape. Moreover, it has caused the alignment of the pins to shift. The needle bar is not productive if the pins are not aligning in straight line. Thus, the needle bar maker applies hitting technique to modify the shape. The hitting position was significantly based on the experience of the bar maker which was started from the middle area of the needle bar. The hitting process gradually straightened the needle bar as the hitting cycle increased. In addition, the gap between the pins' tip decreased and resulted in more straight alignment.

References

1. Humpston, G., Jacobson, D.M. (eds.): Principles of Soldering. ASM international, Materials Park (2004)
2. Huling, J.S., Clark, R.E.: Comparative distortion in three-unit fixed prostheses joined by laser welding, conventional soldering, or casting in one piece. J. Dent. Res. **56**(2), 128–134 (1977)
3. Tomlinson, W.J., Collier, I.: The mechanical properties and microstructures of copper and brass joints soldered with eutectic tin-bismuth solder. J. Mater. Sci. **22**(5), 1835–1839 (1987)

Towards a Theory for Bio–Cyber Physical Systems Modelling

Didier Fass[1] and Franck Gechter[2](✉)

[1] ICN Business School, Mosel Loria UMR CNRS, Université de Lorraine,
7503 Nancy, France
didier.fass@loria.fr
[2] IRTES-SET, EA 7274, 90010 Belfort Cedex, France
franck.gechter@utbm.fr

Abstract. Currently, Cyber Physical Systems (CPS) represents a great challenge for automatic control and smart systems engineering on both theoretical and practical levels. Designing CPS requires approaches involving multi-disciplinary competences. However they are designed to be autonomous, the CPS present a part of uncertainty, which requires interaction with human for engineering, monitoring, controlling, performing operational maintenance, etc. This human-CPS interaction led naturally to the human in-the-loop (HITL) concept. Nevertheless, this HITL concept, which stems from a reductionist point of view, exhibits limitations due to the different natures of the systems involved. As opposed to this classical approach, we propose, in this paper, a model of Bio-CPS (i.e. systems based on an integration of computational elements within biological systems) grounded on theoretical biology, physics and computer sciences and based on the key concept of human systems integration.

Keywords: Bio-CPS · Human system integration

1 Introduction

Currently, researching theoretical principles of Cyber Physical Systems (CPS) represents a great challenge for automatic control and smart systems engineering. Designing CPS requires a multidisciplinary approach involving mathematics, automatic control and applied mathematics and physics. Those disciplines are based on computation and regulation loop paradigms. However they are designed to be autonomous, one cannot neglect that the CPS present a part of uncertainty, which requires interaction with human for engineering, monitoring, controlling, performing operational maintenance, etc. This interaction led naturally to the human in-the-loop (HITL) concept, which is now widespread in literature. Nevertheless, this HITL concept has got several limitations due to the different natures of the systems involved and their different organizations. Indeed, the traditional system of systems engineering point of view stands from reductionism. If this approach is suitable to computational sciences and physics,

© Springer International Publishing Switzerland 2015
V.G. Duffy (Ed.): DHM 2015, Part I, LNCS 9184, pp. 245–255, 2015.
DOI: 10.1007/978-3-319-21073-5_25

it is not well adapted to the human nature. This reductionist approach, i.e. mechanization and computerization of human being, reaches out its own limits and needs a scientific theoretical approach to face with future human machine challenges. In this paper, we propose a model of Bio-CPS grounded on theoretical biology, physics and computer sciences and based on the key concept of human systems integration. Bio-CPS are considered to be an integration of computational elements within biological systems. In a sense, Bio-CPS can be compared to the Cyber-Physical systems, in which the challenge is to make physical systems working along with computer systems. For decades, the Cybernetics has been a huge influence on human-machine systems concepts and development. It is based on information theory, automatic control theory, and algorithm theory. Cybernetics is about regulation and control of a mechanical system behavior. In this context, human-machine interactions are generally seen as an exchange of information between the operator and the controlled object. Hence, designing and developing human machines systems cannot be reduced to a simple information exchange. Using interactive and artificial technologies requires integrating artificial elements and structural design usually by artificial or artifactual functional interactions and its dynamics. Considering this, designing Bio-CPS is a real intellectual challenge since this can be considered as the hyperlink between the biology and the cyber sciences. The development of new interactive systems for many applications such as airplane control, car smart driving assistance, bedside monitoring in intensive care, etc. and their growing implication in our daily life (smartphone, augmented and virtual reality, etc.), involve the necessity to develop theoretical basis for designing Bio-CPS. This design task is hard to cope with. In addition to the classical issues encountered in Cyber-Physical Systems such as the relationship between a continuous time reference on the one side (physical part) and a dynamics based on sequences of state changes on the other (cyber part), Bio-CPS have add some other difficulties linked the differences in the nature of the interactions between system components with their scale relativity. Whereas the interactions between elements are, by nature, local and symmetrical in physical and, by extension, in cyber systems, they are non-symmetrical and non-local in biological systems. This difference in the nature of interaction is one of the main difficulties that have to be overcome. Another important issue is linked to the numerous hierarchical levels involved in biological systems from the cell level to the body level, the Physical or the cyber systems dealing at most with two levels. Finally, if the complexities of these two systems make the interoperability hard to design, the nature of these is also different in both cases. In biological systems the complexity is required in order to make the system more stable. By contrast, in cyber systems engineering, the complexity need to be avoided as far as it is possible because it can bring instabilities. However, cyber systems complexity, even not desired, stems from the numerous interactions between components. Consequently, the main concern in Bio-CPS design is how to make these two kinds of systems coupling together to perform a common task with a high level of confidence. The goal of this paper is to propose a general model aimed at helping the comprehension, the description and the design of Bio-CPS. The proposed design process of such systems integrates human factors and their fundamental ethological principles as the central element so as to obtain reliability and efficiency to the target common task to be performed. The paper will firstly present the main concepts involved and give some definitions linked to Bio-CPS. Then, after a detailed presentation of the related issues and of the possible applications, the paper will present a theoretical framework aimed at characterizing and designing such systems.

2   Concepts and Definitions

2.1   Cyber-Physical Systems and the Time Representation Issue

Cyber-Physical Systems (CPS) are now widespread in literature and can be defined as follows:

Definition 1. *CPS are systems with deep integrations of computational elements with physical processes ([19]).*

To some points of view, it can be seen as an extension of the classical embedded systems which are mainly based on feedback loop concepts. Thus, one can consider the CPS as a mutual interaction between a computational processes, the time-line of which is based on discrete state changes, and a physical process based on continuous time evolution. The main issue of CPS is tied to the difficulty to manage this time-line duality.

Two main CPS conception approaches can be found in literature whether one focuses on the cyber part or on the physical aspects. the "Cyberizing the Physical" approach [19] is based on the integration of computing element into physical process. This approach is generally linked to hybrid systems theories where the time is common to all the parts of the system. However, the model of time is still a problem because the time continuum linked to the physical system needs to be discretized to fit cyber requirements. If this discretization can be sufficient for physics inspired artificial intelligence systems for instance [20], it is not the case for events based systems for which the use a superdense time model is required [22]. This time model is aimed to manage both continuous time-line and the causally related actions.

By contrast, the "Physicalizing the cyber" approach [19] focuses on the integration of physical elements into computer science algorithms. This requires to re-think the abstractions used in classical approaches, which have now to fit physical part constraints and to reduce, as far as possible, the time variabilities and unpredictability due to the use of high level algorithms. Within these approaches the time issue is still the first order element. If the habit in computer science is the optimisation of the algorithms/computer couple so as to obtain the fastest possible behaviour, this point of view is no longer pertinent for CPS. Indeed, the efficiency of the computer side is not linked to the speed of its time response but to the adaptability of this response to the evolution of the physical part. Consequently, instead of being considered as a quality factor, the time becomes a semantic property common to both physical and cyber parts. Thus, the quality measurement of algorithms for CPS is related to adaptability, reliability, robustness, predictability, accuracy or repeatability. For these reasons, novel approaches such as parallel computing [23], distributed computing [24], multi-agent systems [21], etc. are well adapted to CPS issues.

2.2 Complexity, Emergence and Complex Systems

A complex system can be defined as a set of a huge number of interacting entities, the global behaviour of which cannot be predicted by calculations or by an external observer. Generally, the evolution of the system is also unpredictable. Thus, a system is said as complex if the global obtained result (we'll see later in this paper what kind of result can be expected) can only be predicted by experiments and simulations even with a total knowledge of all its components and the rules that gather them. The existence of such systems challenges the reductionist approach [9] which considers that the complex nature of systems can be reduced to a sum or a composition of fundamental principles. The complex system study is an activity widespread among many scientific fields.

Basically, there's a confusion between complicated system and complex system concepts. If one goes back to the etymological origin of these concepts, one will find the following definitions.

Definition 2. *A system is said **complicated** if time and talent are required to understand it well. For instance, a clockwork mechanism is a complicated system. The complicated system organization is deterministic and computable.*

Definition 3. *The term **complex** means that the system is made of many intrications which make impossible the study of a part of it separately while neglecting its other components. Even if some part of a complex system could be computable, it is mainly non-deterministic and unpredictable.*

In [10], a difference between these two concepts is made based on the dynamical nature of the relations between system components. Thus, even if both can be defined as a set of numerous interacting elements, the system components are considered to be fixed in time and space in a complicated system while they can vary dynamically into a complex system.

The complex nature of a system leads to two other concepts: the emergence and the self organizing ability. These concepts are closely tied and complementary. The self organizing ability is often linked to an increase in the order of the system or to a decrease of its entropy without any external control in computation sciences and automation. In [11], the self-organization is defined as a dynamical and adaptive process allowing the system to obtain or to maintain an organizational structure without any external intervention. Therefore if the self organization concept is relevent for interactive systems then it remains inadequate for describing physical systems behaviour.

If the self organization concept is clear and its definition is widely recognized with a certain scientific consensus, this is no truly the case for the emergence concept. Indeed, there exist many different definitions for emergence. In the common mind, the emergence concept is linked to an existing external observer who is able to determine and to analyse the phenomena produced by a process. During the $XIX^{t}h$ century, has been introduced in biology and in philosophy as opposed to reductionism. Then, more recently, this concept lead to a great deal of research work in several scientific domains such as in computer science, [12,15,16,18], in complex systems study [10], in sociology,...

By the same as for the concept of complex system which cannot be studied into a reductionist frame, the concept of emergence share the same kind of problems. In [17] for instance, emergence is reduced to a simple problem of description and explanation. In this case, it is not a system property but a property of the point of view one may have on the system. In [11], a system is defined to present emerging properties when phenomena appear dynamically at a macroscopic level as a result of interactions between system components which occur at a microscopic level. In [13,14], emergence concept is split into three categories:

- The **nominal emergence**: it is linked to the presence of macroscopic properties which can not be defined to be microscopic.
- The **weak emergence**: it can be considered as a sub part of the nominal emergence where the appearance of the phenomena cannot be explained easily. As said in [13], this type of emergence requires the use of simulations and experiments.
- The **strong emergence**: as opposed to the nominal emergence, the strong emergence consider that the observed phenomena on a macroscopic point of view have side effects on both macroscopic and microscopic levels.

Considering these definitions, it is now clear that the self-organizing ability is tied to the organisational structure of the system whereas the emergence of properties or functions is tied to the dynamical aspect of the system.

For us self-organization and emergence are system properties resulting from the interactions between the cyber and physical parts of the system.

2.3   Interactions: The Central Elements in CPS

Interactions are the central elements for modelling CPS . Their nature and their conception trigger the way the coupled global system evolves and how it is able to reach its goal(s).

The general definition of an interaction is the following:

Definition 4. *An interaction is a dynamical relationship between two or more entities based on a set of reciprocal actions.*

Interactions can have different forms. Interactions can be direct,i.e. one entity affects directly another one by an action (collision between two physical elements for instance). This kind of interactions is generally encountered in physical systems. By contrast, interactions can be also indirect, i.e. the action of one entity is propagated to another one by using an intermediate element. This element can be a part of the entities common environment or another part of the system. These interactions are mainly met in social biological systems (ant colonies [1], social spiders, etc.) and can lead to stigmergy [2] (i.e. a form of self-organization/coordination mechanism induced by mutual actions performed on a shared element). Besides this direct/indirect properties, some other properties are crucial for Bio-CPS coupling. Among them, the local and the symmetrical characters of interactions are particularly pertinent.

Definition 5. *An interaction is said to be local when the mutual actions between elements are performed within a short distance. By contrast, an interaction is said non-local when it is performed between elements separated in space with no noticeable intermediate agency or mechanism.*

Among local interactions, we can cite as example the local application of forces in Physics such as the tyre/road interaction while studying vehicle behaviours. Non-local interaction can also be found in Physics (the gravitation law or the Aharonov Bohm effect for instance [3] are common examples) but are mainly present in biological systems ruling the exchanges between organs in human bodies for instance [6]. One other important character of interactions is the symmetrical aspect.

Definition 6. *An interaction is said symmetrical when there is a reciprocity between the elements involved.*

In physical world, interactions are generally symmetrical (the electrical interaction between particles for instance) whereas in biological system the symmetry is not the common rule [5]. However, some research works are starting to use virtual Physics inspired interaction where the symmetric character has been removed. For instance, [7,8] are proposing models of non-symmetric physical interactions between vehicles in platoon in order to increase the stability of the system as compared to symmetric spring damper functions.

3   Bio-CPS Issues and Applications

Today human artefact systems are a design and engineering challenge. From human machine system to sociotechnical, systems automation and interaction ground many technical development. Traditional approaches rely on analytic and a reductionist method. They propose an abstraction of the human based on a mechanical or computational model. The limits of that epistemological metaphor leads to the necessity of a strong paradigm shift.

When one wants to make human and CPS working together so as to accomplish a task, the question of the nature of the relationship has to be addressed. Does it corresponds to an *interaction* or to a *coupling* between two systems? The problem is the fact that the two systems are different by nature. Even if they are embedded into a common physical space (i.e. a place where the physical principles are respected); the are different in their structural and dynamic organization.

The challenge is then to be able first to find out an isomorphic framework for describing the two systems and their integrative coupling with a shared reference frame, and secondly to validate fundamental human cyber-physical systems integration principles.

So the Bio-CPS modelling needs bio-compatible and bio-integrable CPS design and engineering scientific grounding.

3.1   Human and Machine: Different Natures, One Isomorphic Framework

Two Different Natures. The human nature is biological (and anthropological, grounded on the former). The machine nature is artificial and cyber-physical. These evidences constrain to define a new theoretical and experimental framework for describing, designing and synthesizing Bio-CPS.

Thus one of the main issues is to think Bio-CPS as a global system of one higher or of one different level of organization of the human body. CPS may be modelled as an anatomical and physiological extension of the biological system and then as an enhancement of its own and social domain of activity and life.

Interaction. One of the main organizational difference from biological systems and CPS is the interaction nature.

As previously said, the interactions in both cyber and physical worlds are all symmetric and mostly local. Some interactions can be non-local but they are focused on physical side and are not met into cyber-physical set of interactions. The reason of this is embedded in the regulation loop concept which is the main inspiration source for CPS.

By contrast, biological interactions are functional interactions. This theoretical concept of functional interaction (i.e. something emitted by an entity has got an action upon on another entity somewhere) introduced by Chauvet [4–6] explains the specific nature of the human interactions. Their three main properties are : non-symmetric, non local and non-instantaneous.

At this point, one can see the difficulty in making biological systems and cyber-physical systems interacting together so as to perform a common task or to reach one common goal as a global entity. Modelling and engineering a Bio-Cyber Physical system relies on making three complex systems, with different interaction natures and with different time representations, working together.

Until now, the willing of interactions between human and CPS has led naturally to the human in-the-loop (HITL) concept, which is now widespread in literature. Nevertheless, this HITL concept has got several limitations due to the different natures of the systems involved and their different organizations. Indeed, the HITL concept stems from a traditional system of systems engineering point of view linked to reductionism concepts. In that epistemological context

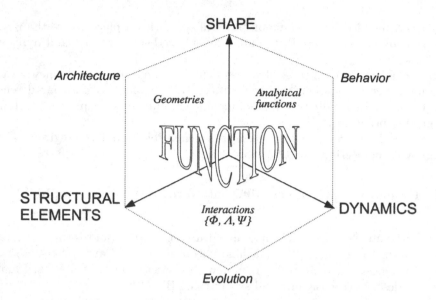

Fig. 1. The Bio-CPS isomorphic framework

modelling or designing human machine interaction is representing interaction as closed symmetrical loop and behavioural process.

After the previous considerations on the nature of human and CPS interactions, it is now clear that the HITL concept has to be override by the introduction of new theoretical foundations. Table 1 presents one classification of biological, cyber and physical systems considering the nature of the interactions and their time representations.

One Isomorphic Framework. First to revise the HITL concept and to shift to our bio-integrative paradigm, we have proposed [25] an isomorphic framework for modelling natural or artificial systems. This conceptual framework describes

Table 1. Classification of systems considering the nature of the interactions and the time representation

	Biological	Cyber	Physical
Symmetricity of interactions	Never	Both symmetric and non-symmetric	Always
Locality of interactions	Mainly non-local	Mainly local	Both local and non-local
Time representation	Continuous (Functional level) Discrete (Structural level)	Discrete or Event based	Continuous

three categories of required main system dimension: structural elements, shapes or forms and dynamics. Taking into account two by two this main classes of system variables, one can describe three specification plan: architecture (structural elements to shape or form specify geometrical structure or system architecture), behaviour (shape or form to dynamics specify analytical functions or functionally analysed) and evolution (structural elements to dynamics specify three main types of functional interactions: physical Φ, logical Λ, biological Ψ).

If one one assume that function does not exist by itself but is the emerging result of integrative organization, this framework grounds our bio-integrative model based Bio-CPS engineering (Fig. 1).

4   Conclusion

After explaining the main issues and the main differences in the natures of biological, physical and cybernetics systems, this paper presents a Bio-CPS framework aimed at helping in conceptualizing, designing and engineering Bio-CPS.

The proposed approach consists in thinking up such systems by considering the CPS system as an extension and/or an enhancement of the human biological nature which requires bio-compatible and bio-integrable scientific and design principles. This approach is a paradigm shift as compared to the classical approaches which reduce the human to only mechanical, logical or computational properties.

As opposed to CPS, where the interactions are only logical and physical, the interactions in Bio-CPS can be considered as multi-modal couplings which involves physical, logical and biological modalities and specific combinations of these.

So as to ensure a complete and coherent coupling between systems in Bio-CPS, one must design and engineer interactions which deal with biological, physical and logical elements. The coupling being made at interaction level, the bio-compatibility must be ensured by the choices made for the structural elements, the dynamics and the form or shape and thus made for the global design of the Bio-CPS.

The approach, proposed in this paper, is epistemologically different from traditional CPS modelling method based only on a functional and behavioural analysis and metaphorical reductionism. Our Bio-CPS modelling is ground on both a structural analytical description and a functional integrative synthesis based on bio-compatibility and bio-integration needs and theoretical principles. In this three-dimensional integrative isomorphic framework - 3D-space of requirements and specifications, the interaction sub-space takes into account both statical and dynamical evolution of integrated Bio-CPS structural systems. The desire and emerging global function results from this integrative structural and dynamics organization. According this modelling approach human is not reduced to a logical or a logical factor or sub-system. CPS to be couple with human must fulfil biological requirements of human nature, its domain of life and activity.

Thus we can plan to model and construct with correctness bio-compatible and bio-integrative CPS. This conception and design of Bio-CPS will ensure not only the coupling interactions but the reliability of the overall integrated function of the artificially extended human body and its domain of life and activity in the time. This is an issue for the design of safety critical systems next-gen CPS for extending and enhancing human capability in health, aerospace, transport and defense.

References

1. Parunak, H.V.: Go to the ant: Engineering principles from natural multi-agent systems. Ann. Oper. Res. **75**, 69–101 (1997)
2. Theraulaz, G., Bonabeau, E.: A brief history of stigmergy. Artif. Life **5**(2), 97–116 (1999). doi:10.1162/106454699568700
3. Figielski, T., Wosinski, T.: On the quantum interference transistor based on the electrostatic Aharonov-Bohm effect. In: Second International Conference on Advanced Semiconductor Devices and Microsystems, pp. 27–30, 5–7 October 1998. doi:10.1109/ASDAM.1998.730158
4. Chauvet, G.A.: Hierarchical functional organization of formal biological systems: a dynamical approach. I. The increase of complexity by self-association increases the domain of stability of a biological system. Philos. Trans. R. Soc. Lond. B: Biol. Sci. **339**(1290), 425–444 (1993). doi:10.1098/rstb.1993.0041
5. Chauvet, G.A.: Hierarchical functional organization of formal biological systems: a dynamical approach. II. The concept of non-symmetry leads to a criterion of evolution deduced from an optimum principle of the (O-FBS) sub-system. Philos. Trans. Royal Soc. Lond. B: Biol. Sci. **339**(1290), 445–461 (1993). doi:10.1098/rstb.1993.0041
6. Chauvet, G.A.: Hierarchical functional organization of formal biological systems: a dynamical approach. III. The concept of non-locality leads to a field theory describing the dynamics at each level of organization of the (D-FBS) sub-system. Philos. Trans. Royal Soc. Lond. B: Biol. Sci. **339**(1290), 463–481 (1993). doi:10.1098/rstb.1993.0042
7. Contet, J.M., Gechter, F., Gruer, P., Koukam, A.: Reactive multi-agent approach to local platoon control: stability analysis and experimentations. Int. J. Intell. Syst. Technol. Appl. **10**, 231–249 (2011). doi:10.1504/IJISTA.2011.040348
8. Ali, A., Garcia, G., Martinet, P.: The flatbed platoon towing model for safe and dense platooning on highways. IEEE Intell. Transp. Syst. Mag. **7**(1), 58–68, Spring (2015). doi:10.1109/MITS.2014.2328670
9. Nagel, E.: The Structure of Science. Harcourt Brace World, New York (1961)
10. Moncion, T., Amar, P., Hutzler, G.: Automatic characterization of emergent phenomena in complex systems. J. Biol. Phys. Chem. **10**, 16–23 (2010)
11. De Wolf, T., Holvoet, T.: Emergence versus self-organisation: different concepts but promising when combined. In: Brueckner, S.A., Di Marzo Serugendo, G., Karageorgos, A., Nagpal, R. (eds.) ESOA 2005. LNCS (LNAI), vol. 3464, pp. 1–15. Springer, Heidelberg (2005)
12. Dessalles, J.-L., Ferber, J., Phan, D.: Emergence in agent based computational social science: conceptual, formal and diagrammatic analysis. Intelligent Complex Adaptive Systems (2008). ISBN:978-1-59904-717-1
13. Bedau, M.A.: Weak emergence. Philos. Perspect.: Mind Causation World Tomberlin **31**, 375–399 (1997). issn:1468–0068, Blackwell Publishers Inc

14. Bedau, M.A.: Downward causation and the autonomy of weak emergence. Principia **6**(1), 5–50 (2002)
15. Bonabeau, E., Dessalles, J.-L., Grumbach, A.: Characterizing emergent phenomena (1): a critical review. Rev. Int. Syst. **9**(3), 327–346 (1995)
16. Bonabeau, E., Dessalles, J.-L., Grumbach, A.: Characterizing emergent phenomena (2): a conceptual framework. Rev. Int. Syst. **9**(3), 347–371 (1995)
17. Memmi, D.: Emergence et niveaux d'explication. Journes Thmatiques de l'ARC (mergence et explication) (1996)
18. Yamins, D.: Towards a theory of "local to global" in distributed multi-agent systems (I). In: AAMAS, pp. 183–190 (2005)
19. Lee, E. A.: CPS foundations. In: Proceedings of the 47th Design Automation Conference, DAC 2010, pp. 737-742 (2010). ISBN: 978-1-4503-0002-5
20. Gechter, F., Contet, J.-M., Gruer, P., Koukam, A.: A reactive agent based vehicle platoon algorithm with integrated obstacle avoidance ability. In: Fifth IEEE International Conference on Self-Adaptive and Self-Organizing Systems SASO (2011)
21. Dafflon, B., Gechter, F., Gruer, P., Koukam, A.: Vehicle platoon and obstacle avoidance: a reactive agent approach. IET Intell. Transport Syst. **7**, 257–264 (2013). issn: 1751–956X
22. Manna, Z., Pnueli, A.: Verifying hybrid systems. In: Grossman, R.L., Ravn, A.P., Rischel, H., Nerode, A. (eds.) HS 1991 and HS 1992. LNCS, vol. 736, pp. 4–35. Springer, Heidelberg (1993)
23. Jozwiak, L.: Automatic architecture exploration of massively parallel MPSoCs for modern cyber-physical systems. In: 17th International Symposium on Design and Diagnostics of Electronic Circuits and Systems, pp. 10, 23–25 April 2014. doi:10.1109/DDECS.2014.6868752
24. Zhou, K., Ye, C., Wan, J., Liu, B., Liang, L.: Advanced control technologies in cyber-physical system. In: 5th International Conference on Intelligent Human-Machine Systems and Cybernetics (IHMSC), pp. 569–573, 26–27 August 2013. doi:10.1109/IHMSC.2013.284
25. Fass, D.: Augmented human engineering: a theoretical and experimental approach to human systems integration. In: Cogan, B. (eds.) System Engineering Practice and Theory, Intech - Open Access Publisher, Rijeka, Croatia pp. 257–276, March 2012. ISBN 979-953-307-410-7

Colorimetry and Impression Evaluation
of Insert Molded GFRP Plate
with Black Silk Fabrics

Kiyoshi Fujiwara[1], Erika Suzuki[2], Tetsuo Kikuchi[2],
Takashi Furukawa[3], Takahiro Suzuki[4], Atsushi Endo[5],
Yutaro Shimode[6], Yuka Takai[4(✉)], and Yuqiu Yang[7]

[1] Mazda Motor Corporation, Hiroshima, Japan
fujiwara.k@mazda.co.jp
[2] Toyugiken Co., Ltd., Kanagawa, Japan
{erika-suzuki,tetuo-kikuchi}@toyugiken.co.jp
[3] HISHIKEN Co., Ltd, Kyoto, Japan
t-furukawa@hishiken.co.jp
[4] Osaka Sangyo University, Osaka, Japan
ytakai9@gmail.com, takai@ise.osaka-sandai.ac.jp
[5] Kyoto Institute of Technology, Kyoto, Japan
shootingstarofhope30@gmail.com
[6] Future-Applied Conventional Technology Centre,
Kyoto Institute of Technology, Kyoto, Japan
shimode-yutaro@xa2.so-net.ne.jp
[7] Donghua University, Shanghai, China
amy_yuqiu_yang@hotmail.com

Abstract. Black silk fabric, a traditional craft produced using the Kyo-Yuzen dyeing technique, is another luxury product. The intention behind the present report is to mold Urushi-like glass fiber-reinforced plastic, using black silk fabric. We first manufactured a glass fiber-reinforced plastic (GFRP) molded plate consisting of various laminate layers, and compared the surface color with Urushi products. Subsequently, we used an impression evaluation to reveal how the glass fiber-reinforced plastic (GFRP) molded plate using black silk fabric was rated. As the results of this study, it was confirmed that; L* and a* value of FRP sample was similar to the Urushi sample, FRP sample was bluer than the Urushi sample according to b* value, and C* value of FRP sample was higher than the Urushi sample. About half of the subject regarded GFRP using black silk fabric with the lightness similar to the Urushi product as Urushi product in the impression evaluation. The sample regarded as the Urushi product makes subject more feel "Beauty", "Sense of luxury and high quality", "Gloss" and "Depth of blackness" than the sample not regarded as the Urushi product. Evaluation point of the subject regarded the FRP sample as the Urushi product showed a strong association between "Beauty" and "Sense of luxury and high quality", between "Beauty" and "Gloss", between "Sense of luxury and high quality" and "Gloss".

Keywords: GFRP · Kyo-Yuzen dyeing · Silk fabric · Urushi · Black · Colorimetry · Impression evaluation

© Springer International Publishing Switzerland 2015
V.G. Duffy (Ed.): DHM 2015, Part I, LNCS 9184, pp. 256–266, 2015.
DOI: 10.1007/978-3-319-21073-5_26

1 Introduction

Plastic products are light, user-friendly, and indispensable to our lives. However, they cannot really be said to give consumers a sense of luxury and high quality. Commodity prices therefore inevitably tend to be kept down, regardless of high functionality. To make plastic products that give consumers a sense of luxury and high quality, we need to know people's sensibilities. A huge range of physical factors affect peoples' sensibilities, including the surface profile, weight and color of a plastic product. Analyzing these factors one by one and recreating the products based on that analysis requires a lot of time.

Japan has products termed traditional crafts which have a long legacy. As traditional crafts are created using traditional processes, carefully selected materials are used and work is often done manually. In line with this, prices are also high. However, traditional crafts give consumers a sense of luxury and high quality that is equal to or higher than the price. Moreover, many traditional crafts provide one with a moment of peace when taking it into one's hand. We think it is therefore a natural development to learn from traditional crafts this sense of luxury and high quality that plastic products are in need of.

The present study focuses on the Japanese traditional craft of Urushi (lacquer) products. Figure 1 shows an example. The black often used in Urushi products has a depth which is regarded as high grade in Japan. In previous study, Urushi product has been evaluated by various analysis methods [1–6]. However there is only a study compared the Urushi product and the plastic injection molding product in the studies compared the Urushi product and the plastic product [7].

Black silk fabric, a traditional craft produced using the Kyo-Yuzen dyeing technique, is another luxury product. The intention behind the present report is to mold

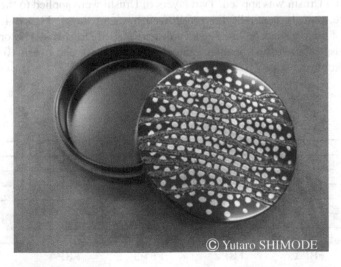

Fig. 1. An example of Urushi product [Incense case with Maki-e decoration "Yukyu no Sasayaki" (made by Yutaro Shimode)]

Urushi-like glass fiber-reinforced plastic, using black silk fabric. We first manufactured a glass fiber-reinforced plastic (GFRP) molded plate consisting of various laminate layers, and compared the surface color with Urushi products. Subsequently, we used an impression evaluation to reveal how the glass fiber-reinforced plastic (GFRP) molded plate using black silk fabric was rated.

2   Method

2.1   Sample

We used glass fiber-reinforced molded plates using black silk fabric and Urushi plates for the samples. For the glass fiber-reinforced molded plate, we used clear resin (2035P, manufactured by U-PICA), glass mats (#230, manufactured by Central Glass), and, as decorative material, blackened silk fabric. Five samples were prepared with the black silk fabric occupying different positions between the layers. Figure 2 illustrates the layered compositions for the glass fiber-reinforced molded plate using black silk fabric. The sample with the black silk fabric in the uppermost layer is labeled FRP1, with the others labeled FRP1-5, depending on the location of the silk fabric. For FRP1, a silk fabric layer was layered on top of a gel coat, with four glass mat layers placed on top of that. The gel coat surface was taken as the sample surface. Curing conditions were 24 h at room temperature. Figure 3 shows the appearance of an FRP sample using black silk fabric.

The Urushi plates were manufactured by a skilled artisan with 36 years' experience. By adjusting the mix of a glossy and a matt Urushi, he prepared Urushi in ten gradations of luster. For the glossy Urushi "Kourin Nuritate Jyohonkuro" (Kourin finishing black, manufactured by Tsutsumi Asakichi Urushi-ten) was used, and for the matt Urushi, Sugurome (oil-free Urushi, manufactured by Tsujita Urushi-ten). A PMMA (Poly-methylmethacrylate) plate measuring 100 mm × 100 mm × 5 mm was used as the base onto which the Urushi was applied. Two layers of Urushi were applied to the top of this PMMA plate, namely a middle layer followed by a top layer. Figure 4 shows the appearance of the Urushi samples. The samples are named Urushi1–10 according to the degree of gloss, with Urushi1 being the sample with the least, and Urushi10 the sample with the most gloss.

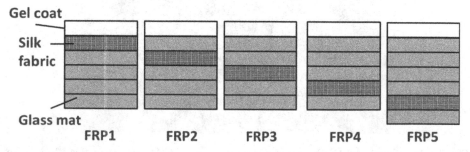

Fig. 2. Layered compositions for the glass fiber-reinforced molded plate using black silk fabric

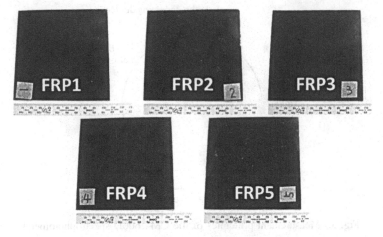

Fig. 3. Appearance of an FRP sample using black silk fabric

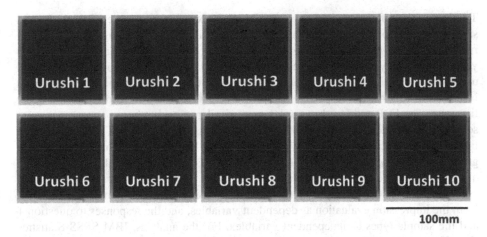

Fig. 4. Appearance of the Urushi samples

2.2 Colorimetry

To clarify the difference between the black of the FRP samples and the Urushi samples, color measurements were taken of the sample surfaces using a CM-2600D spectrophotometer (Konica Minolta, Inc.). Figure 5 illustrates the measurement principles of the CM-2600D spectrophotometer. Using a D65 light source, the sample is exposed to light which is diffused through an integrated sphere. The light received at 8° from the sample's perpendicular plane was measured. Regular reflected light was eliminated. The following aspects were measured: L* (Lightness), a* (Red/Green Chromaticity), b* (Yellow/Blue Chromaticity) and C* (Chroma).

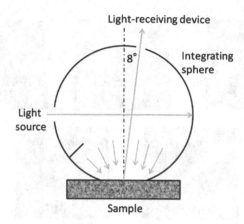

Fig. 5. Measurement principles of the CM-2600D spectrophotometer

2.3 Impression Evaluation

To identify the differences in the way the black is experienced for the FRP and Urushi samples, we performed an impression evaluation using a questionnaire. There were 21 male and female respondents ranging from 21 to 66 years in age (average age 28.5 years, SD = 13.5 years). They were shown the FRP1 and Urushi5 samples in a room lit using fluorescent lighting at a light intensity of 60 lx, and, without having been informed as to what the respective samples were, were asked to respond to the questionnaire. The FRP and Urushi samples most similar to each other in appearance were selected. Respondents were prohibited from touching the samples. The questionnaire first asked to select the sample they thought was an Urushi product, and then asked to grade the respective samples on a 5-point scale for "Beauty", "Sense of luxury and high quality", "Gloss" and "Depth of blackness".

We performed a two-way analysis of variance using the evaluation values obtained from the impression evaluation as dependent variables, and the responses to question 1 and the sample types as independent variables. For the analysis, IBM SPSS Statistics (Var.20) was used. Furthermore, the correlations between the evaluation items were analyzed. In both analyses, the critical p-value was set at 5 %.

3   Results

3.1   Colorimetry

Figure 6 showed the result of L^* in each sample. The lower the position of black silk fabric was in the layer construction of the sample, the higher the L^* value became in the case of FRP1, FRP2 and FRP3. The L^* value of FRP4 and FRP5 was low. The L^* value of Urushi1 was the highest in all Urushi samples. The higher the value of the gloss of Urushi sample became, the lower the L^* value of it became. L^* value of FRP samples were similar to the Urushi samples with the high and middle level of gloss.

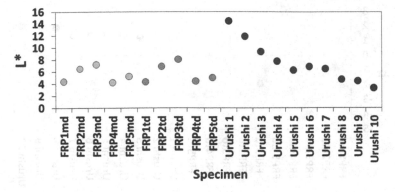

Fig. 6. Results of L*

Figure 7 showed the result of a* in each sample. The higher the a* value became, the more the color became red. The lower the a* value became, the more the color became green. The upper the position of black silk fabric was in the layer construction of the sample, the higher the a* value became in the case of FRP1, FRP2 and FRP3. The a* value of FRP4 and FRP5 was high. The a* value of Urushi1 was the highest in all Urushi samples. The higher the value of the gloss of Urushi sample became, the lower the a* value of it became. Green was strong in both FRP and Urushi samples because it's a* value was negative value. The a* value of FRP sample was similar to the Urushi sample with low level of gloss.

Figure 8 showed the result of b* in each sample. The higher the b* value became, the more the color became yellow. The lower the b* value became, the more the color became blue. The upper the position of black silk fabric was in the layer construction of the sample, the higher the b* value became in the case of FRP1, FRP2 and FRP3. The b* value of FRP4 and FRP5 was high. The b* value of Urushi1 was the lowest in all Urushi samples. The higher the value of the gloss of Urushi sample became, the higher the b* value of it became. Blue was strong in all FRP samples because it's b* value was

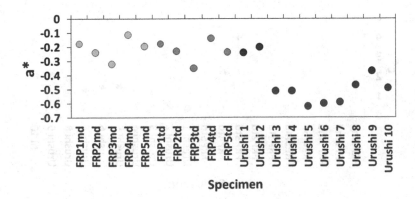

Fig. 7. Results of a*

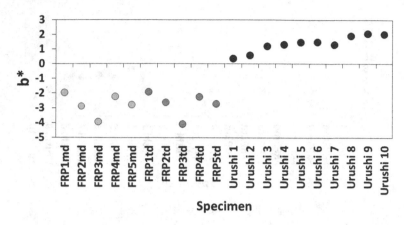

Fig. 8. Results of b*

negative value. On the other hand, yellow was strong in all Urushi samples because it's b* value was positive value.

Figure 9 showed the result of C* in each sample. The upper the position of black silk fabric was in the layer construction of the sample, the higher the C* value became in the case of FRP1, FRP2 and FRP3. The C* value of FRP4 and FRP5 was low. The C* value of Urushi1 was the lowest in all Urushi samples. The higher the value of the gloss of Urushi sample became, the higher the C* value of it became. The C* value of FRP sample was similar to the Urushi sample with high level of gloss, or it was two times as high as the Urushi sample with high level of gloss.

As these results, it was found that the L* and a* value of FRP sample was similar to the Urushi sample, FRP sample was bluer than the Urushi sample according to b* value, and C* value of FRP sample was higher than the Urushi sample. Furthermore, it was found that depth of blackness was not sufficient in the FRP products according to the hearing from Urushi craftspeople.

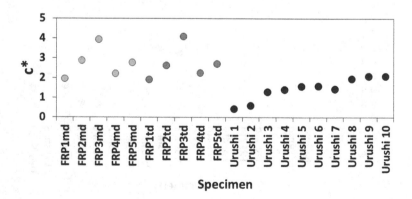

Fig. 9. Results of C*

3.2   Impression Evaluation

Question 1 was "Which sample is Urushi?" 10 subjects selected the FRP sample, and 11 subjects selected the Urushi sample. Figure 10 showed the result of the impression evaluation about "Beauty" of FRP and Urushi sample. Gray bar showed the subject selected the Urushi, and black bar was showed the subject selected the FRP sample in the question 1. All subjects felt the sample regarded as the Urushi product in question 1 more beautiful than the other sample. As a result of an analysis of variance, a main effect was not shown, but a significant interaction was shown (F (1.42) = 10.3, p < .01). Figure 11 showed the result of the impression evaluation about "Sense of luxury and high quality" of FRP and Urushi sample. Figure 12 showed the result of the impression evaluation about "Gloss" of FRP and Urushi sample. Figure 13 showed the result of the impression evaluation about "Depth of blackness" of FRP and Urushi sample. All subjects felt the sample regarded as the Urushi product in question 1 more "Sense of

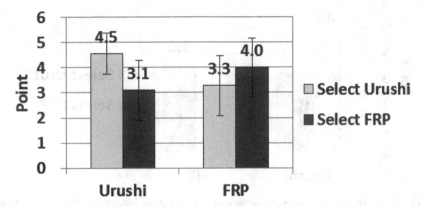

Fig. 10. Result of the impression evaluation about "Beauty" of FRP and Urushi sample

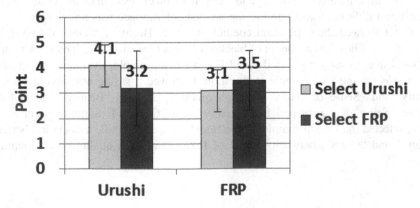

Fig. 11. Result of the impression evaluation about "Sense of luxury and high quality" of FRP and Urushi sample.

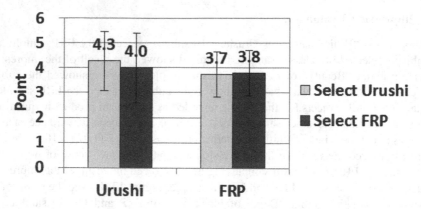

Fig. 12. Result of the impression evaluation about "Gloss" of FRP and Urushi sample

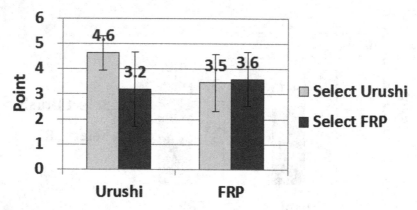

Fig. 13. Result of the impression evaluation about "Depth of blackness" of FRP and Urushi sample.

luxury and high quality", "Gloss" and "Depth of blackness" than the other sample. A significant difference according to the analysis of variance was not shown.

Table 1 showed the correlation coefficient (r) of "Beauty", "Sense of luxury and high quality", "Gloss" and "Depth of blackness" about the sample judged the Urushi in question 1 in each subject selected the FRP and Urushi sample. Evaluation point of the subject selected the FRP sample in question 1 showed a strong association between "Beauty" and "Sense of luxury and high quality", between "Beauty" and "Gloss", between "Sense of luxury and high quality" and "Gloss". Evaluation point of the subject selected the Urushi sample in question 1 showed a middle association between "Beauty" and "Gloss", between "Sense of luxury and high quality" and "Depth of blackness".

Table 1. Correlation coefficient of "Beauty", "Sense of luxury and high quality","Gloss" and "Depth of blackness".

Selected product	Beauty-Sense of luxury and high quality	Beauty-Gloss	Beauty-Depth of blackness	Sense of luxury and high quality-Gloss	Sense of luxury and high quality-Depth of blackness	Gloss-Depth of blackness
FRP	0.816	0.733	0.0895	0.821	0.0877	−0.315
Urushi	0.360	0.549	0.214	0.377	0.422	−0.113

4 Discussions

It is found that b* and C* value of GFRP using black silk fabric was different from the Urushi product as a result of the colorimetry. However, about half of the subject regarded GFRP using black silk fabric as Urushi product in the impression evaluation. Although Urushi crafts is a traditional crafts in Japan, Urushi product is a high quality product now, the use of Urushi product is reduced in public life, and it is little seen by many people. Therefore, it seems that it is difficult to recognize the Urushi product. Interaction of question about "Beauty" in the impression evaluation was significant. It seems that this means the Japanese stereotype which Urushi product is more beautiful than the other material products. Furthermore, it suggests that black board with a lightness equivalent to the Urushi product makes people feel beauty and high quality equivalent to the Urushi product because evaluation point of the subject selected the FRP sample in question 1 showed a strong association between "Beauty" and "Sense of luxury and high quality", between "Beauty" and "Gloss", between "Sense of luxury and high quality" and "Gloss". Therefore, there is a possibility that the GFRP inserted the black silk fabric immediately beneath the gel coat is used as the Urushi-like FRP.

5 Conclusions

This study aimed to mold the glass fiber-reinforced plastics (GFRP) using black silk fabric with the color equivalent to the Urushi product. Colorimetry and impression evaluation about the GFRP using black silk fabric and Urushi board was conducted. As the results of this study, it was confirmed that;

1. L* and a* value of FRP sample was similar to the Urushi sample, FRP sample was bluer than the Urushi sample according to b* value, and C* value of FRP sample was higher than the Urushi sample.
2. About half of the subject regarded GFRP using black silk fabric with the lightness similar to the Urushi product as Urushi product in the impression evaluation.
3. The sample regarded as the Urushi product makes subject more feel "Beauty", "Sense of luxury and high quality", "Gloss" and "Depth of blackness" than the sample not regarded as the Urushi product.

4. Evaluation point of the subject regarded the FRP sample as the Urushi product showed a strong association between "Beauty" and "Sense of luxury and high quality", between "Beauty" and "Gloss", between "Sense of luxury and high quality" and "Gloss".

For the above results, there is a possibility that the GFRP using black silk fabric immediately beneath the gel coat is used as the Urushi-like FRP.

References

1. Shimode, Y., Takahashi, Y., Nakai, A., Kotaki, M., Hamada, H.: Surface characteristics of Urushi products. In: Proceedings of 11th Japan International Sampe Symposium and Exhibition (JISSE-11), TC-6–1 (2009)
2. Shimode, Y., Takahashi, Y., Endo, A., Narita, C., Takai, Y., Nishimoto, H., Yamada, K., Goto, A., Yasunaga, H., Hamada, H.: Surface shape characteristics of shellfish pieces used for Urushi products. In: Proceedings of 12th Japan International Sampe Symposium and Exhibition (JISSE-12), TRA-1 (2011)
3. Shimode, Y., Takahashi, Y., Endo, A., Narita, C., Takai, Y., Nishimoto, H., Yamada, K., Goto, A., Yasunaga, H., Hamada, H.: Optical characteristics of shellfish pieces used for Urushi products. In: Proceedings of 12th Japan International Sampe Symposium and Exhibition (JISSE-12), TRA-3 (2011)
4. Shimode, Y., Takahashi, Y., Endo, A., Narita, C., Takai, Y., Yamada, K., Goto, A., Yasunaga, H., Hamada H.: Optical characteristic of gold powder processed by traditional *Maki-e* technique. In: Proceedings of 12th Japan International Sampe Symposium and Exhibition (JISSE-12), TRA-4 (2011)
5. Shimode, Y., Ohtani, Y., Yasunaga, H.: How do craftspeople distinguish the appearance of natural-lacquerware? Approach by optical image analysis. J. Jpn. Soc. Colour Mater. **84**(3), 81–86 (2011)
6. Narita, C., Endo, A., Shimode, Y., Yamada, K.: Study on the appearance and peel strength of Byakudan-Nuri works. Mater. Sci. Appl. **5**, 81–85 (2014)
7. Shimode, Y., Takahashi, Y., Endo, A., Narita, C., Murakami, M., Takai, Y., Yamada, K., Goto, A., Yasunaga, H., Hamada, H.: Wide angle reflection properties of Urushi (Japanese lacquer) products and black injection molded article. In: Proceedings of 12th Japan International Sampe Symposium and Exhibition (JISSE-12), TRA-2 (2011)

Light Transmission Properties of Insert Molded GFRPs with Different Crape Structure of Silk Fabrics

Kiyoshi Fujiwara[1], Erika Suzuki[2], Tetsuo Kikuchi[2],
Takashi Furukawa[3], Atsushi Endo[4], Yuka Takai[5(✉)],
and Yuqiu Yang[6]

[1] Mazda Motor Corporation, Hiroshima, Japan
fujiwara.k@mazda.co.jp
[2] Toyugiken Co. Ltd, Kanagawa, Japan
{erika-suzuki, tetuo-kikuchi}@toyugiken.co.jp
[3] HISHIKEN Co. Ltd., Kyoto, Japan
t-furukawa@hishiken.co.jp
[4] Kyoto Institute of Technology, Kyoto, Japan
shootingstarofhope30@gmail.com
[5] Osaka Sangyo University, Osaka, Japan
takai@ise.osaka-sandai.ac.jp
[6] Donghua University, Shanghai, China
amy_yuqiu_yang@hotmail.com

Abstract. In this research, the hand lay-up method was focused as one of the decoration molding techniques for the GFRP lighting materials. The hand lay-up method can be more developed in the market of the GFRP lighting material because type of form and reinforced material are free to be selected in this method. Therefore, this research aimed to clearly the light transmission property of the GFRP inserted the Kyo Yu-zen fabric with crape. The cross section structure, light transmission property and luminance distribution of the GFRP samples were analyzed. As the results of this research, it was confirmed that the structure of the GFRP inserted the silk fabric with crape was different in each sample according to a laid direction of the yarn and use of the laid yarn, the GFRP inserted the silk fabric with crape had more profound effect on a dispersion of the light with the luminous intensity and the luminance than the GFRP with only glass mat, and a degree of the dispersion of the light was changed by the structure of the crape, and it was the highest in the Silk4 showed the highest Ra value.

Keywords: GFRP · Hand lay-up · Silk fabric · Crape structure · Light transmission property · Luminance distribution

1 Introduction

Use of glass fiber reinforced plastics (GFRP) as lighting materials has spread. For example, exterior as the roof material of the housing terrace or the carport, interior material as the bathroom door and the indoor partition window as shown in Fig. 1. GFRP lighting materials has been said for appearance – a glass pattern appears – to be

© Springer International Publishing Switzerland 2015
V.G. Duffy (Ed.): DHM 2015, Part I, LNCS 9184, pp. 267–276, 2015.
DOI: 10.1007/978-3-319-21073-5_27

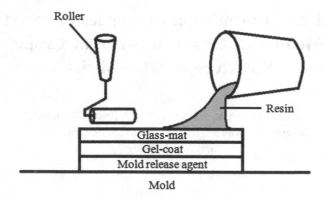

Fig. 1. Hand lay-up method

bad although physical properties, such as mechanical strength, are good. This problem was solved in pattern printing to the surface of the GFRP board with transcriptional molding technique. The ratio of the parallel light/diffusion light of the transmitted light of the GFRP board was shifted to the diffusion light side. From this technique, the glass pattern disappeared by the difference in the refractive index of resin and glass. As a result, the panel which does not have visibility at the same time it lets light pass was realized. On the other hand, LED lighting has the high directivity of light and it is difficult to illuminate all the directions like a filament lamp. As one of the solution for this problem, it is thought that GFRP lighting materials with high light diffusion can be diverted to the housing of LED lighting.

In this research, the hand lay-up method was focused as one of the decoration molding techniques for the GFRP lighting materials. The hand lay-up method can be more developed in the market of the GFRP lighting material because type of form and reinforced material are free to be selected in this method. Therefore, this research aimed to clearly the light transmission property of the GFRP inserted the Kyo Yu-zen fabric with crape. The cross section structure, light transmission property and luminance distribution of the GFRP samples were analyzed.

Previous researches on the embossed or grained FRP can be referred for GFRP inserted the Kyo Yu-zen fabric with crape [1, 2]. Light transmission property and luminance of the FRP have been analyzed [3–5], there are less researches aimed to develop the GFRP lighting materials. Whereat, this research is significant for the development of the GFRP lighting materials.

2 Method

2.1 Materials and Fabrication

The samples were molded by hand lay-up method as shown in Fig. 1. Hand lay-up method has been used for molding composite structures from long ago. It can be performed by only a mold, skill and material. Reinforcing fiber is impregnated with liquid resin and it is laminated on the mold with roller by hand.

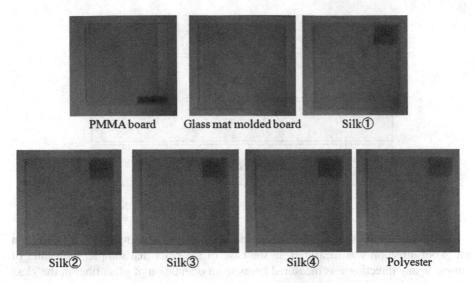

Fig. 2. Photos of insert molded GFRPs with Silk Fabrics

An unsaturated polyester resin (2035P, U-PICA Company. Ltd.) was used as the matrix resin. A glass mat (#230, Central Glass Co., Ltd.) was used as reinforcing material. The crape fabric was used as decorative material. Figure 2 shows photos of samples. A size of the sample was 200 mm×200 mm. The crape fabric was called "Silk1", "Silk2", "Silk3", "Silk4" and "Polyester crape" based on a difference in crape structure or fiber. Each silk fabric structure is as follows;

- Silk1: Fabric woven left-laid and right-laid woofs alternately one by one.
- Silk2: Fabric woven left-laid and right-laid woofs alternately two by two.
- Silk3: Fabric woven left-laid and right-laid woofs alternately two by two.

  A number of the warp is larger than the Silk2.

- Silk4: Fabric woven right-laid woof.

The laminated constitution of samples was shown in Fig. 3. First, glass mat was laminated two layers on the PMMA (Polymethylmethacrylate) board, and it was cured at room temperature for three hours. Then crape fabric was laminated on the glass mat layer, and it was cured at room temperature for twenty-four hours.

2.2   Measurement

In order to reveal influence of lamination of crape on the light transmission property of the sample, the light transmission property and the luminance distribution of the sample were measured.

Cross Section Structure. The cross section structure of the sample was measured by using non-contact three-dimensional measuring device (NH-3SP, Mitaka Kohki Co., Ltd.).

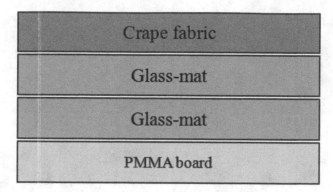

Fig. 3. Laminated constitution of sample

In the case of the sample with silk fabric, a center of the sample in warp direction and woof direction was measured. In the case of the glass mat sample, the canter of sample in any direction was measured because an orientation of glass fiber in the glass mat was random. Measurement range was 50 mm in all samples.

Light Transmission Property. The light transmission property was measured by the light distribution measurement bench as shown in Fig. 4. This instrument consists of biaxial goniometer, douser and spectroscope. The optical path length was 1 m. The light source is a LED light reflector bulb (equivalent to 40 W, white daylight, total luminous flux 280 lm). Sample was placed at a distance of 25 mm from the light source, the transmitted light of the sample was measured.

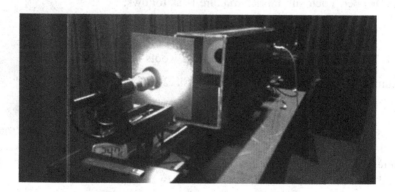

Fig. 4. Light distribution measurement bench

Luminance Distribution. The luminance distribution was measured by two-dimensional luminance colorimeter (CA-2000; Konica Minolta, Inc.) as shown in Fig. 5. Light source was a LED light bulb (equivalent to 40 W, white daylight, total luminous flux 485 lm). Sample was placed at a distance of 500 mm from the light source. The optical path length was 750 mm. Measurement image was divided into 960400 area based on x direction 900 and y direction 980, and 960400 luminance distribution data per one measurement were got in this instrument.

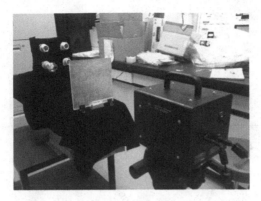

Fig. 5. Two-dimensional luminance colorimeter

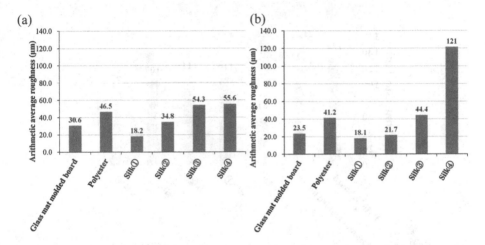

Fig. 6. Arithmetic average roughness; (a) Warp direction, (b) Woof direction

3 Results and Discussions

3.1 Cross Section Structure

Figure 6 shows arithmetic average roughness (Ra) of the sample. Arithmetic average roughness is the depth of mean value of the unevenness. Silk4 in the warp and woof direction showed the highest value in all samples. There wasn't so much of a difference between the value in the warp direction and the woof direction in each sample except for Silk4. It seems that the arithmetic average roughness of Silk4 was large because the fabric was woven by using only right-laid woof.

Figure 7 shows average length (RSm) of the sample. Average length is an average value of the unevenness of the intervals. Silk3 in the warp and woof direction showed the highest value in all samples. It seems that this result was caused by the crape with large width because 4 woofs were woven in Silk3. It is found that the space of the crape in all of the silk fabrics with crape in the woof direction was larger than it in the warp direction.

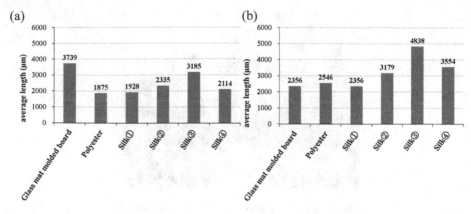

Fig. 7. Average length; (a) Warp direction, (b) Woof direction

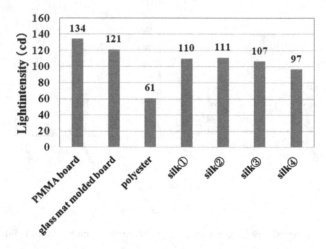

Fig. 8. Results of luminous intensity of the transmitted light

3.2   Light Transmission Property

Figure 8 shows results of luminous intensity of the transmitted light. The luminous intensity of the sample with laminated crape fabric was lower than the sample with only glass mat. In the case of the sample with crape fabric, it was revealed that luminous intensity changed because of the difference of thickness, structure and fiber.

Figure 9 shows results of general color rendering index (Ra). Color rendering index is a value which means the difference between the color under the light source evaluating the color rendering properties and the color under the stated base light source when the color under the stated base light source with respect to each correlated color temperature was regarded as 100. In general, the higher color rendering index is, a light source is similar to the natural light, Ra value of incandescent and halogen bulb is 100. Ra value reduced by laminating crape fabric, but a color shift did not occur. It is found

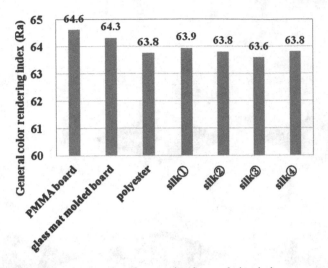

Fig. 9. Results of general color rendering index

that a thickness, structure and fiber of crape fabric didn't significantly affect the Ra value in this research.

3.3 Luminance Distribution

Figure 10 shows luminance distribution of LED bulb, PMMA board, glass mat molded board, and Silk2. Luminance distribution of LED bulb was similar to the one of the PMMA board. Luminance distribution of the glass mat molded board was showed in a wide range, but a luminance value was high in a part range. Luminance distribution of

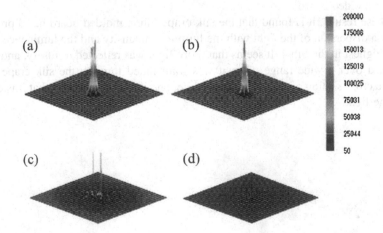

Fig. 10. Luminance distribution of (a) LED bulb, (b) PMMA board, (c) Glass mat molded board, (d) Silk2.

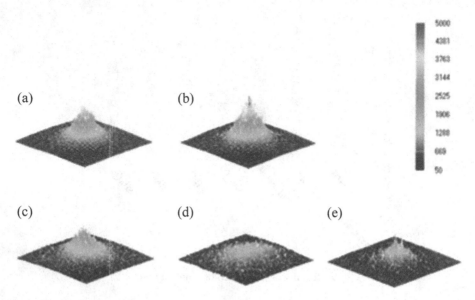

Fig. 11. Luminance distribution of (a) Silk1, (b) Silk2, (c) Silk3, (d) Silk4, (e) Polyester crape

Silk2 was showed in a whole range. In order to know the detail luminance distribution of the laminated crape fabric molding board, a display scale of the luminance distribution figure was changed. Figure 11 showed the luminance distribution of each sample with enlarged display scale. Luminance distributions of Silk1, Silk2, Silk3, Silk4 and Polyester crape was showed in a whole range, the luminance value was high near the light source. The luminance of Silk4 did not increase rapidly near the light source. Figure 12 showed an average luminance. The average luminance of silk crape fabric molded board was decreased by about 40%, and the average luminance of the polyester crape fabric molded board was decreased by about 70% compared with the glass mat molded board.

As these results, it is found that the silk crape fabric molded board has a profound effect on a dispersion of the light with the luminous intensity and the luminance, and it was the highest in the Silk4. It seems that more light was reflected diffusely, and it was transmitted over a wide range when it was transmitted through the silk crape fabric because a cross section of a silk fiber is triangle, and it has the property that it is easy to reflect the light.

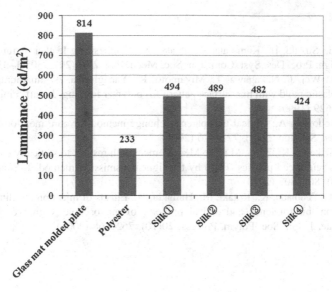

Fig. 12. Average luminance

4 Conclusions

In this research, the hand lay-up method was focused as one of the decoration molding techniques for the GFRP lighting materials. This research aimed to clearly the light transmission property of the GFRP inserted the Kyo Yu-zen fabric with crape. The cross section structure, light transmission property and luminance distribution of the GFRP samples were analyzed.

As the results of this research, it was confirmed that;

- The structure of the GFRP inserted the silk fabric with crape was different in each sample according to a laid direction of the yarn and use of the laid yarn.
- The GFRP inserted the silk fabric with crape had more profound effect on a dispersion of the light with the luminous intensity and the luminance than the GFRP with only glass mat.
- A degree of the dispersion of the light was changed by the structure of the crape, and it was the highest in the Silk4 showed the highest Ra value.

In the case of the GFRP inserted the silk fabric with crape, there is a good possibility that the dispersion of the light is free to be controlled by its structure. Therefore, it seems that the GFRP inserted the silk fabric with crape is expected to be used as a lighting equipment, and it makes the environment more comfortable.

References

1. Minamiji, H., Suzuki, H., Kamibata, J., Ohtake, Y.: Synthesizing leather textures for digital SHIBO design. Proc. Des. Syst. Conf. Jpn. Soc. Mech. Eng. **2010**(20), 3305-1–3305-6 (2010)
2. Noguchi, H., Wei, J., Nakagawa, T., Miyamoto, K., Yanagisawa, A., Imamura, M.: Development of plastic mold with fine surface pattern for polymer forming. J. Surf. Finish. Soc. Jpn. **41**(6), 624–629 (1990)
3. Hana, N., Todoroki, A.: Optical transparency change method for cure monitoring of GFRP. J. Soc. Mater. Sci. Jpn. **56**(8), 771–776 (2007)
4. Fujii, T., Mizikawa, K., Zako, M.: The Measurement with respect to statically characteristics, of fiberglass reinforced plastics (FRP) by the light transmission method. J. Soc. Mater. Sci. Jpn. **19**(204), 803–808 (1970)
5. Murakami, O., Yamada, K., Kotaki, M., Hamada, H.: Effects of injection molding conditions on replication, birefringence and optical property of microscopic V-groove structures for polycarbonate. J. Jpn. Soc. Polym. Process. **20**(10), 762–768 (2008)

Evaluation of Kimono Clothes
in Kyo-Yuzen-Zome using Image

Takashi Furukawa[1]([⊠]), Yuka Takai[2], Noriaki Kuwahara[1],
and Akihiko Goto[2]

[1] Kyoto Institute of Technology, Kyoto, Japan
t-furukawa@hishiken.co.jp, nkuwahar@kit.ac.jp
[2] Osaka Sangyo University, Osaka, Japan
{takai,gotoh}@ise.osaka-sandai.ac.jp

Abstract. "Yuzen" is a traditional but still popular method of dyeing fabrics in Japan. The products using the Yuzen method and manufactured in Kyoto city are called "Kyo-Yuzen." The dyeing method of Yuzen can be dividing into 10 procedures. A specialized craftsman is in charge of each procedure. During the paste application (Nori-oki) procedure, the expert applies a starch paste or a rubber paste to a fabric in order to resist dyeing. The two resist pastes create different effect on the dyed fabric. At market, the fabric with a starch paste application is perceived to have a higher value than that with a rubber paste. In this study, the difference of the viscosity between two materials was clarified, and specimens which craftsman dyed were observed. Then how two materials put on fabrics, and the structures of them were measured. As a result of this research, it was clarified that rubber paste penetrated into fabrics rather than starch paste.

Keywords: Fabric · Resist · Dyeing · Paste · Starch · Rubber

1 Introduction

There are some methods to dye a kimono in Japan such as Yuzen-zome (Yuzen dyeing), Shibori-zome (tie dyeing), Ai-zome (indigo dyeing), and Rou-zome (batik dying). Among these methods, the most widely used dyeing technique is Yuzen-zome. The Yuzen-zome dyed in Kyoto is specifically called "Kyo-Yuzen-zome." Not much literature clarifies the origin of Yuzen-zome; however, the "Genji Hiinagata" published in 1686 indicate the names of Yuzen-zome and Yuzensai, with the descriptions of pattern dying such as Icchin-zome, Chaya-zome,and Edo-zome. Yuzensai Miyazaki is alleged to be a fan painter, Yuzensai Miyazaki, living in Kyoto at that time. Later, Kyo-Yuzen-zome has been supporting the garment industry in Japan together with Kaga-Yuzen and Edo-Yuzen. In the Meiji era, the dyeing technology of the synthetic dye was advanced, and most of the currently used dyes are synthetic dyes. Likewise in the Meiji era, once the technique to dye a fabric using a dyeing stencil was established, a mass production of kimono using Yuzen-zome became possible. The amount of products had been increased and the annual production reached to 16,500,000 bolts in 1971; however, it has been decreased and reached to 840,000 bolts in 2003 along with

V.G. Duffy (Ed.): DHM 2015, Part I, LNCS 9184, pp. 277–288, 2015.
DOI: 10.1007/978-3-319-21073-5_28

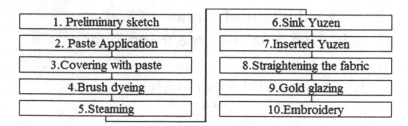

1. Preliminary sketch	6.Sink Yuzen
2. Paste Application	7.Inserted Yuzen
3.Covering with paste	8.Straightening the fabric
4.Brush dyeing	9.Gold glazing
5.Steaming	10.Embroidery

Fig. 1. Flow chart of manufacturing process

the lifestyle change [1]. Regarding the market size of Japanese dress industry, it was 627 billion yen in 2003, but was 400 billion yen in 2008, [2], and has been believed to be lower than 300 billion yen in 2013.

Generally, Kyo-Yuzen-zome can be classified into five types: hand-drawn Yuzen, kata Yuzen (i.e., dyed with paper patterns), screen printed,machine printed,and inkjet dyeing. Among them, the representative example is the hand-drawn Yuzen which whole production procedure is performed by handwork. This shows the uniqueness that each product has its own character. Each craftsman is in charge of each manufacturing procedure. In the process of producing the hand-drawn Yuzen, the outline of the design was dawn on the fabric with a dayflower extract. Then, using the paper tube, a fine line paste or "itome" is applied to the fabric to mask the line, and insert the dyes within the area with the target color. As this method masks the line of the pattern with a paste, it is also called as Itome-Yuzen.

As the flow chart shows in Fig. 1, the dyeing process of hand-drawn Yuzen consists of ten procedures. The first procedure, "preliminary sketch," is to draw a pattern of the design on a white fabric with a dayflower extract. The second procedure called "paste application (i.e., masking)" is a procedure to apply a fine line paste along with the lines of the preliminary sketch to avoid the dyes to bleed other parts when inserting colors on the fabric. Figure 2 shows the scene of a paste application during the paste application procedure. The third procedure, "covering with paste," is to apply a paste on the pattern to avoid the dyes to penetrate the parts of design in brush dyeing. The fourth procedure, "brush dyeing (or hiki-zome)", is a procedure to dye evenly or gradate by a brush, using a combined colors. The fifth procedure, "steaming," is to place the brush dyed

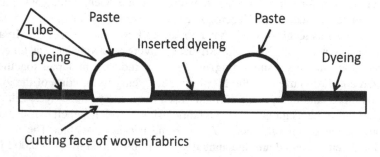

Fig. 2. Model of process about Paste application

fabric in a steamer and steams it at the temperature of about 100°C for 20 to 50 min. By steaming the fabric for 20 to 50 min, the ground color (dye) is stabilized on the fabric. The sixth procedure, "sink yuzen, or mizumoto," is to wash the fabric with water to eliminate the excess dyes, medicaments, and pastes from the fabric on which dyes are completely stabilized. The seventh procedure, "inserted yuzen" is a procedure to give colors to the design by using different types of brushes. The eighth procedure, "straightening the fabric or Yunoshi" is to steam wrinkles out of the fabric to soften the texture. The ninth procedure, "gold glazing" is to add here gold and silver foils and powders on the dyed fabric to make the product gorgeous. The tenth procedure, "embroidery," is to embroider a part of the design with gold and silver threads and other colory embroidery threads, to add elegance and luxuriousness to the product by giving the design volume.

2 Paste Application and the Function

2.1 Paste Application

In Japanese dress industry, inventing and deciding the first design to draw on kimono is considered to influence strongly on the end product. Without a high artistic quality or an aesthetic sense for the design, the product will remain unsold regardless of each procedure of making Kyo-Yuzen-zome was completed in a careful manner. The process to draw a design on a silk fabric is a preliminary sketching. The paste application procedure plays a significant role in changing highly artistic product drawn during the preliminary sketching into a manufactured product. Furthermore, recently, in many cases, instead of drawing the preliminary sketch on the silk fabric, a new method is used; a craftsman places a paper template of kimono with designs under the silk fabric and traces the design during the paste application. Therefore, it is very important to complete the putting a paste procedure by tracing the design accurately while taking the artistic quality of the designs drawn during the preliminary sketch or on the paper template.

  Materials used for a paste application procedure are a starch paste, a rubber paste, and a flour. The typical materials are a starch paste and a rubber paste, which consists of over 99 % of the material used in the process. There is a research on paste application and dyeing technology. In 1984, Kyoto City Senshoku Shikenjou (presently, the Kyoto Municipal Institute of Industrial Technology and Culture) published the "Technology and Techniques of Hand-Drawn Yuzen-Zome" [3], which editor-at-large was the Committee of the Technology and Techniques of the Hand-Drawn Yuzen-Zome. While a starch paste is made from sticky rice, a rubber paste is made by melting a rubber sheet with benzin and gasoline. Currently, more than 90 % of hand-drawn Yuzen which were produced in Kyoto uses the rubber paste.

2.2 Objective of Research

On the other hand, in the Japanese dress industry, it is said that dyeing method using a starch paste during the paste application procedure makes the end products have an impression of softness and depth than using a rubber paste. Consequently, the final product value becomes higher when using a starch paste than a rubber paste; in many cases, the product using the starch paste tends to be sold at a higher price than the rubber paste.

In research on the relation between sensitivity evaluation and price setting, if starch paste is used as a result of evaluating the sample dyed using related [4]. Starch paste and rubber paste of the sensitivity evaluation and price setting in the Kyoto yuzen stain which uses different paste using the questionnaire technique, if high-quality increases and rubber paste is used on the other hand, it turns out that clearness increases. Furthermore, it is clear that the factor's which the starch paste is highly set up in a price rather than rubber paste, and has on a price about price setting it is a high-quality feeling. On the other hand, there are the technology and technique of Tegaki-yuzen dyeing which Kyoto Municipal Institute of Industrial Technology and Culture performed in 1984 also as that of Tegaki-yuzen dyeing technology and technique investigating committee editorial supervision in research on the dyeing and finishing technology of paste application or a kimono. However, researches, such as viscosity about the starch paste used for paste application and perviousness with a fiber bundle, are not made.

So, in this research, the structure dyed using starch paste and rubber paste was solved, and it aimed at clarifying relation between structure of paste application, and an impression difference and price setting. Therefore, the viscosity of starch paste and rubber paste was measured and the difference was clarified. Furthermore, by observing the section and the surface of the product produced using starch paste and rubber paste, when starch paste and rubber paste dyed, the influence which it has to a fiber bundle was investigated.

3 Materials

3.1 How to Manufacture Putting Paste

Starch paste steams and kneads rice cake rice flour and rice bran, and it mixes the solution which melted lime, paints red pigment mix it, and it needs it. Finally starch paste is filtered with the cloth of cotton. Since the antiseptic is not contained, it is easy to decompose starch paste. Therefore, it is necessary to put into a container and to save in a refrigerator. When using it again, warming in hot water must be carried out and heat must be applied. Then, rubber paste cuts board rubber finely and pickles it in benzene or gasoline together with Dan Mull liquid. Furthermore, board rubber melts by mixing the ultramarine of paints and soaking for several days, and it becomes rubber paste. The reason of red pigment mixing and mixing ultramarine with rubber paste is for using the mark color of paste at starch paste.

3.2 Viscosity

In the Kimono industrial world, it is said that it is hard to treat starch paste firmly compared with rubber cement. Therefore, the craftsman who can use starch paste is limited to the ability of a craftsman to use rubber cement every paste of all the members. Then, the viscosity of starch paste and rubber cement was measured.

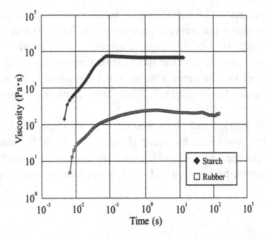

Fig. 3. Viscosity of starch and rubber on shear rate (1/s)

Production of the starch paste and rubber paste which were used for measurement was requested from the craftsman of Paste application, (70 ages, a male, right-handed person) of years-of-experience about 50 year. Indoor temperature is gone into the range of 19 ~ 20°C, in order to carry out to viscosity measurement using a viscosity measuring device (ARES G2) . The viscosity of the starch paste at the time of the shear rate 1 (/s) and rubber cement is shown in Fig. 3. As a result, it was shown that starch paste high viscosity about 30 times compared with rubber paste.

4   Experiment

4.1   Observation of Cutting Faces

Cloth prepared plain weave of the pure silk fabrics made from Nankyu, Inc. Manufacture was requested from the same craftsman using the same starch paste and rubber paste which were used for measurement of viscosity. The temperature which performed process of paste application was about 18°C. The specimen performed by paste application, dyed the thing of the stage (silk has not dyed) which the ground color is not dyeing, the gradual thing which dyes a ground color and has not removed paste, and the ground color, removed two paste, and prepared the thing of the stage which became the end products. Starch and rubber judged the specimen by silk along with warp, and the observation method observed those sections. It carried out to observation using the done type metallurgical microscope (PME3: made by Olympus, Inc.) of a handstand.

4.2   Observation of Woven Surfaces

In order to carry out surface observation of the part was given, a total of three things [six] of three sheets and rubber paste use was prepared [the sample to which three craftsmen (more than all the members craftsman history 50 year, a male, a right-handed person) performed the process] for the thing of starch paste use, respectively. The entire sample of six sheets chose the general pattern in the kimono industrial world called "Paddle bucket". "Paddle bucket" is a comparatively linear pattern, and it performed so that it might be parallel at warp and the woof, respectively. The size of the pattern was made into what has all six the same sheets. All were dyed through the manufacture process of the kyo-yuzen shown in Fig. 1. Each time spent on the paste application was about 30 min.

Cloth is pure silk fabrics and plain weave. It is a sample of these six sheets IOS D6000. A photograph was taken by make (Canon Co, Ltd). In order to suppress the variation in a light source, the indoor fluorescent light was erased and the window facing north was opened, and it adjusted so that outdoor available light might enter.

5   Results

5.1   Observation of Cutting Faces

The cross-sectional picture carried out every paste with starch paste and rubber paste is shown in the Figs. 4, 5, 6 and 7. Figure 4 shows the specimen which performs paste application and is not having the ground color dyed. Figure 5 shows the specimen which mixed dye with starch paste and rubber paste, and performed the same process. Starch paste has blue rubber paste in reddish brown, and this is because the adhe-sion degree of paste and a fiber bundle becomes clearer. Starch paste did not permeate a fiber bundle rather than rubber paste, but adhesion area of rubber paste was larger than Figs. 4 and 5, and it turned out that it has permeated deeply into a fiber bundle. Figure 6 shows the specimen before performing dyeing of paste application and a ground color and removing paste continuously. Adhesion area of rubber paste was larger than starch paste, and it turned out that it has permeated deeply into a fiber bundle. Figure 7 is a sectional view of the same stage as the end products continuously. The part which removed starch paste and rubber paste was enclosed white. Starch paste did not per-meate a fiber bundle deeply, but the dye which dyed the ground color has permeated the back side (back side of a dyeing side) which performed paste application. On the

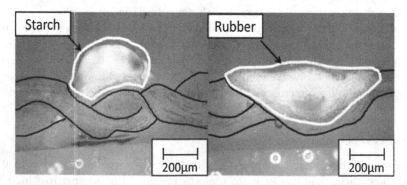

Fig. 4. Cutting faces of fabrics about Starch paste and Rubber paste before dyeing

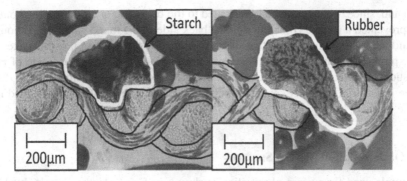

Fig. 5. Cutting faces of fabrics about Starch paste and Rubber paste mixed black dyestuff before dyeing.

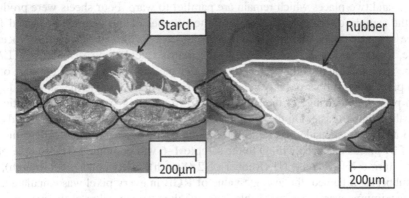

Fig. 6. Cutting faces of fabrics about Starch paste and Rubber paste before washing after dyeing

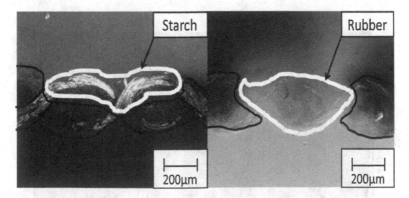

Fig. 7. Cutting faces of fabrics about Starch paste and Rubber paste after washing and steaming

other hand, since rubber paste had permeated to the back side of cloth, it turned out that it has prevented a ground color entering the back side of the marks of paste. Although it was said in the kimono industry that starch paste had resist-printing power weaker than rubber paste, and tends to turn around a ground color from the reverse side of cloth, from such cross-sectional observation, rubber paste permeated the fiber bundle deeply and the resist-printing effect kept from being mixed when a ground color is dyed more became clear.

5.2 Observation of Woven Surfaces

The sample used for surface observation is shown in Fig. 8. In the sample dyed with starch paste and rubber paste, the part which surrounded four parts enclosed with circle at a time by circle using selection and picture processing software (Photoshop, Microsoft Corp. make), respectively was cut off. Two cut-off places are perpendicular to warp, and two places which remain are parallel to warp. Four sheets were produced from the sample of one sheet. Therefore, the number of the pictures produced from surface observation is 24. And in order to detect a RGB value from the processed picture, it outputted to the cell of Excel using matrix calculation software (MATLAB).

The average value of the RGB value of the picture which cut off the part of the starch paste 1 and rubber paste 6 are shown in Fig. 9 in the sample measured in Fig. 8. Starch paste had a change of the RGB value from a dyeing side to an achromatic side looser than rubber paste. On the other hand, the change of rubber paset from a dyeing side to an achromatic side was rapid. Furthermore, the average of the RGB value of a total of 24 places enclosed with O to the sample 1–6 was computed. The sample of six sheets – turn – N1 (Starch), N1 (Rubber), N2 (Starch), N2 (Rubber), N3 (Starch), and N3 (Rubber) – it named, the average value of RGB in every pixel was calculated, and those maximums were detected. Table 1 shows the average value of the maximum of the RGB value of starch paste and rubber paste about the sample of six sheets. As a result of comparing the average of the maximum of starch paste and rubber paste, the difference was seldom seen by the maximum, but the starch paste of standard deviation

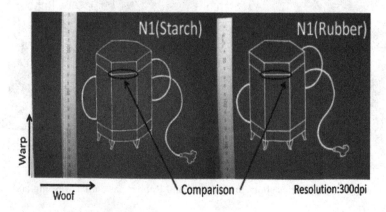

Fig. 8. Specimen for observation of woven surfaces

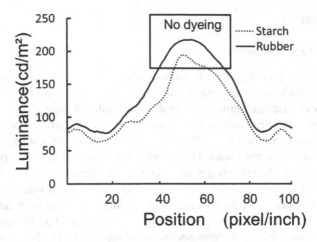

Fig. 9. Average of luminance in N1 specimen

Table 1. Comparison of each average

	Borderline	
	Starch	**Rubber**
N1	8.78	1.83
N2	8.16	1.53
N3	7.09	1.76
N4	5.10	2.22
N5	10.69	1.59
N6	7.06	1.44
N7	14.24	1.08
N8	5.46	1.46
N9	4.73	0.61
N10	8.06	0.86
N11	8.03	0.72
N1～N11	7.95	1.37

$***$

$(*** : P < 0.001)$

and a coefficient of variation are larger than rubber paste. It turned out that the maximum of a RGB value varies.

The dyed part (part by which resist printing was carried out with paste) rubber Paste to uniform being dyed firmly and the white of silk remaining firmly compared with starch paste starch paste, According to resist-printing power being weak, a ground color enters into the portion of the remains of a fine line in some places, and the white of silk does not remain completely. From such a thing, it is thought that the variation of rubber paste in an achromatic side is larger than starch paste.

6 Discussion

6.1 Cutting Face and Surface

Two materials to a fiber bundle that rubber paste is "clear" in "superior quality" at sensitivity evaluation, and starch paste has set up price setting highly compared with rubber paste in this research how In order to investigate whether it pasted up and has affected the fiber bundle, cross-sectional observation and surface observation were performed. As shown in the Figs. 4, 5, 6 and 7, starch paste has not permeated a fiber bundle compared with rubber paste. On the other hand, rubber paste has permeated the fiber bundle firmly. Although it is generally said in the kimono industrial world that the starch paste must take care and it must dye it from the reverse side of cloth by that around which dye turns (it spreads) when resist-printing power is weak and carries out Brush dyeing rather than rubber paste, it can be said that it is in agreement with understanding from this and cross-sectional observation. Furthermore, since the resist-printing effect is high compared with starch paste and rubber paste in which giving impression evaluation that starch paste is high-quality and rubber paste is clear has been reported by research of sensitivity evaluation can dye the boundary of a dyeing side and an achromatic side more vividly, it is in agreement with impression evaluation called a clear feeling. The feature of starch paste has high viscosity, resist-printing power falls compared with rubber paste, and the boundary of a dyeing side and an achromatic side does not dye vividly. Therefore, when starch paste is used from this, it is thought that it is in agreement with the result of sensitivity evaluation that a high-quality feeling can be obtained by the impression evaluation to the product of completion.

Furthermore, the sample which performed paste application by three craftsmen was prepared. The same pattern was dyed one craftsman using starch paste and rubber paste. As shown in Fig. 9, as a result of carrying out surface observation of the part in the end products, starch paste had a loose change of the RGB value compared with rubber paste. In order to investigate this result in detail, out of the sample of six sheets, four places and a total of 24 places were chosen, respectively, and surface observation was performed. As a result of calculating an average and standard deviation of each maximum, and a coefficient of variation, the difference was not seen so much by average value, but the big difference was seen by standard deviation and the coefficient of variation. Rubber paste shows from this that variation is uniformly dyed the RGB value of an achromatic side few compared with starch paste.

That is, when rubber paste is used, it is shown that the boundary of a dyeing side and an achromatic side is uniform, and it is shown that rubber paste has the feature which it can be uniform and can be dyed vividly. On the other hand, starch paste has large variation to the maximum of a RGB value, and the boundary of a dyeing side and an achromatic side does not dye vividly, but it can be said that this result is high-quality and relevance with the result which can set up a price highly is suggested.

6.2 Dyeing Model

The result of having performed cross-sectional observation and surface observation according to material is made into a mimetic diagram, and is shown in Fig. 10.

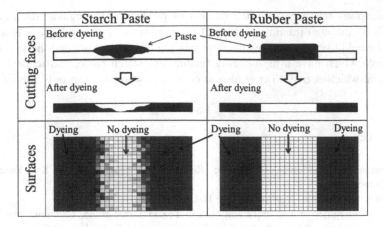

Fig. 10. Relationship between fabrics, pastes and dyeing

Cross-sectional observation and surface observation to starch paste does not permeate a fiber bundle compared with rubber paste, and its boundary of a dyeing side and an achromatic side is not clear. On the other hand, the resist-printing effect of rubber paste is high, it is uniform and the marks of paste application remain vividly. It is thought that there will be relevance with the result that starch paste is high-quality and rubber paste is clear, from the feature of starch paste and rubber paste.

7 Conclusion

In this research, it became clear that starch paste has viscosity about 30 times as high as rubber paste. From cross-sectional observation, starch paste was understood that the resist-printing effect is which has little osmosis in a fiber bundle lower than rubber paste. Moreover, as for the starch paste, the boundary of a dyeing side and an achromatic side varies, and it became clear from surface observation that the boundary of rubber paste of a dyeing side and an achromatic side is uniform and that it is clear. Since the number of the samples produced for surface observation is six, I would like to examine whether a sample is increased and the same result is brought by this research from now on. Moreover, although the part perpendicular to warp and parallel was chosen, I would like to also perform observation of a bias part to warp.

Furthermore, comparison with the way a model performs paste application of a fine line type, and the dyeing method in which mass-production called model Yuzen other than Tegaki-yuzen is possible is also required. Moreover, although it is possible in the kimono industrial world to use it if rubber paste has a skillful degree for about one year, in order to master starch paste, it is said that it generally takes for about ten years. Furthermore, although the craftsman who can use starch paste can also use rubber paste, the craftsman only treating rubber paste cannot use starch paste.

That is, since the number of craftsmen which can use starch paste is limited, there is very little production with starch paste than rubber paste, and the starch paste of the ratio which uses starch paste in the number of production in Tegaki-Yuzen is about 10 %. Then, although training of the craftsman who can use starch paste is a future subject, I would like to make low the development of rubber paste and the viscosity of starch paste which have a high-quality feeling like starch paste, and to develop the starch paste which is easy to treat also to craftsmen who can treat only rubber paste.

References

1. Kyo-yuzen Kyodoukumiai Rengoukai: Research of production in Kyo-Yuzen and Kyo-Komon (2012)
2. Yano Keizai Kenkyujo, Kimono Sangyo Hakusho (2009)
3. Research Committee of Technique and Skill in Tegaki Yuzen-zome, Technique and Skill in Tegaki Yuzen-zome, Kyoto Municipal Institute of Industrial Technology and Culture, pp. 67–100 (1984)
4. Furukawa, T: Relationship between Kansei Evaluation and pricing Decision to Kyo-Yuzen-Zome with Different Pastes, Japan Socuety of Kansei Engineering (2013)

Effects of Spray Gun Handling of Automobile Repair on Carrier of Car Mechanic

Shigeru Ikemoto[1], Kenta Morimoto[2], Yuka Takai[2(✉)], Akihiko Goto[2], and Hiroyuki Hamada[1]

[1] Kyoto Institute of Technology, Kyoto, Japan
ikeike1489@gmail.com, hhamada@kit.ac.jp
[2] Osaka Sangyo University, Osaka, Japan
s625700@ya.osaka-sandai.ac.jp,
{takai,gotoh}@ise.osaka-sandai.ac.jp

Abstract. The goal of this research is development of learning system for automobile repair. In this study, the purpose is characteristics of spray gun handling of automobile repair painting expert. Spray gun movements of 55 craftsmen's were measured by using motion capture system. The spray gun movements of expert were longer length, longer time, higher speed, and narrower swing range, compared to that of non-expert. As a result, spray gun handling of expert is longer running length, longer time, higher speed, narrower spray gun swing range compare with non-expert.

Keywords: Automobile repair · Paint · Spray gun handling · Motion capture

1 Introduction

The work of painting and coating in the automobile industry used to be done by manpower, from prototype production and mass production to repairs. Nowadays, these tasks formerly done by manpower are replaced with automatic production. Prototypes are produced by computer graphics and mass production is done by robots. But repair work must be tailored to customers' requirements, so manpower is essential. However, the number of engineers engaged in painting and coating is decreasing recently and the labor quality also is declining, so there is difficulty in passing on repairing techniques.

Generally, the engineers involved in painting and coating acquire the skills in colleges or vocational schools. But most schools do not allocate sufficient time for painting and coating practice. Thus, most new workers have no choice but to "watch and copy" the techniques of senior skilled engineers. However, it is not easy to acquire the optimal work skills corresponding to each customer's request, because the required skills are different every time.

In Japan, people aged around 60 years old called "baby boomers" have reached retirement one after another, including many skilled engineers. With this social background, it is necessary to sever the decline of quality of engineers, and design a method to help unskilled engineers to acquire the necessary skills quicker and more accurately.

© Springer International Publishing Switzerland 2015
V.G. Duffy (Ed.): DHM 2015, Part I, LNCS 9184, pp. 289–298, 2015.
DOI: 10.1007/978-3-319-21073-5_29

Currently, the ways that non-skilled coating engineers learn coating skills are from corporate or paint manufacture training, or practical guidebooks specified for coating techniques. This situation has not changed for decades. However, using the recent remarkable development of information technology, it is feasible to design a new method for learning coating techniques. We think motion analysis using 3D digital motion analysis equipment is one solution. Behavior analysis technology has been incorporated into acquisition methods of techniques in many fields. This method is effective in learning behaviors [1–10]. For instance, Murata et al. conducted a motion analysis of pitching motion in baseball and proposed a better throwing motion [2]. Marco et al. conducted an analysis of athletes in different postures on the jump phase in a downhill race and clarified the characteristic motions of the skilled skier [9]. In the succession of skills, the characteristic motion analysis of skilled technicians has been conducted in the fields of cooking, sewing, nailing, glass heat forming, and first aid chest compression procedure.

The purpose of this study is to develop the learning materials for unskilled workers to acquire necessary painting and coating techniques. As a first step, this paper intends to clarify the characteristic motions of experts. We measured the motions of the expert and non-expert during a spray gun operation by the 3D digital motion analysis equipment and analyzed the results.

2 Method

2.1 Experimental Outline

We had craftsmen who do work related to metal plate coating do coating work, and we recorded and analyzed the running of the spray gun with a three-dimensional motion capture system.

2.2 Experimental Environment

The experiment was part of an exhibition of metal plate coating that was done in Osaka Prefecture in February 2013, and was done in a period of 2 days. The guests of the exhibition were those who have to do with metal plate coating in auto repair and their family.

2.3 Participants

The participants of the experiment were the guests who came to the metal plate coating exhibition. Beforehand the participants were informed that the motions would be recorded and after the recording, immediately the results would be publicized. Of the participants of the experiment, those who were under-aged or those whose number of years of experience were not asked were omitted from the subjects of analysis. The subjects for analysis were 55 people. Out of them, those with more than 5 years of experience were counted as "experienced" and those with under 5 years of experience were counted as "inexperienced." For the experienced people, there were 11 who had more than 5 years of experience but less than 10, there were 17 people with more than 10 years experience but less than 20, there were 4 people with more than 20 years of experience but less than 30, and one person with more than 30 years of experience, making a total of 33 years. With the inexperienced people, there were 11 people with no years of experience, 6 people with more than 1 month but less than 1 year of experience, and 4 people with more than 1 year of experience but less than 5 years, making a total of 22 people. The participants with no years of experience did not completely lack previous knowledge of coating, but were people who do work with metal plate repair and value estimations, and have a connection with auto repair.

2.4 Materials and Tools

In this research, to omit the necessary time to replace the object for coating, the coating was done by having water inside the spray gun. The object for coating was a white-colored board likened to the door panel of an automobile, and board was marked off by 900 mm vertically and 900 mm horizontally with the inside of the marking as the object for coating.

2.5 Experimental Motion

The participants were instructed to coat the board using a spray gun. Specifically, the instruction was "please move the spray gun in the way you usually use it for coating." Before the measurement the participants were told that the run-ning of the spray gun would be measured, and that the ability to "spray horizontally without moving verti-cally" and the ability to "move the spray gun in one steady speed" would be measured and analyzed.

2.6 Record

An infrared reflective marker was put on in one place at the top of the spray gun and was made as target position. For the gathering of the coordinates of the target position, an optical three-dimensional automatic motion analysis device MAD 3D SYSTEM (made by Motion Analysis) was used, and the sampling frequency was set at 120 Hz. The state during the recording is shown in Fig. 1. For the frame of reference, the direction of right and left was the x axis, forward and backward the y axis, and upward and downward the z axis.

2.7 Analysis

Usually, the running of the spray gun for coating is done by going back and forth with the whole coating object on level with the ground. At this time the first part that gets coated is the upper portion of the coating object. In Fig. 2 the tracks left on the xz surface of the target position of the spray gun is shown. In this research, for the distance and time of the running of the spray gun, all of the tracks were to be ana-lyzed.

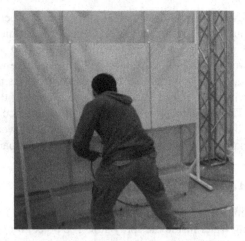

Fig. 1. Photo of measurement

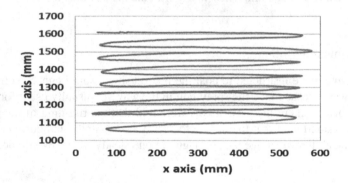

Fig. 2. An example of trajectory in xz plane

For the comparison between the experienced people and inexperienced people, an examination of the difference in average value was made. The significant standard was set at 5 %. And for the observation of the relationship between number of career experience and the results the moving of the spray gun, a cross-correlation function was done. The significant standard was set at 5 %.

3   Results

3.1   Spray Gun Handling Length

Figure 3 shows the running length of the spray gun by expert and non-expert. For the spray gun running length, the target for analysis was set for when the spraying began until the spraying stopped. The length of the expert compared with the non-expert was significantly longer. The length of the expert was 1.49 times longer than that of the non-expert.

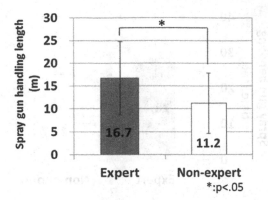

Fig. 3. Spray gun handling length of expert and non-expert

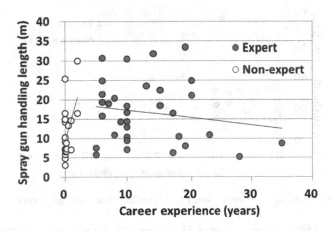

Fig. 4. Relationship between spray gun handling length and career experience

Figure 4 shows the relationship between the spray gun running length and the career experience. With the expert as the number of career experience became longer the running length tended to become shorter. However with the non-expert as the number of career experience became longer the running length of the spray gun became longer. In the non-expert, the spray gun handling length was moderately and positively correlated with the career experience ($r = .530$, $p < .05$).

3.2 Spray Gun Handling Time

Figure 5 shows the running time of the spray gun by expert and non-expert. For the spray gun running time, the target for analysis was set for when the spraying began until the spraying stopped. The time of the expert compared with the non-expert was longer. The time of the expert was 1.20 times longer than that of the non-expert.

Figure 6 shows the relationship between the spray gun running time and the career experience. With the expert as the number of career experience became longer the

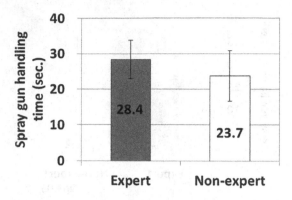

Fig. 5. Spray gun handling time of expert and non-expert

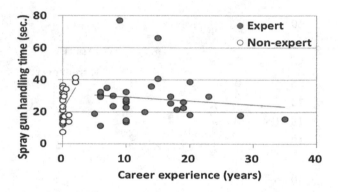

Fig. 6. Relationship between spray gun handling time and career experience

running time tended to become shorter. However with the non-expert as the number of career experience became longer the running time of the spray gun became longer. In the non-expert, the spray gun handling time was moderately and positively correlated with the career experience ($r = .422$, $p < .05$).

3.3   Spray Gun Handling Speed

Figure 7 shows the running speed of the spray gun by expert and non-expert. For the spray gun running speed, the target for analysis was set for when the spraying from 1st stroke to 6th stroke. The speed of the expert compared with the non-expert was significant higher. The speed of the expert was 1.32 times higher than that of the non-expert.

Figure 8 shows the relationship between the spray gun running speed and the career experience. With the expert as the number of career experience became longer the running speed tended to become lower. However with the non-expert as the number of career experience became longer the running speed of the spray gun became higher. In both of the expert and the non-expert, the spray gun handling speed was not correlated with the career experience.

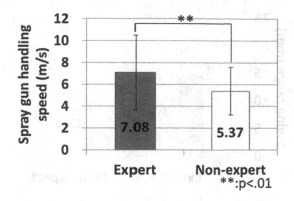

Fig. 7. Spray gun handling speed of expert and non-expert

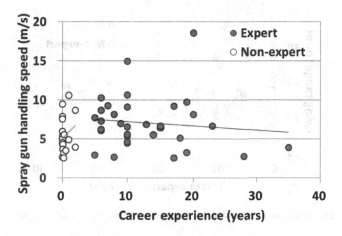

Fig. 8. Relationship between spray gun handling speed and career experience

3.4 Spray Gun Swing Range

The spray gun handling is regarded as good for not shaken up and down and to parallel handling. Figure 9 shows the spray gun swing range by expert and non-expert. For the spray gun swing range, the target for analysis was set for when the spraying from 1st stroke to 6th stroke. The spray gun swing range of the expert compared with the non-expert was narrower. The spray gun swing range of the non-expert was 1.10 times larger than that of the expert. Average standard deviation of the spray gun swing range of expert and non-expert were 6.09 mm and 7.32 mm, respectively. A scattering of swing range of non-expert was larger than that of expert.

Figure 10 shows the relationship between the spray gun swing range and the career experience. With the expert as the number of career experience became longer the swing range tended to become larger. However with the non-expert as the number of career experience became longer the swing range of the spray gun became narrower. In both

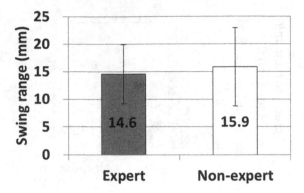

Fig. 9. Spray gun swing range of expert and non-expert

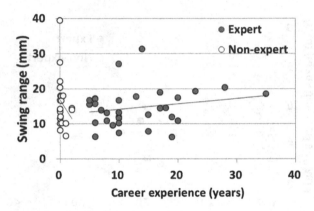

Fig. 10. Relationship between spray gun swing range and career experience

of the expert and the non-expert, the spray gun handling swing range was not correlated with the career experience.

4   Discussions

The running of the spray gun of the experts compared to the non-experts had more distance, was longer in time, and was faster. It is important to cover a long distance in order to perform the coating with evenness, but on the other hand it leads to too much usage of paint, so from the perspective of cost preservation shorter is better. The relationship between the number of years of experience of the experts becoming longer and the distance of the spray gun running becoming shorter shown in Fig. 4 suggests that as the progression of proficiency of technique takes place, so does the ability to perform the coating in the shortest distance possible with evenness.

From the perspective of cost preservation, it is good for the time of the running of the spray gun to be short. The reason is that the cost of work in auto repair is calculated based on the length of time of the work, and not the quality of the work.

So the non-experts need to build enough technique to be able to do coating beauti-fully and in a short period of time. As it is shown in Fig. 6, as the number of years of experience became longer, the time of spray gun running became longer, and it is considered that the reason for there to be a tendency to become shorter is that when the number of years of experience is short the job itself is focused on, and once the performance level is maintained then the adjustment of the time of running the spray gun is possible. The same tendency is shown for the running speed of the spray gun.

The spray gun's running speed that is recommended by paint makers, etc. is 2–3 m/s. In this research the target persons for the analysis all ran the spray gun faster than 2 m/s. As shown in Fig. 8, as the number of years of experience became longer, the running speed of the spray gun tended to become faster and slower. It suggests that once experience is had to allow one to maintain a certain performance level then they can maintain the best running speed. Furthermore, out of the target persons for analysis 43 people ran the spray gun over 4 m/s. It suggests that there was a separation in the education of the work and the work itself.

The space for vertical motion of the spray gun is small, and to run the spray gun parallel to the ground without shifting vertically leads to an even coating. Furthermore if the space of vertical motion of the spray gun is small, then the running distance becomes shorter, which is good from the perspective of cost preservation. However, if the time of work is prioritized, a certain amount of vertical shifting would have to be forgiven. As it is shown in Fig. 10 this is thought to be one of the rea-sons why as the number of years of experience becomes longer, the space of vertical shifting becomes less and more.

5   Conclusions

The purpose of this study is to clarify the characteristic motions of experts on spry gun handling for automobile repair. As a result, spray gun handling of expert is longer running length, longer time, higher speed, narrower spray gun swing range compare with non-expert. The reason for there to be a tendency to become shorter is that when the number of years of experience is short the job itself is focused on, and once the performance level is maintained then the adjustment of the time of running the spray gun is possible.

Acknowledgment.   This work was supported by PROTO RIOS INC. and JSPS KAKENHI Grant Number 26882052.

References

1. Suzuki, A., Furuta, S.: A study of motion analysis of hand-sewing with a computer system-A comparison in the motion of Unshin between skillful and unskillful subjects. Jpn. J. Ergon. **30**(5), 323–329 (1994)
2. Murata, A., Iwase, H.: On skillful pitch of baseball pitchers -Comparison of pitching motion between skilled and nonskilled pitchers-, **36**(6), 299-309 (2000)

3. Hayashi, T., Yanagisawa, Y.: Comparison of the movement of knives cutting food between expertsand non-experts by motion analysis techniques. J. Cooking Sci. Jpn. **37**(3), 299–305 (2004)
4. Sano, S., Ueda, T., Terada, T., Izumi, Y., Nishijima, S.: Fundamental study of evaluation method of nailing by the3D motion analysis for improving the skill. J. Life Support Eng. **20**(1), 3–8 (2008)
5. Umemura, H., Ishikawa, J., Endo, H., Abe, K., Matsuda, J.: Analysis of expert skills on burner works in glass processing. Jpn. J. Ergon. **47**(4), 139–148 (2011)
6. Choi, W., Takahashi, K.: Quantitative analysis of iaido proficiency using characteristic parameters of body movement. Res. J. Budo **45**(1), 35–45 (2012)
7. Onodera, T., Kuriyama, H., Takamura, N., Aoki, S., Irie, T., Marumo, M.: Research on skill transfer support system experienced technician. In: Proceedings of 29th Fuzzy System Symposium, WF2-3, pp. 947-950 (2013)
8. Okada, M., Kayashima, S.: Motion instruction of first aid chest compressions using pseudo-reference and its evaluation. Trans. Jpn. Soc. Mech. Eng. Ser. C **79**(800), 1090–1101 (2013)
9. Mazzola, M., Aceti, A., Gibertini, G., Andreoni, G.: Aerodynamics and biomechanical optimization of the jump phase in skiing, through a simulation-based predictive model. In: Proceedings of the 5th International Conference on Applied Human Factors and Ergonomics AHFE 2014, pp. 7245–7254 (2014)
10. Tsurumaru, N., Hirata, I.: Optimal shape of a welding torch for easing worker burden. Jpn. J. Ergon. **50**(Suppl.), S128–S129 (2009)

Visual Evaluation of "The Way of Tea" Based on Questionnaire Survey Between Chinese and Japanese

Soutatsu Kanazawa[1], Tomoko Ota[2], Zelong Wang[3($\boxtimes$)],
Rutchaneekorn Wongpajan[3($\boxtimes$)], Yuka Takai[4], Akihiko Goto[4],
and Hiroyuki Hamada[3]

[1] Urasenke Konnichian, Kyoto, Japan
kanazawa.kuromon.1352.gentatsu@docomo.ne.jp
[2] Chuo Business Group, Tokyo, Japan
Tomoko.ota@k.vodafone.ne.jp
[3] Kyoto Institute of Technology Advanced Fibro-Science, Kyoto, Japan
simon.zelongwang@gmail.com
[4] Department of Information Systems Engineering, Osaka Sangyo University,
Osaka, Japan
gotoh@ise.osaka-sandai.ac.jp

Abstract. In this paper, "The way of tea" process conducted by expert, non-expert and beginner was investigated. Firstly, final tea made by expert, non-expert and beginner applying three kinds of tea whisks were taken into photos. Afterwards, random ranked tea photos were employed as visual evaluation questionnaire and subjective ranking material. In order to compare and characterize "The way of tea" process difference, 10 Japanese and 10 Chinese participates were chosen as evaluation subjects. Consequently, it can be concluded that both Japanese and Chinese are able to distinguish expert's tea as top rank easily because of sufficient small bubble size on the tea surface.

Keywords: The way of tea · Visual evaluation · Japanese tea · Questionnaire survey · Chinese and japanese

1 Introduction

"The Way of Tea" is called the "Japanese tea ceremony", which is a special ceremonial art preparation and presentation of "Matcha"(a kind of green tea powder) to entertain the guests, through the tea ceremony people will achieve temperament, improve the cultural quality and aesthetic view. The essence of "The Way of Tea" is meant to demonstrate reverence and respect between host and guest, both of them can truly experience the artistic conception and taste the most primitive taste of green tea during tea-tasting activity and service process with the tallest state of the etiquette.

"Urasenke" is one of the three main genres of "Japanese tea ceremony", which is derived from "Sen-Rikyu". The other two main genres are "Omotesenke" and "Mushakojisenke". The different tea genres have different tea making skills after diversified

© Springer International Publishing Switzerland 2015
V.G. Duffy (Ed.): DHM 2015, Part I, LNCS 9184, pp. 299–306, 2015.
DOI: 10.1007/978-3-319-21073-5_30

development. However "The Way of Tea" of each genre is consisted of many specific and strict procedures, whose basic skill just only handed over by oral instructions by expert.

Therefore, in order to create a favorable atmosphere between the tea master and guest the tea masters have to study and practice for a long time to master and understand the whole tea ceremony [1, 2]. However, until now the scientific evaluation for the process analysis of "The way of tea" is limited [3]. But above all, it's very difficult for every master to inherit the essentials of tea ceremony essentials to the next generation without an effective way.

In this research, expert, non-expert with different experience years and beginners were employed as the behavior subjects. The three types of different tea whisks as the same with previous research, "Yabunouchi", "Kankyuan", "Ensyu" were used to make tea. Through visual perceiving directly on final product, we would like to clarify the relationship between bubble distribution/size and process characterization.

As well known, no matter use what kind of tea whisks, the final bubble distribution was one of most important features for a tasty tea, which depend on the bubble size, distribution and so on. On the other hand, the bubble forming process was also reflected the characteristics of the tea whisks' performance. It is notify that expert can master the performance of three types of tea whisks than non-expert and beginner, and made excellent cups of tea with sufficient small bubble. Therefore, evaluation subjects were easily to distinguish the tea photos of expert and then give a high rank.

In a word, the purpose of this study is through visual evaluation to clarify "The way of tea" process characteristic in order to provide a suggestion to help learner easier to understand and keep the perfect tea impression in mind (Fig. 1).

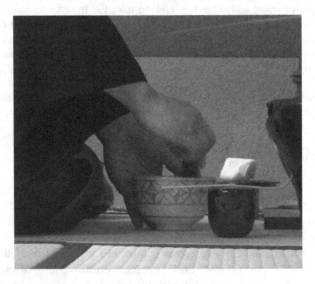

Fig. 1. The way of tea

2 Experiment

2.1 Participants

A Japanese tea master (expert), a non-expert and four other beginners from Kyoto were employed as the tea conductor participant. Especially, expert participant had more than 30 years experience in "the way of tea", who can keep the motion of scooping water and ensure the added water weight in the bowl nearly the same for each tea making process.

2.2 Evaluation Subjects and Objects

Three types of Japanese tea whisks were prepared for participants to make the tea as "Yabunouchi", "Kankyuan", "Ensyu", which were the three most popular tea whisks in Japan as shown in Fig. 2. And the made teas were taken into photo and 15 pieces were used for following visual evaluation process. Finally, 10 Japanese and 10 Chinese were required to asset the tea and give a total rank.

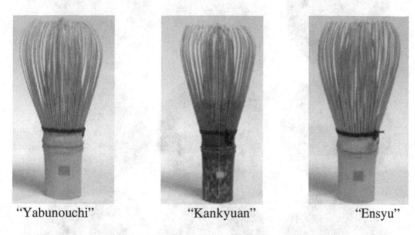

"Yabunouchi"   "Kankyuan"   "Ensyu"

Fig. 2. Three types of Japanese tea whisks

2.3 Experimental Process

Every participant was required to make 3 cups of tea by previous three kinds of tea whisk one by one, during the process 1.5 g of "Matcha" tea power and approximate 56 g of hot water were dumped into the bowl following with hard mixing behavior, and finished tea were taken into photo by single-lens reflex camera (D40x Nikon CO. Ltd) immediately to record the bubble distribution and bubble size on the tea surface. Selected tea photos for visual evaluation were illustrated in Fig. 3.

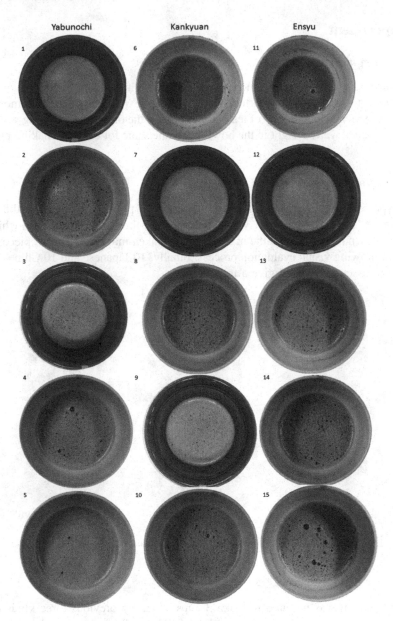

Fig. 3. Random scheduled tea photos

3 Results and Discussions

As illustrated in Fig. 4, ranked tea photos in top 3 and bottom 3 were voted by 20 evaluation subjects landside. Comparing with rank bottom 3 group, rank top 3 group showed lighter tea green color with rich and creamy small bubbles on the surface. On the opposite, bottom rank 3 group showed dark green color with inconformity bubble size.

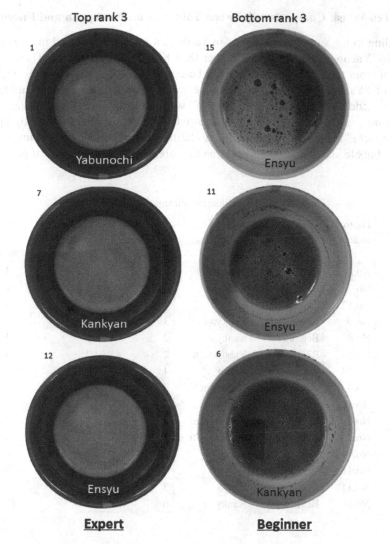

Fig. 4. Ranked tea photos in Top 3 and Bottom 3

3.1 Tea Aesthetic Comparison Between China and Japan

Japanese tea ceremony originated from China, which has its own formation, development process and specific connotation with the charming of oriental culture. Learning tea ceremony could cultivate people's aesthetic and moral values. According to the rank of tea photos, both Chinese and Japanese evaluation subjects showed the same vote of top 3 and bottom 3 groups. It was consider that tea culture and tea aesthetic were same between two countries even along with spreading, so the tea process characteristic also can be concluded to be the same.

3.2   Tea Whisk Comparison Between Yabunouchi, Kankyuan and Ensyu

According to the summarized results in Table 1, it is obvious to find that expert's tea made by Yabunouchi was ranked higher than Kankyuan and Ensyu. The shape was different from three kinds of tea whisks, based on previous study conclusion, the tea whisk of "Yabunouchi" was presented the wider distribution of small bubbles. And bubbles made by "Kankyuan" and "Ensyu" were almost concentrated in the range of $0.2 \sim 1$ mm^2. In a word, the bubbles showed smaller size after mixing by applying "Yabunouchi" tea whisk. Therefore, it is clarified that tea made by Yabunouchi with smaller bubble size could be accepted and favored by larger numbers of people.

Table 1. Evaluation summarized results

Rank list	Photo code	Tea maker	Applied tea whist	Japanese vote number	Chinese vote number	Total vote number
1st	No.1	Expert	Yabunouchi	6	3	9
2nd	No.7	Expert	Kankyan	6	1	1
3rd	No.12	Expert	Ensyu	4	2	6
4th	No.9	Non-expert	Kankyan	3	1	4
5th	No.8	Beginner	Kankyan	2	1	3
6th	No.5	Beginner	Yabunouchi	2	2	4
7th	No.13	Beginner	Ensyu	4	1	5
8th	No.4	Beginner	Yabunouchi	2	3	5
9th	No.10	Beginner	Kankyan	3	1	4
10th	No.3	Non-expert	Yabunouchi	2	2	4
11th	No.2	Beginner	Yabunouchi	3	2	5
12th	No.14	Non-expert	Ensyu	3	1	4
13th	No.15	Beginner	Ensyu	2	3	5
14th	No.11	Beginner	Ensyu	3	4	7
15th	No.6	Beginner	Kankyan	6	4	10

3.3   Easy Identification of Expert's Tea During Visual Evaluation

Based on the counting results of ranked photos, it is obvious to find that except top 3 and bottom 3 groups other tea photos identification is very difficult for subjects evaluation, therefore, middle rank tea photos showed variable votes. However, expert could master skillful technique to make tea by any kind of tea whisk and produce richer and smaller bubbles on tea surface. So expert's tea has easy identification with obvious characteristics, which help for visual evaluation.

3.4   The Influence of Bubble Size and Distribution for Visual Evaluation

As showed in Fig. 5, vote people number for ranked tea photos were listed clearly. It is worthwhile to note that top 3 and bottom 3 ranked photos were voted with nearly over half of total people, however vote number for the middle rank tea photos is less and lack of persuasion. That is to say, people subjects were easily to identify the best and worst but difficult to judge the middle rank. As previous discussion, bubble size in ranked tea photos upper ones had smaller bubble on tea surface, which obtained better confirmation from evaluation subjects. It demonstrated that when bubble fineness reaches to a certain limit could support beauty assessments directly. In other words, expert is able to make rich small bubbles on tea surface stable, so evaluation subjects could easily identify expert's tea. However, non-expert could not keep stable tea making technique, and beginner do not understand the bubble making technique and its important points. So during visual evaluation, their teas product photos are difficult for identification.

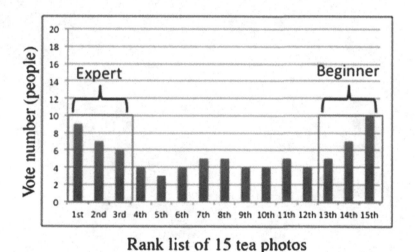

Fig. 5. The number of vote people for corresponding rank listed photo

4   Conclusions

In this paper, process analysis on technique of "The way of tea" was investigated by visual analysis on expert, non-expert and beginner' tea work. It is found that expert's tea was easier to be ranked in the top with obvious tea bubble characteristic. Furthermore, tea whisk's behavior was also clarified that Yabunouchi could produce more fitness bubble and obtained more people's favor. In a word, when bubble fineness reaches to a certain limit tea work was easier to be evaluated and confirmed directly.

References

1. Tujimoto, N., Ichihashi,Y., Iue, M., Ota, T., Hamasaki, K., Nakai, A., Goto, A.: Comparison of bubble forming in a bowl of thin tea between expert and non-expert. In: Proceeding of 11 th Japan International SAMPE Symposium and Exhibiton (2009)
2. Goto, A., Endo, A., Narita, C., Takai, Y., Shimodeand, Y., Hamada, H.: Comparison of painting technique of Urushi products between expert and non-expert. In: Advances in Ergonomics in Manufacturing, pp. 160–167 (2012). ISBN: 978-1-4398-7039-6
3. Aiba, E., Kanazawa, S., Ota, T., Kuroda, K., Takai, Y., Goto, A., Hamada, H.: Developing a system to assess the skills of japanese way of tea by analyzing the forming sound: a case study. In: Human Factors and Ergonomics Society International Meeting. (2013)

A Study of the Tacit Knowledge on the Design of Kimono Patterns from Japanese Painting

Masashi Kano[1](✉), Hiroyuki Akaji[1], Noriaki Kuwahara[2], and Hiroyuki Hamada[2]

[1] Kano-ko Co., Ltd., Kyoto, Japan
{masashi, akaji}@kano-ko.com
[2] Kyoto Institute of Technology, Kyoto, Japan
{nkuwahar, hhamada}@kit.ac.jp

Abstract. One of the most important characteristics of the *Nishijin obi* (a traditional Japanese textile product) has been to express unique aesthetics in Japanese paintings by making full use of weaving techniques for imparting a three-dimensional effect. However, weaving today tries to distinguish itself merely through colors and patterns, losing the true depth inherent in weaving. An obi can emphasize the beauty of a kimono through its simple design, and a kimono can bring out the personality of the person dressed in it. The types of weaving that enable such design are the three main weaving styles of *Nishijin*-weaving. We will present the basics of these techniques, and how they are applied in order to realize the obi design that expresses unique aesthetic in Japanese paintings.

Keywords: Kimono · Nishijin obi · Nishijin-weaving · Weaving structure · Three-dimensional effect · Japanese painting

1 Introduction

There are three major producing areas of Japanese kimono woven fabric production, Nishijin, Hakata and Kiryu. Among them, Nishijin produces around 80 % of all the fabrics produced. The trend recent years in Japanese clothing is to regard obi (a broad sash tied over a kimono) as secondary to kimono. This trend reflects the decline of tradition and skills in weaving that is closely tied to obi production.

In Nishijin obi-making tradition, the craftsmen create volume in pattern using their highly developed weaving skill, in order to express sense of "*Ma*" (Aesthetic of empty spaces between objects) or "*Iki*" (understated stylishness) developed by the *Rimpa*-school. The *Rimpa* refers to the art sect, craftsmen and their art works, originated in late Momoyama-period (late 16th century) and continued until modern time, who employed highly original visual styles. Established by Hon'ami Koetsu (1558–1637) and Tawaraya Sotatsu (early 17th century), It has influenced European Impressionists or contemporary Japanese painting and design, and there are many examples of obis and kimonos inspired by *Rimpa*. However, weaving today tries to distinguish itself merely through colors and patterns, losing the true depth inherent in weaving.

© Springer International Publishing Switzerland 2015
V.G. Duffy (Ed.): DHM 2015, Part I, LNCS 9184, pp. 307–315, 2015.
DOI: 10.1007/978-3-319-21073-5_31

With this situation in mind, the authors of this study have been trying to pass on the weaving techniques to the next generation, as well as creating additional values more suitable to contemporary lifestyle [1, 2]. An obi can emphasize the beauty of a kimono through its simple design, and a kimono can bring out the personality of the person dressed in it. The obi design of Kano-ko Co., Ltd. is characterized by its creativity in expressing "Aesthetic of *Ma*" and "*Iki*" within the limited space of an obi, sometime getting its clue from Japanese painting. The types of weaving that enable such design are the three main weaving styles of Nishijin-weaving, namely (1) Plain weave, (2) Twill weave, and (3) Satin weave. In this paper, we will present the basics of these techniques, and how they are applied in order to realize *Kano-ko*'s obi designs.

2   Basics of Three Main Weaving Structures

2.1   Plain Weave (*Hira-ori* or *Aze-ori*)

The plain weave is the simplest structure in weaving, and its examples can be found all over the world. Its structure consists of the equal amount of warp and woof (warp and woof ratio = 1:1). It is not three-dimensional, and it can be seen as plain and simple fabric, but both its process and necessary machines are also simple, making it easier to produce. Most of plain weave products are for casual wear. It can only express relatively simple patterns, and its texture is rough, meaning it does not feel lush *Tsuzure* weave is advanced styles of plain weave. It is characterized by its invisible warp. It can said to be a luxurious version of plain weave (Fig. 1).

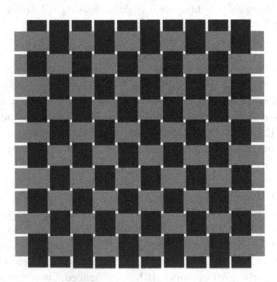

Fig. 1. Structure of Hira-ori

2.2   Twill Weave (*Shamon-ori*)

It is commonly called *Nishiki-ori* among producers. Its structure's warp and woof ratio is 2:1. In Nishijin, as well as others, luxurious products such as hand-woven fabrics are usually twill weave, though it is getting increasingly rare. Known for its glossy and tasteful appearance, this luxurious fabric is often used for formal wear. Especially for the *Hikibaku* technique used in Nishijin for a long time (technique that applies lacquer on the paper made from Oriental paperbush, pasting gold or silver sheet, cut them into filaments and then weave them with the weft into fabric), twill weave is more suitable than plain weave. By making fabric with double layer and then pressing down the surface layer with gold leaf, the *Hikibaku* can be more directly expressed. In formal obi, the volume which is the characteristic of *Hikibaku* method can be fully utilized by using this technique. There are many variations in twill weave. There are three different ways in just how to bind *Hikibaku* method (Fig. 2).

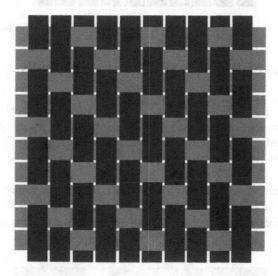

Fig. 2. Structure of Shamon-ori

2.3   Satin Weave (*Shusu-ori*)

Shusu (satin), *Donsu* (brocade) or *Tsuzure* Satin. Most of them are known as *Gomai Shushi* (5-harness satin) of which structure consists of warp and woof in the ratio of 5:1. It is extremely glossy and smooth, and has strong presence even when in plain color. Many satin used in Nishijin fabric is this *Gomai Shushi*, and used in special occasions such as obi for *Furisode* kimonos (Long-sleeved kimono for women, worn in ceremonial occasions). Satin produced by Kano-ko is 8-harness satin and there is 8 times more warp than woof. The fabric used for making *Mawashi* (a type of loincloth worn by a sumo wrestler) in Sumo is 32-harness satin which has far more warp than this 8-harness satin, but 8-harness is the limit for weaving patterns (Fig. 3).

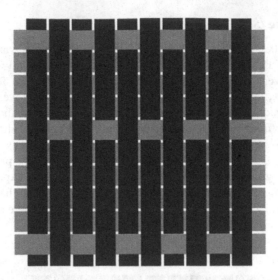

Fig. 3. Structure of Shushi-ori

3   Applications of Weaving Structures and Results

3.1   Applications of Plain Weave (*Hikibaku*)

There are equal amount of warp and woof in plain weave, meaning there are many tome (binding: binding edge with a thread) for weaving in *Hikibaku* paper filaments. Therefore, *Hikibaku* method in plain weave is almost like sinking the filaments into the structure of fabric.

Shiyu: Represents rain with threads in order to express dainty and fragility by intentionally sink in *Hikibaku* and emphasize the weave of threads. The selection of which weave and technique to realize the desired pattern and color is an essential aspect of obi making (Fig. 4).

Fig. 4. Shi-u: application of Hira-ori

3.2   Applications of Twill Weave (*Hikibaku*)

In case of twill weave, weaving in *Haku* (paper filaments) gives it more sensual appearance than plain weave. This is because by binding *Hikibaku* with *Karami-ito* separate from the weaving structure, the paper filaments are more exposed, resulting in the emphasis of the filaments shiny surfaces.

Rimpa Utai-hon (Songbook of the Rimpa school): These are obis that employed patterns from book covers by Tawaraya Sotatsu for songbooks (in this case Noh theatre text) by Hon'ami Koetsu. Even though its design has large plain parts, giving it simple and calm presence, it is a fabric that maximally utilizes the *Hikibaku* method in twill weave in order for it to function as an obi for formal occasions. This obi is favored even by the imperial household, proving its elegance, splendor and perfection as a fabric (Fig. 5).

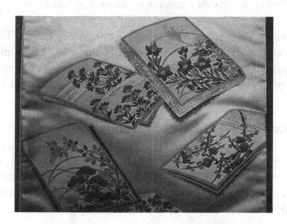

Fig. 5. Rinpa-utai-hon: application of Shamon-ori

3.3   Application of Satin Weave (8-Harness Satin)

Satin is commonly woven in what is called 5-harness satin, with warp and woof in ratio of 5 to 1. *Kano-ko* however, developed its original 8-harness satin in order to realize satin that is thinner and more lustrous. Production of 8-harness satin requires usage of more and thinner threads than usual. Therefore, we started with carefully selecting highest-quality threads with no damage. Using thinner and more warp means more time-consuming process. Moreover, because a lot more warp is visible, even the smallest damage in threads will be obvious, making it a faulty product. It is an extremely delicate fabric. It demands high concentration from both the producer and craftsmen, especially the weaver. However, the quality and yield ratio are increasing after many years of production, and we are currently developing more diverse colors and patterns.

Ryusui-kanoko (Deer hide pattern arranged like running water): The completed 8-harness satin shows formal beauty through the luster seen only in the highest quality fabrics. At the same time, it is thinner and lighter than usual satin, making it suitable

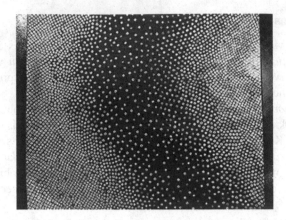

Fig. 6. Ryusui - kanoko: application of Shushi-ori

also for casual wear. This is a new horizon for kimono fabric. This product was presented as a good example of highest grade Nishijin satin kimono fabric to Ms. Margarida Barroso, wife of then the President of the European Commission Mr. José Manuel Barroso, who was present at G8 Hokkaido Toyako Summit (Fig. 6).

4 Systematization of Weaving Methods

Because in weaving, elements such as the pattern one wants to create, color or material are complexly interconnected, it is not realistic to strictly systematize it in relation to the weaving method and desired products. However, the direction of how and what to produce can be more or less decided when considering the characteristics of the three main weaving methods.

In plain weave, its structure is primitive and simple. In addition, its structure consists of equal number of warp and woof. Meaning its merit is its strength. Consequently, plain weave is used to produce thin fabric for summer obi.

In case of plain or twill woven fabric, the fabric color can easily be changed with the color of woof thread. In case of twill weave, it is difficult to make *Hikibaku* visible due to its dense woof threads, though there is a technique that leave only the section with *Hikibaku* unbound in order to keep it exposed. This however is only possible when weaving with handloom. Thus, it is necessary to pursue different techniques with material and type of loom following the application of each weaving method.

Because twill weave can create fine texture, through techniques such as combining it with *Ukiori*, it is suitable for the basis of formal obi. The technique that uses twill weave's *Karami-ito* is the best for fully utilizing the power of *Hikibaku*.

We know that since satin is a fabric that makes good use of warp threads, it becomes particularly beautiful when expressing a pattern that flows vertically. A pattern with ample empty space is more desirable as it shows the quality of the fabric. It is indeed an expensive and delicate fabric, with many difficulties during the production process, but this gives it the direct beauty of the fabric itself, which is the unique quality of satin fabric.

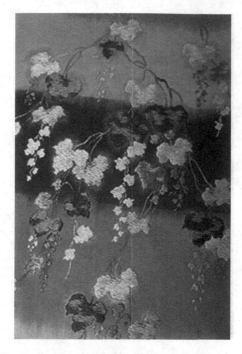

Fig. 7. Sou-tatsu-Tsuta-Fumi (Color figure online)

5 Analysis of Obi Design Examples

5.1 Sotatsu Tsuta-mon (Ivy Pattern Sotatsu Style)

Figure 7 shows a pattern based on "Ivy Lane folding screen" by Tawaraya Sotatsu. The original painting is of course a two-dimensional picture on a folding screen. Hence turning it in to a voluminous weaving requires more than merely copying the original, but also good sense, experience and technical innovation. In addition to what is called *Kara-ori* (Chinese-style weaving) which let threads float in order to create volume in pattern, it uses a technique called *Somikomi* (staining) which creates the appearance of mixing colors by layering many thick threads. In Japanese painting, there is a technique called *Tarashikomi* which intentionally make paint to blot in order to create a blur. This *Somikomi* technique is employed in order to create similarly delicate blur on the fabric. Moreover, there is very subtle gold leaf around the leaves which create slightly blurry shade around them, making individual leaf to stand out. The ivy pattern does not cover the entire obi, but placed with ample space, or "*Ma*" between them. This usage of empty space in design is akin to the style of Japanese painting tradition exemplified in the works of *Rimpa* as well as the understanding of space in Japanese tea ceremony. In this way, the products of Kano-ko deeply invoke Japanese tradition and history despite their modern sense of color. As a result, this obi not only reproduced the greatness of the ivy picture by Sotatsu, but it revived it as contemporary version of Sotatsu-ivy through accomplished craftsmanship.

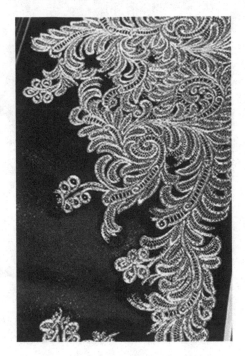

Fig. 8. Dynasty filet (Color figure online)

5.2 Dynasty Lace

This obi (Fig. 8) is an example of recreating the appearance of lace in weaving. It appears as though the lace is glued on the fabric even though it is a woven pattern. The design is developed from the research on French lace from the time of Louis the 14th, the Sun King. Anyone who sees this fabric for the first time is astonished by its beauty, opulence and the three-dimensionality of its pattern that could have been made by embroidery. However, it soon becomes clear that this obi too employs the mastery placement of empty spaces around the lace pattern that bring it out. If the lace pattern is simply turned into woven fabric, even the most beautiful pattern becomes flat and lacks the sense of luxury. The glossy part around the lace with golden halo is black *Hikibaku*. The filament that is woven into the fabric as though they are melting into it emits the sense of depth unachievable in simple monochrome fabric. These *Hikibaku* are bound just before the lace, making the edge of lace to appear matt compared to the glossiness of *Hikibaku* around it, creating the effect of shading around the lace, making the lace to have the appearance of volume. Its thinness, softness, lightness as well as the glossiness, volume and opulence that can only be seen in the highest quality fabric are the results of the traditional skill developed in Nishijin throughout the years. It is also the fruition of the union between beautiful design and the highest standard of weaving skill. Figure 9 shows the magnified view of the lace. The golden and slightly coarser parts are *Hikibaku*. You can see that by not putting *Hikibaku* on the edge of the lace, it creates shadow-like visual effect.

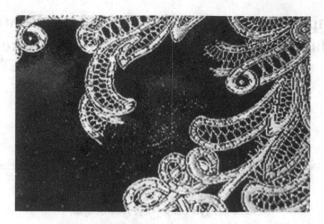

Fig. 9. Magnified view (Color figure online)

6 Conclusion

We believe that the traditional weaving skill passed on in Nishijin for hundreds of years will be carried on for a long time, and each generation will discover its own innovative applications. It is important to protect people, works, knowledge and craftsmanship in order to preserve the wonderfully diverse weaving method, rather than only leaving cheap and easy products behind.

References

1. Masashi, K., et al.: The basics and applications of the three main weaving methods in Nishijin-ori – Toward systematization of obi weaving technique. Presented at the 58th Congress of the Society of Materials Science, Japan (2014)
2. Masashi, K., et al.: Toward ease in tying and reducing exhaustion during kimono usage through making obi lighter. Presented at Joint Meeting of Chugoku, Shikoku and Kansai Branches of Japan Ergonomics Society (2014)

Comparison of KEMOMI Technique Between Master Craftsman and Unskilled Worker

Shinichiro Kawabata[1]([✉]), Zhilan Xu[1], Akihiko Goto[2],
and Hiroyuki Hamada[1]

[1] Graduate School of Science and Technology,
Kyoto Institute of Technology, Kyoto, Japan
s-kawabata@solitongrp.com, rararangrang@gmail.com,
hhamada@kit.ac.jp
[2] Department of Information System Engineering,
Osaka Sangyo University, Daito, Japan
gotoh@ise.osaka-sandai.ac.jp

Abstract. The Nara FUDE, made of several kinds of fibers with different properties, can achieve quality. However, the insufficiency of the mix process of the fibers may lead to the unstable quality of the final product. Fiber bundle of about 400 pieces of brush were mixed by hand at one time, which was called 'KEMOMI'. In this study, subjects with three different experiences were chosen (Master worker with 17 years of experience, Intermediate worker with 8 years of experience, Unskilled worker with 8 month of experience.). Refer to the method of the analysis of 'KEMOMI', three colours were in the rested fiber bundle, two kinds of filaments painted red and blue on the opposite of the taper side as well as the non-painted white colour. In order to analyse the progress degree of KEMOMI, binary coded processing was carried out on the picture taken every elapsed time during 'KEMOMI'.

Keywords: Nara FUDE · KEMOMI · Traditional handicraft · High quality brush · Master work

1 Introduction

Nowadays, traditional handicrafts are faced with serious problems such as decrease in demand as a result of the changing of the lifestyle and the decrease of the successors. Carrying out the motion analysis as well as the process assessment on the manufacture of the traditional crafts is of great meaning. Among them, there are also companies that have achieved the production with low cost but high quality from the heritage of the traditional craft skills. Soliton corporation is one of them and has made the flexible use of the traditional handicraft by making parts of the process automatized. And soliton corporation has succeed in the quantification of the worker's motion from an independent view, which did not mean only bringing the process in to automation but also managing to reappear the handy motion of the craft worker.

In the case of adopting of the automation, 30 times improvement in the production of that of the previous method can be realized, that made it possible for the new products to compete against the cheap products imported from oversea. However

© Springer International Publishing Switzerland 2015
V.G. Duffy (Ed.): DHM 2015, Part I, LNCS 9184, pp. 316–323, 2015.
DOI: 10.1007/978-3-319-21073-5_32

automation will not be brought into the whole processes, and the important process is still controlled by human hand, aiming at the manufacture of products with wisdom and human feelings, which is identified as products with high quality. This study has thrown a light upon the unknown process of the handicraft manufacture. The Nerimaze method, as a symbol of the Nara FUDE, refers to that a bundle of fiber for only one calligraphy brush will be took out and inverse into the water and shape into the desire shape, meanwhile the receipt and the size will also be changed according to the characteristic of the calligraphy brush. More than 10 kinds of natural fiber will be adopted from animals to make the calligraphy brush with suitable rigidity and good ink maintenance property. The adopting period of the fiber as well as the body section of the animal may bring great influence to the finishing process. Thus the ancient calligraphy brush craft had been thinking about the slight difference, such as flexibility, strength and length, between the natural animal fibers and put them together in a fantastic way according to the sufficient experience and long years' effort. In this way, the Nara FUDE was designed and manufactured.

Fibers are not able to demonstrate the performance only by mixing the filaments with different characteristics, synergy of high performance only begins to appear when filaments are uniformly distributed. As a result, different fibers were chosen and mixed together in order to produce the brush with high quality. However if those different fibers are not mixed sufficiently, the quality of the final product will not be stable. By the process of 'KEMOMI', all kinds of the fibers were mixed according a certain ratio, and distributed evenly. In this study, with the using of the binary coded method on the 'KEMOMI' process simulating the Nerimaze method of Nara FUDE, subjects with three different experiences were chosen (Master craft's man with 17 years of experience, Intermediate worker with 8 years of experience, Unskilled worker with 8 month of experience.), the degree of the process of 'KEMOMI' was carried out and analyzed. Information and the essential points got from the analysis results, can give a support to correct direction and plays an important role in the training of the unskilled worker.

2 Method

2.1 Operation Condition of the KEMOMI Process

In this study three types of PBT filaments listed below was used to manufacture the brush.

(1) 520 M-0.14 Round shaped (TORAY MONOFILAMENT CO., LTD.)
(2) SOW-W-0.10 Round shaped (Suminoe Textile Co., Ltd)
(3) 521 M-0.15 Star shaped (TORAY MONOFILAMENTCO., LTD.)

Three kinds of PBT filaments after "KEGUMI" was mixed 40 g each in this experiment. Two kinds of filaments were painted red and blue on the opposite of the taper side, which allows checking the mixing degree by eyesight. The bundle of filament was made and the process of "KEMOMI" was taken place. The Fig. 1 is illustrating the scene of the 'KEMOMI' process by worker.

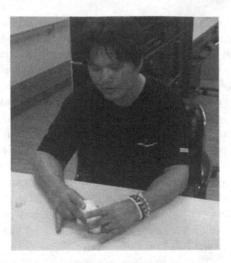

Fig. 1. Scene of 'KEMOMI' process

In this study test subject with three different experiences was chosen (Master worker with 17 years of experience, Intermediate worker with 8 years of experience, and unskilled worker with 8 month of experience). The subject work will judge the 'KEMOMI' process degree independently by check the color of the bottom of the fiber bundle. Ten times of 'KEMOMI' process were repeated, and the white threshold percentage was calculated and the process time was recorded (Fig. 2).

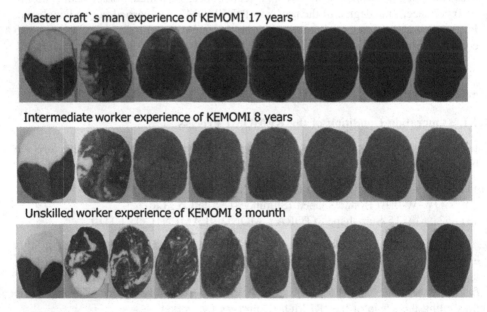

Fig. 2. States of fiber bundle from bottom sight

2.2   Analyzing Method of the 'KEMOMI' Process

To analysis the progress degree of KEMOMI, binary coded processing was carried out. For the first step, the experiment for deciding the optimal threshold value used for analysis was conducted. In this study binary coded processing was operated by using unimodal binary coded processing method. The picture image of the base of the fiber bundle was taken every elapsed time during "KEMOMI", also with one minute extra time. The images of the master worker as an example are shown in Figs. 3 and 4. Ten times of 'KEMOMI' process were repeated for every subject.

In order to determine the optimal threshold value for analysis, picture image of the last lapsed time which is thought as the most progressed "KEMOMI" process was used for the first step of analysis. The image was cut to 320 × 240 pixel size for binary coded processing. To analyze the "KEMOMI" progress, distribution of the white fiber was focused and threshold value used for next analysis step was computed when the number of lumps of a white pixel becomes the maximum in the final minutes of KEMOMI. The optimal threshold value presupposed as the same value from which the number of lumps of the white pixel became the maximum.

The second analysis was carried out to analyze the share of a white pixel in fiber bundle using this threshold. The image of every elapsed time was partitioned to Upper, Left, Right parts for analysis and each image was analyzed based on a similar threshold computed in the first step, and the occupancy rate of the white pixel at every elapsed time was calculated. There by the progress degree of "KEMOMI" process became possible to be measured. As the Fig. 3 is showing, the changing of the state of the fiber of different kind in the case of the master worker can be seen by human eyes. In this way the optimal threshold value can be collected and calculated.

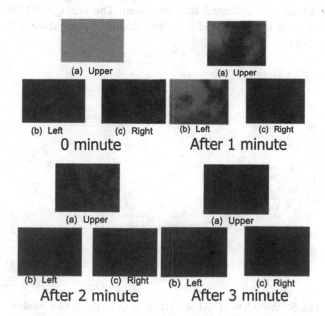

Fig. 3. The fiber mixing state of the master worker in the first 3 min

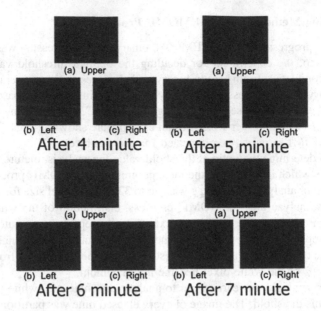

Fig. 4. The fiber mixing state of the master worker from 4–7 min

3   Results and Discussion

3.1   Result of the Master Worker

In this part, the optimal threshold values of all the parts the upper side the left side as well as the right side were collected and calculated. The average 'KEMOMI' process time for master worker is 6.9 min and the white threshold percentage is 13.98 % as the Fig. 5 showing below.

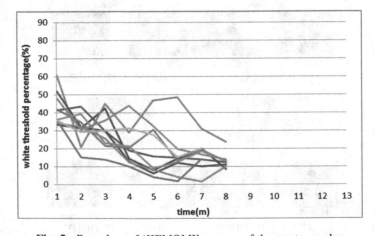

Fig. 5. Procedure of 'KEMOMI' process of the master worker

3.2   Intermediate Worker B (8 Years' Experience)

For the intermediate worker with 8 years' experience, the average 'KEMOMI' time is 7.9 min and the white threshold percentage is 11.16 % as the Fig. 6 showing below.

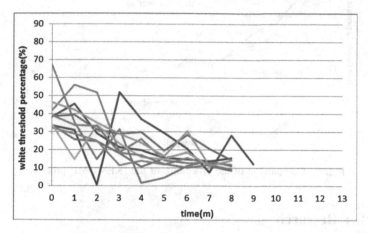

Fig. 6. Procedure of the 'KEMOMI' process of the Intermediate worker B

3.3   Unskilled Worker A (8 Month' Experience)

While for the unskilled worker with experience of only 8 months, the average 'KEMOMI' time is 11.8 min and the white threshold percentage is 14.02 % as the Fig. 7 showing below.

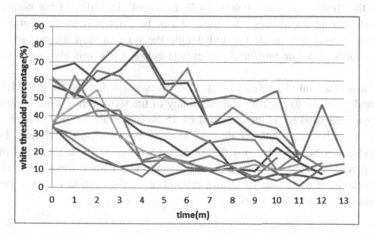

Fig. 7. The procedure of the 'KEMOMI' process of the Intermediate worker A

The results of average of the process time of the three subjects were illustrate in the Fig. 8. According to the degree from the calculation, the efficiency deviation of process of the three subjects was $F = (2,27) = 7.19$, $p > 0.05$, which means there were actually difference among the three subjects.

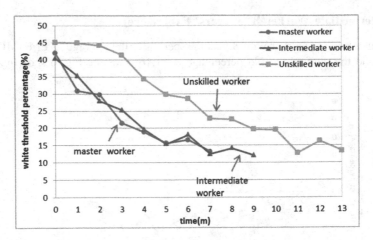

Fig. 8. Comparison of the procedure of the 'KEMOMI' process

4 Further Research

The average 'KEMOMI' process time for master worker is 6.9 min and the white threshold percentage is 13.98 %; for the intermediate worker with 8 years' experience, the average 'KEMOMI' time is 7.9 min and the white threshold percentage is 11.16 %; while for the unskilled worker with experience of only 8 months, the average 'KEMOMI' time is 11.8 min and the white threshold percentage is 14.02 %. From that all of three subjects can judge the 'KEMOMI' process degree and control the white threshold percentage below 15 % by check the color of the bottom of the fiber bundle during the process. Besides, it can be known from the figure that the intermediate worker can not judge and decide the time to stop the process and cost more time although white threshold percentage below 15 % was also achieved just as the master.

Thus, it is essential to judge and stop at the very point that the 'KEMOMI' process was finished, in order to improve the efficiency of the work time. What's more, in the case of unskilled worker A, the standard of 15 % was realised, however, it was still necessary to analyse the data for decreasing the operation time in future. From the figures it also can be seen that, for the unskilled worker A, the decrease of the white threshold percentage was slow in the first three minutes. Thus it was supposed to carry out the research on the comparison and difference on the motion between the master worker and the intermediate worker.

5 Conclusions

In this study, the "KEMOMI" process was researches and experiments were carried out among subject workers with experience of different years. This research managed to make the process judging by experience and institution into quantification standard. Obviously the result from the research can be a useful direction in training the unskilled workers in shorter time and thus try to solve the problem and make a contribution to the cultivation of the successor of the traditional handicraft industry.

References

1. Asada, M., Sakata, M., Shiono, T., Koshino, T., Yoshikawa, T., Takai, Y., Goto, A., Hamada, H.: Characteristics of motion during plaster model stuffing. In: Proceedings of 12th Japan International SAMPE Symposium and Exhibition, POS-5, pp. 1–6 (2011a)
2. Asada, M., Sakata, M., Shiono, T., Takai, Y., Goto, A.: Observation of surface structure of KYO-KAWARA (Ceramic material for roof component) fabricated by traditional skillful technique. In: Proceedings of the ASME International Mechanical Engineering Congress and Exposition, vol. 3, pp. 655–659 (2011b)
3. 小田原晶子・佐藤ひろゆき・杉江朋彦・森迫　清貴・塩野剛司・北島佐紀人・仲井朝美・濱田泰以.複合材料としての京壁.日本複合材料学会誌,vol. 35, no. 1, pp. 27–32 (2009)
4. 柴田勘十郎・仲井朝美・榎本晃朗・後藤彰彦・濱田泰以.京弓作製時における材料の見極めに関する研究.日本材料学会学術講演会講演論文集,vol. 60, pp. 49–50 (2011)
5. 柴田勘十郎・奈須慎一・久米雅・仲井朝美・濱田泰以.接着剤の違いにおける京弓の変形挙動と弓力の関係. Dynamics and Design Conference 2009,"422-1"–"422-4" (2009)
6. Tsuji, K., Takai, Y., Goto, A., Sasaki, G., Ohta, T., Hamada, H.: Human motion of weaving "Kana-ami" technique by biomechanical analysis. In: Advances in Ergonomics in Manufacturing, pp. 178–186. CRC Press (2012a). Chap. 19
7. Tsuji, K., Narita, C., Endo, A., Takai, Y., Goto, A., Sasaki, G., Ohta, T., Hamada, H.: Motion analysis of weaving "Kana-ami" technique with different years of experience. In: Proceedings of the ASME International Mechanical Engineering Congress and Exposition, IMECE2012-88809, pp. 1–6 (2012b)
8. Hamada, A., Ohnishi, A., Tanaka, T., Kume, M., Nakai, A., Yoshida, T
9. Biomechanical analysis of an-wrapping motion of the Kyogashi sweets expert. 京都光華女子大学短期大学部研究紀要, vol. 48, pp. 57–70, December 2010

Inside the User's Mind – Perception of Risks and Benefits of Unknown Technologies, Exemplified by Geothermal Energy

Johanna Kluge[✉], Sylvia Kowalewski, and Martina Ziefle

Human-Computer Interaction Center, RWTH Aachen, Campus-Boulevard 57,
52074 Aachen, Germany
{kluge,kowalewski,ziefle}@comm.rwth-aachen.de

Abstract. In the context of large scale projects public acceptance is indispensable for a sustainable roll out and broad implementation of technology. Especially when those projects deal with the implementation of relatively unknown technologies like geothermal energy. To find out what communication need the general public has, knowledge about the underlying cognitive attitudes toward the technology as well as the mental representation is important. In this context especially uncertainties about the consequences and risks are of importance. In this study we get a deeper understanding of the mental representation of geothermal energy by uncovering acceptance-relevant cognitions which were assessed by interviews with open answer format. Results show, that especially the communication about risks and possible disadvantages should be integrated in an adequate information strategy.

Keywords: Technology acceptance · Geothermal energy · Communication strategy · Information strategy

1 Introduction

Due to the climate change and the need to find alternatives to fossil fuels, renewable energy forms are very important for our society. Although the acceptance of renewable energies in general is rather high, several studies revealed that when it comes to concrete projects, people start to oppose them [1, 2]. Especially unknown technologies often lead to feelings of distrust and to a decreasing acceptance in society [3, 4]. Thus, adequate and timely information and communication strategies for large-scale projects - such as geothermal projects - is an important part in social acceptance [5, 6]. As several studies showed, the lack of adequate communication between project managers of large-scale technologies and the local residents is one major reason for a lack of acceptance [7, 8]. Project managers often face the difficulty that they don't have the knowledge about how to communicate and which content is adequate for the general public [9]. Especially in the context of complex technologies, communication between experts and non-experts is difficult, because there is no shared base of knowledge and technical terms. Perceived risks of lay peoples might not be "real" or "valid" out of the perspective of a person with

© Springer International Publishing Switzerland 2015
V.G. Duffy (Ed.): DHM 2015, Part I, LNCS 9184, pp. 324–334, 2015.
DOI: 10.1007/978-3-319-21073-5_33

a high domain knowledge [10]. Experts thus are often not able to evaluate the information need of the public [11].

Hence, for the development of adequate information strategies, the understanding of underlying mental models of energy technologies, in this case geothermal energy, is essential. It is assumed that the internal representation shapes unconsciously (risk) perceptions and, in consequence, the overall acceptance of the technology. By exploring people's internal representation of geothermal energy, we get a deeper understanding of the image of geothermal energy in the public, as well as about the need for information and communication. To get insights into the mental representation of geothermal energy and to uncover implicit meanings and hidden drivers for user acceptance, a free answer format study design is methodologically very important [12–14]. As several studies have shown, the public level of knowledge about geothermal energy is low [15–17]. This makes it difficult to uncover relevant acceptance patterns without shaping the perception by giving information, as this would be the case for example in questionnaires. Therefore, we examined the perception of geothermal energy in this study by a free answer format interview guideline.

With this approach we aim at deeper insights into the mental representation of geothermal energy, uncovering barriers and perceived benefits, which can be used as a information base for a communication strategy that considers the perception of geothermal energy in the general public [18, 19].

2   Conceptual and Methodological Approach

To prepare a communication strategy that is adequate for the public, a deeper understanding of the information need is indispensable [4, 5]. Traditional research methods such as questionnaires might not be suitable in the case of an unknown technology. By choosing questions with given answer format and giving directional input, answers are shaped in a concrete direction.

Thus, a first step for a communication guideline has to be the uncovering of existing mental representations of geothermal energy. As we know, mental models shape the perception and thus the acceptance, it is important to understand when trying to develop an adequate communication strategy. Insights into the mental representation of geothermal energy can be collected whenever participants have the possibility to freely associate what might come into their mind in connection to a specific technology. The benefit of that method is to get an unobstructed view of the perception of benefits and risks of geothermal energy because people are free to answer questions in their words and verbal elaborateness of their own choosing.

Both the language usage, the verbal associations but also the specific choice of words and the level of detail in which the participants answer, might give information about the cognitive representation of geothermal energy. From the specificity of answers, conclusions can be drawn about the level of knowledge and public perception of geothermal energy. The latter might help to plan and to tailor further research studies, but also to develop an adequate communication strategy which is based on the actual demand for communication and information in the public.

In the here presented interview study, participants were asked for perceived risks and benefits but also about the meaning of transparency in communication of large-scale technologies and what transparent communication should be like.

Altogether, 159 people took part in this study, aged between 18 to 64 years. Single answers were combined to parent categories for evaluation. For validity reasons, three independent evaluators accomplished the categorization. As found, the categorizations were in high accordance, hinting at a high validity of findings.

3   Results

The results are presented visually in order to reach a high transparency. We chose "word clouds" for a graphical representation of the frequency of response. Different shades indicate different categories.

In each of the questions we first report on outcomes of the whole sample, followed by an analysis of user diversity, taking age and gender into account.

3.1   Perceived Disadvantages

Looking at the answers to the question what disadvantages people think geothermal projects present, we see three main answering categories: costs, unknown risks and earthquakes (Fig. 1).

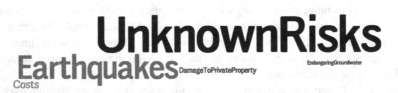

Fig. 1. Perceived disadvantages of geothermal energy (N = 104)

Answers can be divided in thematic subgroups. One group of perceived disadvantages is, that geothermics could lead to damages for the environment. The fear of environmental damages was mentioned in general but also more specifically people referred to the fear of earthquakes and damage to the groundwater. Another group of perceived risks is the fear of disadvantages for oneself or the community. This includes concerns about noise pollution, costs and damage to private property.

Overall the level of detail of the answers was not very high. Also, a quite negative image was revealed, dominated by distrust in the technology itself, its controllability and its economical and ecological value.

Regarding age differences, there are different perceptions of disadvantages of geothermal projects. A closer look shows, that older people referred more to unknown risks, while the younger tend to distrust the economical benefit (Fig. 2).

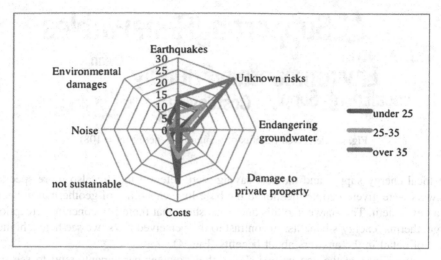

Fig. 2. Age differences in perceived disadvantages of geothermics in percent (N = 104)

Looking for gender differences, we see that women and men perceive risks nearly the same way. An exception is the fear of environmental damages, which is not mentioned by men (Fig. 3).

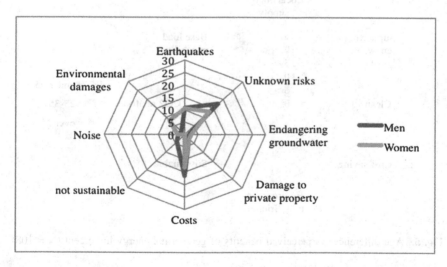

Fig. 3. Gender differences in perceived disadvantages of geothermics in percent (N = 104)

3.2 Perceived Benefits

Regarding the perceived benefits, mostly the ecological benefits of renewable energies in general were mentioned. The general support of renewables is mentioned most often, followed by environmental friendliness and sustainability. Also economical aspects as

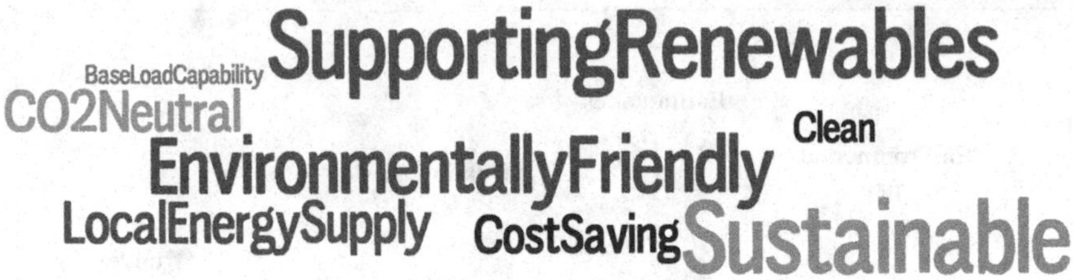

SupportingRenewables
BaseLoadCapability
CO2Neutral
Clean
EnvironmentallyFriendly
LocalEnergySupply
CostSaving
Sustainable

Fig. 4. Perceived benefits of geothermal energy (N = 108)

the local energy supply and the cost saving were referred to. But also more specific answers were given. People mentioned the base load capability of geothermal projects as a key benefit. The answers to this questions show that there is a concrete perception of geothermal energy's benefits. In contrast to the perceived risks, we see here a higher level of detail in the answers about benefits (Fig. 4).

A closer look at the age groups shows that younger participants tend to see the benefit of geothermal energy mainly in the sustainability, while the middle-aged group most frequently mentions the property of geothermic as an alternative to fossil fuels (Fig. 5).

Local energy supply
Base load capability
CO2 neutral
Sustainable
Environmentally friendly
Cost saving
Clean
Supporting renewables
30
25
20
15
10
5
0
under 25
25-35
over 35

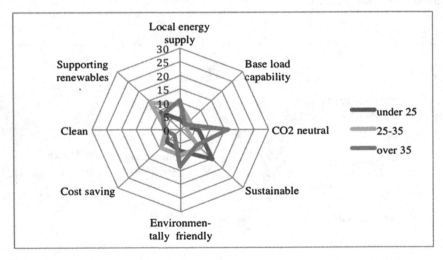

Fig. 5. Age differences in perceived benefits of geothermal energy in percent (N = 108)

The older group focuses on the local energy supply.

Comparing men and women we can observe, that men focus on the economical benefits and the advantage of a local energy source, while women's perception focuses more on the sustainability and the eco-friendliness (Fig. 6).

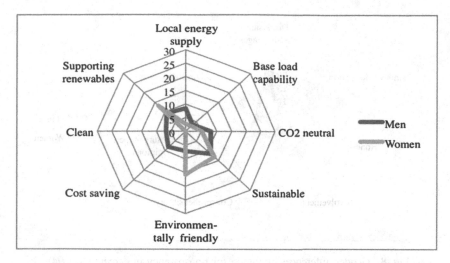

Fig. 6. Gender differences in perceived benefits of geothermal energy in percent (N = 108)

3.3   Perceived Transparency in Communication About Geothermal Energy

Being asked what transparency in communication means to them, participants associated most often the disclosure of risks, expert reports, and costs. Another often mentioned aspect of transparency is the involvement of the public in the decision-making process and information in time. Also mentioned were honesty and comprehensibility (Fig. 7).

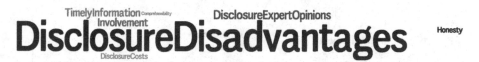

Fig. 7. Named characteristics of transparent communication (N = 94)

We see that the idea of transparent communication is very concrete in contrast to the perceived risks. The answers emphasize the wish for open communication about disadvantages, and a feeling of control by getting insights into expert opinions. Comparing men and women it can be seen from Fig. 8 that the wish for the disclosure of disadvantages is not gendered, thus is not different between men and women. An exception is the wish for disclosure of the costs and the wish for comprehensibility, which is not mentioned by women.

Contrasting the age groups (Fig. 9) it was found that the older group more often mentions honesty as an important factor for transparent communication.

Concluding, overall results show, that lay people have a high communication need. As the findings regarding perceived disadvantages clearly showed, the perception of

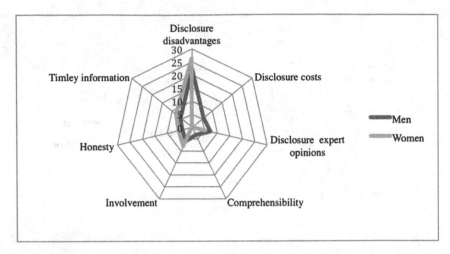

Fig. 8. Gender differences in criteria for transparency in percent (N = 94)

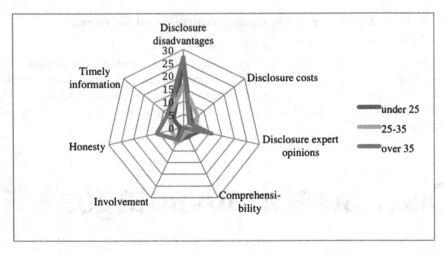

Fig. 9. Age differences in criteria for transparency in percent (N = 94)

the public is dominated by a high uncertainty about possible (negative) consequences of a geothermal project for the environment, but they also assume economical risks and unforeseeable consequences for them personally. The most often mentioned aspect *"unknown risks"* illustrates the unsharp fear of uncontrollability and perceived information lacks about risks and disadvantages.

The idea of transparent communication is very concrete. It shows the wish for information about the disadvantages of geothermics. This reflects also the need and the request for information about possible disadvantages.

4 Discussion

Acceptance is indispensable for the acceptance of large-scale projects - especially in the renewable energy sector which is important with regard to the climate change and the need to find alternatives to fossil fuels [20, 21]. For social acceptance in the general public and a successful implementation of renewables, communication and information strategies are a key factor [22]. Project leaders often face the problem not to know how to communicate with a non-expert, heterogeneous target group [11]. One condition for an optimal communication guideline is therefor the understanding of the mental picture the public has of a certain technology and its implementation. In this study we got deeper insights into the mental model of geothermal energy and the way users form their opinions.

It is noteworthy that associations in this context are mostly negative (if not explicitly asked for benefits) and center about risk and uncontrollability in terms of economic or environmental issues. Outcomes mirror findings of Huits et al. [22], which conclude that "worrisome environmental and societal problems related to energy use have spurred the development of more sustainable energy technologies" (p. 526). In their comprehensive paper they analyze psychological factors that impact acceptance in the energy sector. Authors argue: "the resistance can result from perceived hindrance and safety risks, but resistance can also arise because people think that collective resources could have been spent in a better way, or the cost-benefit ratio is too low" (p. 526).

It is an interesting finding that the acceptance-related negative cognitions are both, specific for geothermics and at the same time, quite unspecific and generic. While the perceived risk for earthquakes, for example, is specifically related to geothermal energy technology, the broad aloofness towards economic or environmental related risks represent more unspecific fears that were also reported for other energy technologies [23, 24], but appear in completely different contexts, such as V2X technologies [25], information and communication technologies [26, 27], or, even medical technologies [28, 29].

Future studies will have to find out in how far these generic concerns deal with the innovation openness of persons towards novel developments in the technological sector and the fact that unpopular technologies naturally evoke concerns. Bell [30] concludes in this context that "each generation is reimagining the dangerous impacts of technology on mind and brain. From a historical perspective, what strikes home is not the evolution of these social concerns, but their similarity from one century to the next, to the point where they arrive anew with little having changed except the label" [30, http://www.slate.com].

From the results we can draw insightful guidelines for communication and information strategies. With this study we identified the topics that should be integrated in a communication concept. Especially the communication about risks and disadvantages could be identified as a major topic for communication. The lack of information about possible consequences of the technology leads to distrust and insecurity and thus to a decrease in acceptance. In particular, the frequently mentioned fears of unknown risks underline the need for explanation of possible negative consequences of a geothermal project. Another important perceived risk was the fear of earthquakes. This is common to other studies that found out, concerns about geothermal technology often concentrate on the fear of seismic activity [31].

Based on our results we can draw conclusions about the wording of communication as we know in which terms people talk about geothermal energy. Taking that into account leads to a better understanding of information given to the public, because it helps to prevent misunderstandings caused by the use of technical terms or differing understanding of terms. For example the participants didn't mention seismic activity, but used the term earthquakes.

Also we could identify first results about the communication specific to the target group. We found age and gender specific focuses in the perception of disadvantages and benefits. Results show that there is need and request for information and communication strategies in the context of geothermal energy projects. For a successful implementation of geothermal projects, these strategies should discuss risks and benefits [32].

Continuing this line of research future studies have to evaluate the findings referring to the choice of topic, type of information, and wording regarding their practicability and validity for further guidelines for communication. Also, deeper insights into the relevance of age and gender specific communication for an adequate information strategy are necessary.

Acknowledgements. This research project (TIGER) is funded by the German Federal Ministry for Industry and Energy (BMWi, no. FKZ 0325413A). The research team owes gratitude to the ministry project coordinator Sarah Wurth for her helpful support in organizational as well as research issues.

References

1. Vittes, M.E., Pollock III, P.H., Lilie, S.A.: Factors contributing to NIMBY attitudes. Waste Manag. **13**(2), 125–129 (1993)
2. Groothuis, P.A., Groothuis, J.D., Whitehead, J.C.: Green vs. green: Measuring the compensation required to site electrical generation windmills in a viewshed. Energy Policy **36**(4), 1545–1550 (2008)
3. Zaunbrecher, B.S., Kowalewski, S., Ziefle, M.: The willingness to adopt technologies – a cross-sectional study on the influence of technical self-efficacy on acceptance. In: Kurosu, M. (ed.) HCI 2014, Part III. LNCS, vol. 8512, pp. 764–775. Springer, Heidelberg (2014)
4. Zaunbrecher, B., Ziefle, M.: Social acceptance and its role for planning technology infrastructure – A position paper, taking wind power plants as an example. In: 4th International Conference on Smart Cities and Green ICT Systems (SMARTGREENS 2015) (2015)
5. Kowalewski, S., Borg, A., Kluge, J., Himmel, S., Trevisan, B., Eraßme, D., Ziefle, M., Jakobs, E.-M.: Modelling the influence of human factors on the perception of renewable energies. Taking geothermics as an example. In: Amala, B., Dalgetty, B. (eds.) Advances in Human Factors, Software and System Engineering, pp. 155–162 (2014)

6. Trevisan, B., Eraßme, D., Hemig, T., Kowalewski, S., Kluge, J., Himmel, S., Borg, A., Jakobs, E.-M., Ziefle, M.: Facebook as a source for human-centred engineering. Web Mining-based reconstruction of stakeholder perspectives on energy systems. In: Ahram, T., Karwowski W., Marek, T. (eds.) 5th International Conference on Applied Human Factors and Ergonomics, pp. 5688–5699 (2014)

7. Kluge, J., Kowalewski, S., Ziefle, M.: What can we learn from the geothermal energy sector for communication concepts for large-scale projects? In: 2nd International Conference on Human Factors and Sustainable Infrastructure (2015)

8. Kowalewski, S., Kluge, J., Ziefle, M.: Investigating public preferences when implementing large scale technologies. In: International Conference on Human Computer Interaction (2015)

9. Zoellner, J., Schweizer-Ries, P., Wemheuer, C.: Public acceptance of renewable energies: Results from case studies in Germany. Energy Policy 36(11), 4136–4141 (2008)

10. Zaunbrecher, B., Beul-Leusmann, S., Ziefle, M.: Laypeople's perspectives on electromobility. A focus group study. Internet of Things Summit - IOT360. In: International Conference on Mobility and Smart Cities 2014. Springer, Berlin (2014)

11. Bostrom, A., Morgan, M.G., Fischhoff, B., Read, D.: What do people know about global climate change? 1. Mental models. Risk Anal. 14, 959–970 (1994)

12. Rouse, W.B., Morris, N.M.: On looking into the black box: Prospects and limits in the search for mental models. Psychol. Bull. 100(3), 349 (1986)

13. Hill, R.C., Levenhagen, M.: Metaphors and mental models: Sensemaking and sensegiving in innovative and entrepreneurial activities. J. Manag. 21(6), 1057–1074 (1995)

14. Ziefle, M., Bay, S.: Mental models of a cellular phone menu. Comparing older and younger novice users. In: Brewster, S., Dunlop, M. (eds.) Mobile HCI 2004. LNCS, vol. 3160, pp. 25–37. Springer, Heidelberg (2004)

15. Dowd, A.-M., Boughen, N., Ashworth, P., Carr-Cornish, S.: Geothermal technology in Australia: Investigating social acceptance. Energy Policy 39(10), 6301–6307 (2011)

16. Cataldi, R.: Social acceptance of geothermal projects: problems and costs. In: Proceedings of the European Summer School on Geothermal Energy Applications, Oradea/RO, pp. 343–351 (2001)

17. Kubota, H., Hondo, H., Hienuki, S., Kaieda, H.: Determining barriers to developing geothermal power generation in Japan: Societal acceptance by stakeholders involved in hot springs. Energy Policy 61, 1079–1087 (2013)

18. Morgan, M.G.: Risk Communication: A Mental Models Approach. Cambridge University Press, New York (2002)

19. Leiserowitz, A.: Communicating the risks of global warming: American risk perceptions, affective images, and interpretive communities. In: Moser, S., Dilling, L. (eds.) Creating a Climate for Change: Communicating Climate Change and Facilitating Social Change, pp. 44–63. Cambridge University Press, Cambridge (2007)

20. Batel, S., Devine-Wright, P., Tangeland, T.: Social acceptance of low carbon energy and associated infrastructures: A critical discussion. Energy Policy 58, 1–5 (2013)

21. Wüstenhagen, R., Wolsink, M., Bürer, M.J.: Social acceptance of renewable energy innovation: An introduction to the concept. Energy Policy 35, 2683–2691 (2007)

22. Huijts, N.M.A., Molin, E.J.E., Steg, L.: Psychological factors influencing sustainable energy technology acceptance: A review-based comprehensive framework. Renew. Sustain. Energy Rev. 16(1), 525–531 (2012)

23. Wallquist, L., Visschers, V., Siegrist, M.: Lay concepts on CCS deployment in Switzerland based on qualitative interviews. Int. J. Greenhouse Gas Control 3(5), 652–657 (2009)

24. Bidwell, D.: The role of values in public beliefs and attitudes towards commercial wind energy. Energy Policy 58, 189–199 (2013)

25. Schmidt, T., Philipsen, R., Ziefle, M.: From v2x to control2trust - Why trust and control are major attributes in vehicle2x technologies. In: International Conference on Human Computer Interaction (2015)
26. Arning, K., Kowalewski, S., Ziefle, M.: Health concerns vs. mobile data needs: Conjoint measurement of preferences for mobile communication network scenarios. Int. J. Hum. Ecol. Risk Assess. **20**(5), 1359–1384 (2014)
27. Kowalewski, S., Arning, K., Minwegen, A., Ziefle, M., Ascheid, G.: Extending the engineering trade-off analysis by integrating user preferences in conjoint analysis. Expert Syst. Appl. **40**(8), 2947–2955 (2013)
28. Ziefle, M., Schaar, A.K.: Gender differences in acceptance and attitudes towards an invasive medical stent. Electron. J. Health Inform. **6**(2), e13, 1–18 (2011)
29. Klack, L., Wilkowska, W., Kluge, J., Ziefle, M.: Telemedical vs. conventional heart patient monitoring – A survey study with German physicians. Int. J. Technol. Assess. Health Care **29**(4), 376–383 (2013)
30. Bell, V.: Don't touch that dial. A history of media scares, from the printing press to facebook (2010). http://www.slate.com/id/2244198
31. Brian, M.: Vertrauensbildung durch zielgerichtete Kommunikation. bbr – Sonderheft Geothermie 2013, S. 72–74 (2013)
32. Fairbanks, J., Plowman, K.D., Rawlins, B.L.: Transparency in government communication. J. Pub. Aff. **7**(1), 23–37 (2007)

Factor of Feeling "Hannari" from Kimono Images

Kumiko Komizo[✉], Noriaki Kuwahara, and Kazunari Morimoto

Kyoto Institute of Technology, Kyoto, Japan
kkumikok@gmail.com

Abstract. A separation from the kimono in Japanese society has an effect which has serious implications not only for the clothing industry, but for the continuation of traditional Japanese culture. However, for clothing, the lure of the kimono's beauty only remains in a modern age as "attire for special occasions." This paper attempts to define and classify one part of the kimono's appeal, the Japanese expression, "hannari-kan," or "feelings of elegance." Considering online shopping, we used a display device to show many kimonos for consideration and ratings, to collect data and quantify "hannari". We also assessed brightness and color in relation to "hannari" ratings.

Keywords: Kimono · Obi · Aesthetics · Brightness · Color

1 Introduction

As the kimono stopped being used for daily activities during the Showa era, its functionality, social context, and the economic activity generated by kimono manufacturers also declined. Now, the kimono is rarely worn, except for weddings, graduations, or other ceremonies, on special occasions if the wearer so chooses. The kimono industry follows a course of decline. The kimono industry has been decreasing even in Nishigin, the seat of kimono production, where looms, businesses, and staff peaked in 1975. The purchase expense rate for kimono and obi against the entire apparel purchase expense has fallen to 20 % of 1975 levels in 2011. Kimono consumption has dropped from 1 every 3 years in 1975 to 1 every 40 years in 2011. Obi consumption has fallen from 1 every 5 years in 1975 to 1 every 56 years [1]. These statistics show a separation from the kimono in Japanese society, an effect which has serious implications not only for the clothing industry, but for the continuation of traditional Japanese culture. However, for clothing, the lure of the kimono's beauty only remains in a modern age as "attire for special occasions." This paper attempts to define and classify one part of the kimono's appeal, the Japanese expression, "hannari-kan," or "feelings of elegance."

The word "Hannari" has a long history, with the first recorded usage in the Gyokujinsho in 1563 [2]. "Hannari" originated in the Kyoto geisha district, but has since spread throughout Japan. When it originated, "hannari" was an adjective meaning "chic" or "sophisticated," but the meaning has changed with time and the spread of the word. It now gives a different impression whether the speaker is referring to a person or an object. It is difficult to properly assess "hannari" without properly clarifying what

© Springer International Publishing Switzerland 2015
V.G. Duffy (Ed.): DHM 2015, Part I, LNCS 9184, pp. 335–344, 2015.
DOI: 10.1007/978-3-319-21073-5_34

makes something "hannari." There are few examples of research about "hannari" which do not first attempt to clarify the possible sources of "hannari" to quantify it and draw conclusions. This study attempts to do the same, applying "hannari" strictly to kimono. Considering online shopping, we used a display to show many kimonos for consideration and ratings, to collect data and quantify "hannari". We also assessed brightness and color in relation to "hannari" ratings.

2 Experimental Methods and Conditions

2.1 Psychological Quantity

Our research assistants were shown images of 20 kimonos and asked to rate them on a 5-tiered scale using 20 sets of adjectives expressing "hannari" selected by specialists. The kimono specialists were 7 members of the Kyoto Institute of Technology Textile Society, who selected a total of 114 images of kimonos from the Kyo-yuzen Silk Cooperative Association. In each set of five, researchers were told to rate two kimonos as "strongly hannari," two as "not hannari," and one as "in-between," as in Fig. 1 and Table 1. We also compiled a list of 100 sets of adjectives related to "hannari," based on words found in writings related to kimono and silk fabrics. These included such scales as "soft or firm" and "feminine or masculine". We then asked the kimono specialists to choose 20 pairs of words from that list that best matched the feeling of "hannari."

Our research members were 58 men and women, aged in their 10's to 89, with no symptoms of color blindness (37 men, 21 women). This sample included 7 members of the Textile Collection Museum & Archives Research Committee, students, working adults, and housewives. All members of the study had heard the term "hannari" used

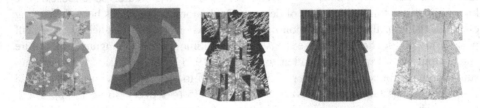

Fig. 1. Images of kimono selected by kimono specialists

Table 1. Sample ranking of kimono in sense of hannari

Rating	Choice	
Strong Sense of "Hannari"	1	5
Weak / No Sense of "Hannari"	2	4
Neither Strong Nor Weak	3	

before. Research took place in a dark room, without natural lighting. Images of kimono were displayed on a 2560 × 1440 pixel Apple Thunderbolt Display. Participants were asked to maintain a distance of 50 cm from the screen (Fig. 2).

2.2 Physical Quantity

2.2.1 Measuring Brightness

In order to evaluate the relationship between image brightness and sense of "hannari," we measured the brightness of each image. We divided each image into 10,000 parts (100 × 100), and measured the brightness of each part. Figure 3 shows an example of the division of an image.

To restrict the influence of external factors, we measured the brightness in a dark room. The camera used was a Nikon D7000. The lens used was an AF-DX NIKKOR 18–200mf/3.5–5.6G ED VR II. The software used was RISSA-DCJ/ONE. Shutter speed was set to 1/10th of a second.

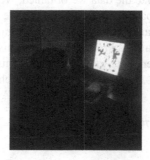

Fig. 2. Ranking kimono in sets of 5 in a dark room

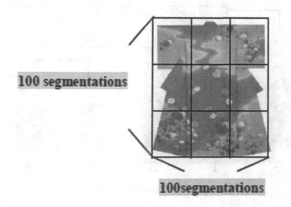

Fig. 3. Illustration of dividing an image into 10,000 parts

2.2.2 Color Measurement

To measure the effect of color on sense of "hannari," we measured the color of each kimono image. The color measurement was conducted at the same time of brightness measurements according to the methods described in 2-2-1. We divided each of the kimono images into 100 parts, translating the X and Y color values into u' and v' values, with u' on the horizontal axis and v' on the vertical axis. We used the CIE1976UCS color space to plot our results.

3   Results

3.1   Psychological Quantity

In order to better view participants' responses about the strength of "hannari" of a given image, we took the average values and plotted them on a scale as shown in Fig. 4. In the graph, we can see that the kimonos shown are ranked 5–1–3–4–2 in terms of "hannari". As kimonos 5 and 1 were chosen as the "most hannari" examples, and kimonos 4 and 2 were "least hannari," we can see that our results match the specialists' opinions.

When using SPSS to analyze the data we obtained, we performed a factor analysis. In order to evaluate what impact each factor had on the sense of "hannari," we performed a multiple regression analysis on the scores of each factor. Table 2 shows the factor loadings of each factor after a Promax rotation. This figure allows us to extract 3 factors. The first factor we were able to discern using this method is "fluffiness." The second factor is "gorgeousness," and the third factor is "chic". These 3 factors allow us to get a regression formula of what represents "hannari".

$$y = 0.579x_1 + 0.269x_2 - 0.012x_3 - 0.094$$

x_1 = **Fluffiness**
x_2 = **Floweriness**
x_3 = **Luxuriousness**

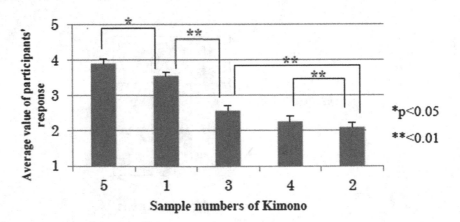

Fig. 4. Averaged sense of "hannari"

Table 2. Factor loadings

Antonym of Adjective			Factor		
			1	2	3
Fluffy	—	Rugged	**.860**	.477	.466
Soft	—	Hard	**.819**	.444	.468
Feminine	—	Masculine	**.775**	.757	.468
Pale	—	Strong	**.742**	.290	.317
Warm	—	Cold	**.702**	.419	.423
Relaxing	—	Stressful	**.670**	.066	.372
Rounded	—	Straight	**.578**	.155	.192
Gorgeous	—	Un-gorgeous	.500	**.932**	.496
Flashy	—	Conservative	.332	**.886**	.459
Glamorous	—	Unglamorous	.447	**.832**	.537
Pretty	—	Cool	.718	**.751**	.438
Graceful	—	Ungraceful	.459	**.686**	.617
Calm	—	Chaotic	.094	**-.582**	-.010
Elegant	—	Inelegant	.503	.430	**.778**
Sophisticated	—	Barbaric	.298	.328	**.776**
High Quality	—	Poor Quality	.497	.642	**.721**
Refined	—	Coarse	.605	.409	**.698**
Trendy	—	Untrendy	.341	.523	**.581**
Traditional	—	Untraditional	.133	.045	.184
Japanese Style	—	Not Japanese	.081	.012	.153

The selection method of factors based on "Maximum likelihood estimations"
Rotation rules: Promax method with normalization of kaiser

3.2 Physical Quantity Results

3.2.1 Results of Brightness Analysis

Figure 5 shows the relationship between average brightness and sense of "hannari". Brightness is tracked on the horizontal axis, and average "hannari" is tracked on the vertical axis. The sense of "hannari" gets stronger as it approaches 4. The most "hannari" kimonos, 5 and 1, both had high average brightness values. The least "hannari" kimonos, 2 and 4, had comparatively low values. The data yields a correlation coefficient of 0.93, which strongly suggests that kimonos with higher average brightness evoke a stronger sense of "hannari."

Next, we used the standard deviation in brightness across the entire kimono to help us judge contrast. The standard deviations, plotted against "hannari," are shown in Fig. 6. This yields a correlation coefficient of –0.67, showing a negative correlation.

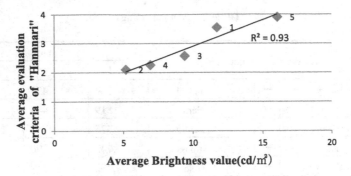

Fig. 5. Average brightness vs. sense of hannar

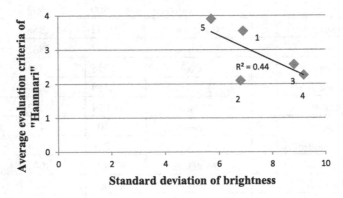

Fig. 6. Standard deviations of brightness vs. sense of hannari

The more "hannari" kimonos, 5 and 1, had smaller standard deviations than the least "hannari" kimonos, 2 and 4. This data suggests that kimonos with lower contrast, or less scattered brightness, are more likely to be considered "hannari."

To investigate the relationship between "hannari" and the frequency distribution of brightness, we plotted the frequency distribution in Fig. 7. The image segmentation domains are on the vertical axis, and the horizontal axis shows the data divided into parts of 2 candela/m2. The most "hannari" kimonos, 5 and 1, have lower peaks in their distributions, while both ends of the distribution are flared. Also, the least "hannari" kimonos, 2 and 4, have higher peaks and one-sided distributions. When examining the relationship between sense of "hannari" and the peakedness and degree of distortion in the frequency distributions, we can see that the degree of distortion and "hannari" have a correlation of –0.79, indicating that the smaller the degree of distortion in the distribution, the more likely the kimono will have a strong sense of "hannari" (Fig. 8).

3.2.2 Color Measurement Results

Measurements were taken at the same time as brightness measurements. Kimono images 1–5 were divided into 10,000 regions, labeled with X and Y values, and assigned u′ and v′ values as below.

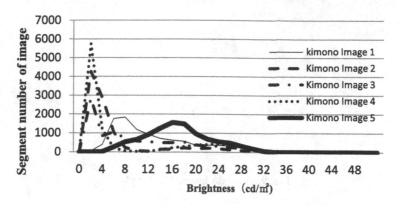

Fig. 7. Brightness frequency distribution vs. hannari

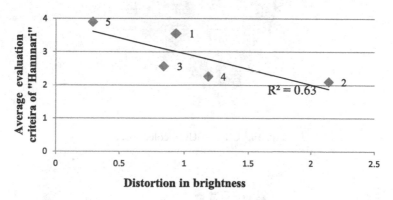

Fig. 8. Distortion in the frequency distribution & hannari

$$u' = \frac{4x}{4x + 15y + 3z} = \frac{4x}{-2x + 12y + 3} \qquad v' = \frac{9y}{x + 15y + 3z} = \frac{9y}{-2x + 12y + 3}$$

These values were plotted in terms of the CIE1976 UCS color space, as in Figs. 9 and 10. In order to evaluate the relationships between $u'v'$ values, and "hannari," we calculated the average $u'v'$ values, the standard deviations, the median, maximum, and minimum. Of these, the average values and standard deviations had the strongest relationship to sense of "hannari."

The distribution range of the color plots included in all the kimono images used in this research are shown as the color space in the Fig. 11. The correlation coefficient between the sense of "hannari" and the average value of u' was 0.50, revealing a slight correlation. As the average value of u' became more, the sense of "hannari" was likely to increase (Fig. 12). As seen in the color space in Fig. 11, it suggested that a cream color contributed more to the sense of "hannari" than light-green.

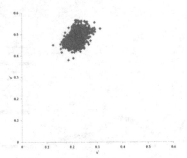

Fig. 9. Kimono image 1 color plot

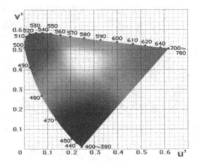

Fig. 10. CIE1976UCS color space

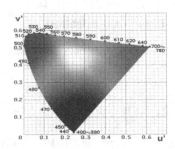

Fig. 11. The rectangular zone of the data of kimono images 1–5 (Color figure online)

The correlation coefficient between the average value of v′ and the sense of "hannari" was 0.56 (Fig. 12). It suggested that a cream color contributed more "hannari" than blue. The correlation coefficient between the standard deviation u′ and the "hannari" was –0.68, and the standard deviation of v′ was –0.86. This suggested that the kimono images with less color variations showed a stronger sense of "hannari" (Fig. 13).

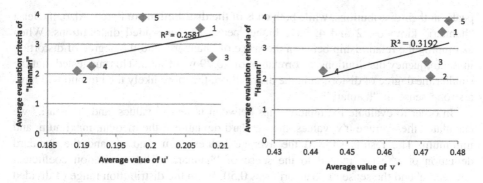

Fig. 12. Correlation between the average u′ and v′ value and sense of "hannari" (Color figure online)

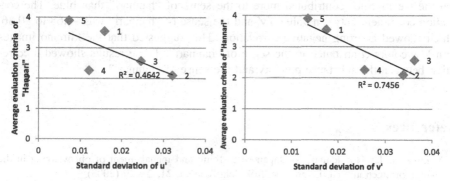

Fig. 13. Correlation between the standard deviation u′ and v′ value and sense of "hannari" (Color figure online)

4 Discussion

We conducted a factor analysis to find the factors that comprised the sense of "hannari" from the perspective of psychological quantity. The results show that three factors constitute the "hannari"; the first factor is "fluffiness", the second factor is "gorgeousness" and the third factor is "chic". These 3 factors allow us to get a regression formula of what represents a sense of "hannari". The coefficient value of the first factor, "fluffiness", was almost twice that of the second factor, "gorgeousness". This suggested that the sense of "fluffiness" strongly affected the "hannari". With quantification results of the "hannari" having been achieved, "hannari" is expected to be utilized in product developments.

Moreover, in order to clarify the correlation between the sense of "hannari" and substance quantity, we examined the relationship between the brightness of kimono images and the sense of "hannari". The results showed that the higher the degree of distribution in the brightness, the more likely the kimono will have a strong sense of "hannari". Investigating the relationship between the "hannari" and the frequency distribution of brightness showed that the most "hannari" kimonos, 5 and 1, have lower peaks in their distributions, while both ends of the distribution are flared. Also, the least "hannari" kimonos, 2 and 4, have higher peaks and one-sided distributions. When examining the relationship between the sense of "hannari" and the degree of distortion in the frequency distributions, a correlation of –0.79 was found. This suggested that the smaller the degree of distortion in the distribution, the more likely the kimono will have a strong sense of "hannari".

In order to evaluate the relationships between u' and v' values, and "hannari," we calculated the average $u'v'$ values, the standard deviations, the median, maximum, and minimum. The results showed the average values of u' and v', and the standard deviation of v' were related to the sense of "hannari." The correlation coefficient between u' and the sense of "hannari" was 0.50. From the distribution range of divided color regions of the kimono images in the Fig. 11, we can assume that cream colored kimonos contribute more to the sense of "hannari" rather than light green ones. The coefficient between v' value and the sense of "hannari" was 0.56. Figure 11 suggested that the cream color contributed more to the sense of "hannari" than blue. The correlation coefficient between value $u'v'$ and the sense of "hannari" was –0.68 to –0.86, which showed a strong negative correlation. This suggested that the kimono images with less colors contributed to the sense of "hannari". These results showed a correlation between the substance quantity and the sense of "hannari".

References

1. Yokoyama, T.: The demand for Japanese clothing and management of obi weaving in the nishijin production area. J. Jpn. Soc. Silk Sci. Technol. **21**, 23–29 (2003)
2. Maeda, T.: Japanese Etymology Dictionary, p. 934. Shogakukan Inc., Japan (2005)

Human Machine Epistemology Survey

Rémi Nazin[1,2]([⊠]) and Didier Fass[2,3]

[1] PErSEUs (EA 7312), Université de Lorraine, Nancy, France
[2] LORIA - MOSEL, Nancy, France
{remi.nazin,didier.fass}@loria.fr
[3] ICN Business School Nancy, Nancy, France

Abstract. Pluridisciplinar convergence is a major problem that had emerged with human-artefact Systems and so-called "Augmented Humanity" as academical fields and even more as technical fields. Problems come mainly from the juxtaposition of two very different types of system, a biological one and an artificial one. Thus, conceiving and designing the multiple couplings between them has become a major difficulty. Some came with reductionnist solutions to answer these problems but since we know that a biological system and a technical system are different, this approach is limited from its beginning.

Using a specifically designed questionnaire and statistical analysis we determined how specialists (medical practitioners, ergonomists and engineers) in the domain conceive themselves what is a human-artifact System and how they relate to existent traditions and we showed that some of them relate to the integrativist views.

1 Introduction

1.1 The Integrative Way of Looking at Things

Designing human-artefact Systems within the current technological context impose to adress safety and reliability issues at the same time[1].

Some theoretical apparatus are currently in use to support the design of human-artefact Systems but either they are "incomplete[2]" of they adopt some form of reductionism. This situation tends to lead researchers and engineers to build their own composite theories on demand thus being exposed to underlying contradiction which represents a critical safety issue.

Therefore, a unified but comprehensive way of conceiving what is a human-artefact System is necessary. This way is that of integration as intellectual approach which explains the functionning of a given system by those of its components and their organization. As the philosopher once said this could be regarded as a *"new name for some old ways of thinking"*[3] but the important word in the definition is **system**. What we mean by **system** is linked to

---

R. Nazin—Supported for a PhD by the Direction Générale de l'Armement.
[1] Particularly in the medical domain.
[2] They can answer only a fraction of the problems.
[3] William James as a subtitle for his *Pragmatism*.

© Springer International Publishing Switzerland 2015
V.G. Duffy (Ed.): DHM 2015, Part I, LNCS 9184, pp. 345–356, 2015.
DOI: 10.1007/978-3-319-21073-5_35

the general system theory (GST) [1] and designate a complex of objects whose interactions give new properties to the whole.

Apart from its systemical dimension, the integrative way of looking at human-artefact Systems requires to be a truly trandisciplinary paradigm. That means that it should allow us to understand the systems from their physical to their social and logical dimensions via their biological or artificial dimension, without getting out of our framework.

1.2 The Generic System

In his article [8], Fass built a new definition of a generic and isomorphic framework for describing systems. This system is defined by its dimensions of requirement (shape, dynamics and elements) and of specification (architecture, evolution and behaviour). The interesting point about specifications is their ability to characterize the functional identity of the modeled system including its behaviours and evolutions. It should be noted that this definition of a system is perfectly coherent with the theory of Bertalanffy [1] and share with it the fact that the system has no $\tau \acute{\epsilon} \lambda o \varsigma$[4] but is equifinal[5].

For more considerations upon the epistemological implications of this redefinition the reader can consult the Master thesis of the main author[6].

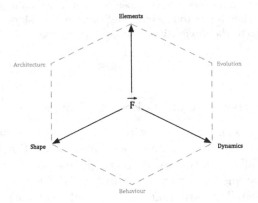

Fig. 1. The generic system and its dimensions. Plain lines represents requirements, dotted lines represents specifications. We can see that specifications are produced by the intersection of requirements and that the function is obtained from the global behaviour of the system.

---

[4] $\tau \acute{\epsilon} \lambda o \varsigma$ is the ancient greek for "completion" and is commonly used to describe the target state of a system as a metaphysical attribute.

[5] An equifinal system tend to a characterstical state from several initial states and various routes.

[6] [11].

1.3   The Link Between Theory and Practice

In order to demonstrate that there is some space available for our framework in the scientifical panorama, we had to adress a difficult problem. Medical practitioners, engineers and ergonomists have indeed little or no knowledge in epistemology because it is not part of their technical education. Being uneducated in a discipline does not mean having no idea about it, it does rather mean having ideas which are not necessarily organized in a consistant way.

There is an obvious link between theory and practice in the sense that some theoretical ideas that are not directly from one's field of expertise[7] can impact his practice. These theoretical ideas are entangled in a more or less coherent way into an underlying theoretical background. This background is not spontaneously created but is built during the education, experience and scientific general culture.

It is therefore impossible to ask our population to which tradition they find themselves the most affiliated. This situation imposes us then to probe their underlying theoretical background as a scientific ideology.

We first established a list of the main traditions used to conceive human artefact Systems. This list is constituted by behaviorism, cognitivism, connexionnism and cybernetics. For comparison, we added a brand new "tradition" called *integrativism* which reflects our point of vue upon the nature of human hachine Systems (Table 2).

It should be duly noted that, although the structure is inherited from our definition of a generic system, the content of the list is not arbitrary but comes from our bibliographical researches.

We then listed the respective theoretical positions upon the major items of the domain if possible[8].

From the bibliography, we could build a table to compare what we call *canonical traditions* (Table 1). A canonical tradition reflects the core principles of a scientific movement about a given subject, the actual positions taken by an individual may not be exactly the same as the canonical tradition which he is related because of the existence of different currents inside a given tradition. This is why we focus on the core principles which are the one that allows to distinguish some groups inside our population.

2   Hypothesis

The survey (Fig. 2) was designed to test the following hypothesis in a qualitative manner.

(h0) The population is divisible into different coherent groups in terms of their sets of answers.
(h1) If (h0) is verified, at least one coherent group can be related to a canonical tradition.

---

[7] e.g. "consciousness is alike of a computer program" for a medical doctor.
[8] Meaning there is a position.

Table 1. Canonical traditions on the nature of human-machine systems (part 1)

	Behaviourism	Cognitivism	Connexionism
Individual			
Body	Sensory organs + Effector organs + Nervous system	Biological computer + Sensory organs	Neural network + Body
Mind	Subvocal language + Memory	Centralized symbolic information processing + Memory	Emergent patterns in the network
Architecture	Mechanistic	Centralized modules	Network
Constitution	Conditioning	/	Reinforcement
Element	Spatial sub-unit	Module	Connex part of the network
Behaviour	Articulated response to stimulus	Problem solving	Computation
Cognition	Articulated response to stimulus	Rule based symbols manipulation	Adequate pattern activation
Perception	Stimulus recognition	Information acquisition	Information acquisition
Action	Articulated response to stimulus	Information treatment result	Computational result
Evolution	Mechanistic processes	Algorithmic sequences	Activation sequences
Interaction	Action and reaction in the environment	Data treatment	Input/Output
Memory	Faculty of the mind	Faculty of the mind	Patterns of activation
Function	None	Related to a module	/
Communication	Inter-individual	Information theory	Physico-chemical signal
Environnment	Stimulus source	Source of information and problems	Source of information and problems

Table 2. Canonical traditions on the nature of human-machine systems (part 2)

	Cybernetics	Integrativism
Individual		
Body	Feedback regulated systems	Self-associated metastable systems [5]
Mind	Decentralized information processing + Memory	Consciousness (In a jamesian way) [6]
Architecture	Feedback loops network	Biological
Constitution	/	Stabilizating self association [2]
Element	Feedback loop	Fonctionnal sub-unit
Behaviour	Return to equilibrium	
Cognition	/	Categorization by thalamo-cortical reentry [7]
Perception	Environmental disturbance	Integration of sensitive data [9]
Action	Recherche d'quilibre	Domain of stability and viability
Evolution	Return to equilibrium	Sub-system interactions
Interaction		Transductive coupling [3,4]
Memory	/	Recategorization [6]
Function	Regulation	Resulting from the activity of the system
Communication	Information theory	Functional interaction [5]
Environnment	Source of perturbations	Hypersystem

(h2) If (h1) is verified, there is no necessary link between the field of expertise and the membership to a coherent group.

(h3) If (h2) is verified, there is a coherent group related to integrativism.

3 Materials Used

- The Inria enquiry plateform runs LimeSurvey 2.05+[9].
- Statistical treatments of the answers were made with R 3.0.2[10] on OS X 10.9.
- Correlation graphs were made with Gephi 0.8.2[11] on OS X 10.9.

---

[9] https://www.limesurvey.org.
[10] http://www.R-project.org.
[11] https://gephi.github.io.

4   Method

From our hypothesis, we see that the purpose of the study was to show the existence of some sets of scientifical beliefs which are not directly provided by a domain of expertise and that these sets are shared by people form very different domains. To do this, a qualitative analysis must be conducted.

4.1   Survey

To examine our hypotheses, we selected some items in our grid of canonical traditions and we transformed them into affirmative propositions. To eliminate every potential bias, we randomized the initial order of the propositions. What we wanted to measure was the degree of agreement of our subjects upon a series of these propositions. For reasons of convenience, we choose to limit the length of the questionnaire to 25, keeping the completing-time under 20 minutes. For measuring the agreement, we used the typical format of a five item Lickert scale [10][12].

We completed the questionnaire with some demographic items such as sex, age and professional occupation[13]. These questions allowed us to refine our results and to test (h4). Using the LimeSurvey plateform, we guaranteed the anonimity of our subjects by not registering their ip adress and not using cookies. The transcription of the questionnaire is available in Fig. 2.

The questionnaire was available to all public trough the dedicated Inria plateform[14] during a 15 days period. The plateform uses a encrypted connection and thus reinforce the anonimity of our subjects. In addition to the common traffic of the plateform, we broadcasted the questionnaire through selected diffusion lists and communities:

– [tousloria] features all the people of the LORIA.
– [ergoihm] features a great variety of ergonomicians and specialists in HCI.
– [info-ic] feature the community of researchers in knowledge engineering.
– La Société de réanimation de Langue Française.

5   Statistical Analysis

5.1   Principal Component Analysis

Principal Component Analysis (PCA) is a factorial analysis method. Its main strength is its ability to describe an individual-variables matrix without any

---

[12] Strong disagreement, simple disagreement, without idea, agreement, strong agreement.

[13] This item has been used as an open question in regard of the means of transmission of the questionnaire. We wanted to touch a maximal variety of subjects and the use of predetermined categories could have exluded a part of our general population.

[14] https://sondages.inria.fr.

statistical hypothesis. As a factorial analysis method, it is not impacted by the size of the population either.

We applied this method to our groups of population by testing the θ_0 hypothesis that the absence of principal component significantly distinguishable in a population is a sign of the existence of some groups inside it. This hypothesis is opposed to θ_1 that the existence of a significant principal component in a group allows to define a group of answers greatly influenced by some determined variables and by then that the group is homogenous.

5.2 Hierarchical Clustering and Classification

This method allows to divide a group into several more homogenous groups in regard of the variation of the eigenvalue. It produces a hierarchical tree of clusters which can be analyzed by other methods described below.

5.3 Graphs of Correlation

As all our variables corresponding to answers are of the same type, it is possible to apply a χ^2 test[15] for each couple of them. We can thus build a correlation matrix and a correlation graph. The correlation graph represents the network of reciprocal influences of the answers in a given group. Each node represents an answer and each edge represents a correlation between two nodes[16].

This tool is interesting because it is more easily readable than a matrix and has graph properties such as connectivity. The more connected is the correlation graph, the more consistent is the group of answers. Then a graph with no connectivity at all represent the case of random answering and a graph fully connected represent the case of a group who has answered all the questions with the same answer.

6 Results

6.1 Description of the Population

After closing of the questionnaire, we had 150 complete sets of answers divisible in three categories (medical practitioners: 36, ergonomists: 59, others: 55). This division of the population doesn't impact the study in so far as it is used in the very end of it in order to obtain the final results displayed in Fig. 4.

Concerning our medical population, its size is of 36 which allowed us to consider our goals as achieved and it validate the population since the size of the general population is sufficient. The "other" category means to represent the non expert part of the population and its number is explained by the large opening of the survey via the plateform.

---

[15] With a p-value of 5 %.
[16] The qualitative dimension of the correlation is not of interest here in so far as we want to represent the absolute influence of each variable on the others.

1. What is our age ?
2. What is your sex ?
3. What is your profession ?

4. A machine may be compared to an organ.
5. Perceptual information treatment is the main function of the brain.
6. Behaviour is solely a reaction to exterior stimulus.
7. It is possible to predict the behaviour of an individual regardless of its body.
8. Reasoning could be considered as the result of a logical calculus.
9. It is possible to study an individual disregarding its interactions with the environment.
10. A living cell may be compared to a machine.
11. Mind est reducible to symbol manipulation.
12. A model which describes the augmented human must necessary be of biological inspiration.
13. An organ can be compared to a machine.
14. Behaviour cans be described as a problem resolution situation.
15. Environnement can be viewed solely as a stimuli source.
16. It is possible to understand the behaviour of an individual regardless of its nervous system.
17. Brain can be described as a computer.
18. We can describe the fonctionnement of an organism by a group of functions.
19. Augmented human is limited to enhance its natural functions.
20. Perception is a passive acquisition of information.
21. Capacity enhancement is the begining of a robotization of humanity.
22. Restoring a damaged biological function is enhancement.
23. Logic can account for the whole mind.
24. Sensorial information is tranformed during perception.
25. Information from the environnment can be regarded as a stimulus.
26. It is possible de reduce the beahviour of a neuron to that of a logical operator.
27. Enhanced humanity is linked to new functions.
28. Capacity enhancement impose deep modifications in the subject.

Fig. 2. Questionnaire used in this research

In the global population, we find two men for a woman and the majority of the subjects has an age between 18 and 55 years with a spike between 25 and 30 years. In the light of socio-demographic researches concerning the scientific population in France, this enables us to qualitatively validate the representativity of the general population.

6.2 Results

i. Statistical analysis (see Fig. 4) show that 25 % of the subjects can not be attached to a canonical tradition. This is explained by the fact that these subjects have not provided sufficiently structurated sets of answers or have provided idiosyncrasical structured sets of answers. This result was fully expected because of the nature of our population, the reader has to remember here that

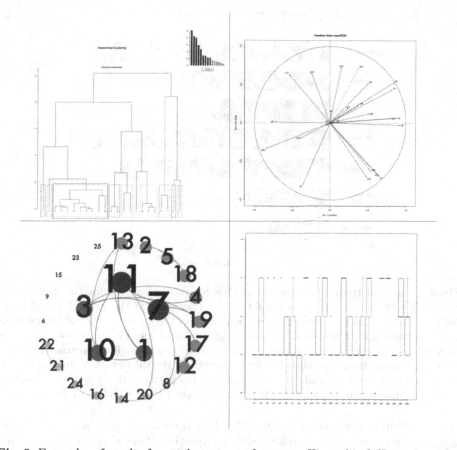

Fig. 3. Examples of results for a coherent set of answers. Hierarchical Clustering: The upper left part of the figure shows the result of a hierarchical clustering in one of our sets of answers. Hierarchical clustering is based on the euclidean distance between indviduals considered as a vector with their answers as coordinates. The highlightened group is the group used for this example. Principal Component Analysis: The upper right part of the figure shows the PCA results. PCA allows to describe a set of observed variables with a number of new variables called principal components by projecting them in a factorial plan. Two points which are not in the immediate proximity with the circle are not considered because of the projection. The more variables are near the circle, the more there is a principal component which can explain the distribution of the answers and the more coherent is the group. Correlation Graph: The lower left part of the figure shows the correlation graph. This graph is builded upon the correlation matrix of all the answers. This graph allows us to determine in a set of answers which one are the most influential in the sense that modifying one of them is susceptible to modify the entire set. The five more influential answers are displayed in the inner circle. Boxplots: The lower right part of the figure shows the boxplots for a set of answers. As we are in the case of a coherent set, we can see that for some answers there is a consensus. In complement to the correlation graph, these boxplots allow us to qualitatively determine what are the most important answers for the considered group.

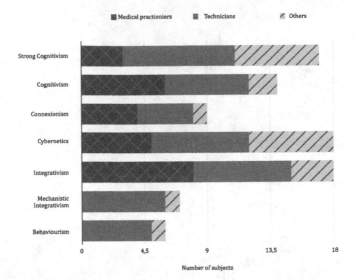

Fig. 4. Canonical traditions repartition. This figure displays the final results of the survey. It gives us a qualitative insight of the clustering of the general population. Subjects non related to a canonical tradition (25 % of the answers) are not represented here because they do not form a coherent group. Is is interesting to note that the "others" category is never a majority of a tradition which leads us to conclude that there is not some tradition related to non expertise of the subject. It is also important to note that there are no medical practitioners in the mechanistic integrativism and in the behaviourism which are two traditions who doesn't have a biological dimension.

the participants were asked to quantify their accordance with a set of propositions which are not from thier field of expertise. This is coherent with the fact that some of them have no structurated approach about our domain. The counterpart of this is the fact that 75 % of our population can be attached to a canonical tradition.

ii. Clustering (see Fig. 3) shows that (h0) is verified in so far as, when dividing the general population, the level of structurality tends to increase significatively.

iii. Fig. 4 shows that seven different groups can be found inside our general population. Thus we can validate (h1). It is interesting to note that there is no dominant tradition.

iv. Appart for two canonical traditions (behaviourism and mechanistic integrativism), the three categories are represented in each tradition. Moreover, medical practitioners are absent from behaviourism and mechanistic integrativism which are two traditions which are deconnected from biological considerations. No professional category has the exclusivity of a tradition or is secluded in one of them. We can then validate (h2).

v. We have related some subjects with integrativism by the way of our grid of canonical traditions. Medical practice contains already an integrative dimension in its modes of thinking thus permitting us to validate (h3) because integrativist tradition is not that of only medical practitioners.

7   Conclusions

There is not a unique way to conceive what is a human machine system, even inside a given domain of speciality. This also means that, when designing human machine systems, important choices must be made concerning which conceptual framework are used because they can't be interchanged and are not necessary intercompatible.

A grounding framework is meaningful and influences the professional practice of the subject without being a part of it. It is based upon the nature of the objects of the subject's practice. We call that set of ideas *ad hoc conceptual considerations*.

Ad hoc conceptual considerations are an important part of science and engineering because they participate to the practice from a more or less conscious position and are then important to consider in so far as their possible lack of consistancy can potentially lead to serious safety issues.

Although the usual traditions are present inside the catalog of *ad hoc conceptual considerations*, a significant part of the population is relatable to the integrativist tendancy which is not already structured around a theory. As we have shown in [11], integrativism is presently more a way to look at things than a structurated scientifical doctrine. It is nonetheless a good starting point to build a comprehensive and coherent paradigm in human related sciences and engineering taken as a whole field of expertise with its own scientifical principles, methodologies and values.

References

1. Bertalanffy, L.V.: General System Theory: Foundations, Development, Applications. George Braziller Inc, Canada (1969)
2. Chauvet, G.A.: Hierarchical functional organization of formal biological systems: a dynamical approach. I. The increase of complexity by self-association increases the domain of stability of a biological system. Philos. Trans. R. Soc. Lond. Ser. B Biol. Sci. **1290**, 425–444 (1993)
3. Chauvet, G.A.: Hierarchical functional organization of formal biological systems: a dynamical approach. II. The concept of non-symmetry leads to a criterion of evolution deduced from an optimum principle of the (O-FBS) sub-system. Philos. Trans. R. Soc. Lond. Ser. B Biol. Sci. **1290**, 445–461 (1993)
4. Chauvet, G.A.: Hierarchical functional organization of formal biological systems: a dynamical approach. III. The concept of non-locality leads to a field theory describing the dynamics at each level of organization of the (D-FBS) sub-system. Philos. Trans. R. Soc. Lond. Ser. B Biol. Sci. **1290**, 463–481 (1993)

5. Chauvet, G.: Comprendre l'organisation du vivant et son évolution vers la conscience. Vuibert, Paris (2006)
6. Edelman, G.M.: Bright Air, Brilliant Fire: On the Matter of the Mind. BasicBooks, New York (1992)
7. Edelman, G.M.: Wider than the sky: the phenomenal gift of consciousness. Yale University Press, New Haven (2004)
8. Fass, D.: Augmented Human Engineering: A Theoretical and Experimental Approach to Human Systems Integration. Systems Engineering-Practice and Theory., pp. 257–276. INTECH, Rijeka (2012)
9. Gibson, J.J.: The Ecological Approach to Visual Perception. Houghton Mifflin, Boston (1979)
10. Likert, R.: A technique for the measurement of attitudes. Arch. Psychol. **22**(140), 1–55 (1932)
11. Nazin, R.: Quels fondements épistmologiques pour l'humain machine? Université de Lorraine, Master Thesis in Cognitive Science (2014)

A Study on Learning Effects of Marking with Highlighter Pen

Hiroki Nishimura[✉] and Noriaki Kuwahara

Kyoto Institute of Technology, Kyoto, Japan
arc-nnlervmenve@arc-edu.com, nkuwahar@kit.ac.jp

Abstract. For learning students including elementary, junior high school and high school students, improvement of academic performance is one of the most important learning objectives. Types of problems in every subject are versatile and it is essential to find key points and keywords in sentences as well as questions under any situation. In order to find these key points and keywords, information on sentences as well as questions should be organized which can lead to increased attentional capacity as well as cognitive capacity. Various kinds of writing materials are used by the learners, and especially highlighter pens which are used by many learners for marking, when they are used for marking as means of organizing information, can have effects on the improvement of academic performance by the visual effects as well as through marking works.

Therefore, the purpose of this study is to clarify the effects of marking with a highlighter pen as a means to recognize necessary information. The Japanese language word problems, arithmetic computation problems and English problems were used and the amount of memory and the number of correct answers were measured to verify the effects.

Keywords: Highlighter pen · Memory · Attentional capacity · Academic performance

1 Introduction

Recently, there are many kinds of writing materials used by learners (elementary school students, junior high school students, high school students, university students) such as pencils, mechanical pencils, and ball-point pens. Presently, highlighter pens are produced and sold to color letters for highlighting which are widely used by students such as elementary school students, junior high school students, high school students, and university students when studying various subjects to enhance learning effects. Marking with highlighter pens is especially used to highlight important points in textbooks or study guides and has become a general learning means.

Purposes of learning for learners are various, but one of the major purposes is to acquire high scores in daily or regularly done written examinations, improve own academic performance level and acquire high scores to pass entrance examinations of preferred high schools or universities.

Currently, test types presented to the learners are often written tests and questions are given in various forms such as cloze test, multiple-choice, or narrative.

© Springer International Publishing Switzerland 2015
V.G. Duffy (Ed.): DHM 2015, Part I, LNCS 9184, pp. 357–367, 2015.
DOI: 10.1007/978-3-319-21073-5_36

However, in any form, it is essential to accurately recognize necessary words, keywords and important points to get right answers.

There have been studies dealing with visually favorable fluorescent colors or simple memory tests to examine the effect of marking with a highlighter pen. Reference [1] Also studies have been done about the effects of silent reading upon memory prose or understanding and memory of arithmetic word problems. References [2, 3] However, it has been unknown how specific marking methods in various subjects would influence attentional capacity, cognitive capacity or memory ability or calculating ability as well as contribute to improve academic performance.

Therefore, in this study, learning effects given to learners by marking key words and important points with a highlighter pen were verified by experiments using tests of story reading in the Japanese language, four-function computation in arithmetic and third person singular present S in English.

2 Experimental

2.1 Test Subjects

Tables 1, 2 and 3 show the number of subjects and data in each experiment. The subjects were from 4th grade of elementary school students to 3rd grade junior high school students who went to a cram school. In experiment I (marking experiment of the Japanese language), the number of subjects was in total 50, among them who used markings was 28 and the number of subjects who did not use markings was 22.

In experiment II (marking experiment of arithmetic), the number of subjects was 45.

In experiment III (marking experiment of English), the total number of subjects was 54. The number of subjects in group A was 28 and the number of subjects of group B was 26. In each experiment, subject sex and grade were selected in random order.

Table 1. Experiment I marking experiment of the Japanese language (attribute)

| Marking Experiment of the Japanese Language (attribute) | | | | | |
| With marking | | | Without marking | | |
Grade	The number of subjects	Ratio of male students and female students	Grade	The number of subjects	Ratio of male students and female students
The fifth grade at an elementary school	1		The fifth grade at an elementary school	0	
The sixth grade at an elementary school	2	male:18	The sixth grade at an elementary school	8	male:8
The first grade at a junior high school	9		The first grade at a junior high school	6	
The second grade at a junior high school	8		The second grade at a junior high school	5	
The third grade at a junior high school	8	female :10	The third grade at a junior high school	3	female :14
Total	28		Total	22	

Table 2. Markings experiment of arithmetic (attribute)

Markings Experiment of Arithmetic (attribute)		
Grade	The number of subjects	Ratio of male students and female students
The fourth grade at an elementary school	1	
The fifth grade at an elementary school	5	
The sixth grade at an elementary school	3	male:26
The first grade at a junior high school	19	
The second grade at a junior high school	15	
The third grade at a junior high school	2	female:19
Total	45	

Table 3. Experiment III marking experiment of English (attribute)

Marking Experiment of English (attribute)					
Group A Marking (without marking + with marking)			Group B Marking (without marking + without marking)		
Grade	The number of subjects	Ratio of male students and female students	Grade	The number of subjects	Ratio of male students and female students
The first grade at a junior high school	4		The first grade at a junior high school	7	
The second grade at a junior high school	11	male17	The second grade at a junior high school	9	male : 10
The third grade at a junior high school	13	female : 11	The third grade at a junior high school	10	female : 16
Total	28		Total	26	

2.2 Highlighter Pens Used for Experiments

Figure 1 shows highlighter pens (Sugata Co. Ltd.) used by the subjects for experiments.

Pens are packaged in a 6-piece set. The subjects used a fixed color or colors to mark necessary sections when needed. Kinds of highlighter pens were not specifically selected. A set affordable by the subjects of elementary school students, junior high school students, and high school students was chosen. The 6-piece set can be purchased at ¥108.

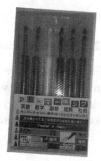

Fig. 1. Highlighter pen

2.3   Experimental Method

Experiment I Marking Experiment of the Japanese Language.

In experiment I, an experiment of memory ability after silently reading the Japanese language sentences (1744 letters) was carried out. The subjects were students who went to the cram school and the usual study rooms of the cram school were used for the experiment. The subjects were separated in a group who used highlighter pens for marking while silently reading and a group who did not use highlighter pens for marking while silently reading. Time of the silent reading was 5 min for each group and the reading could be repeated as many as possible. Marking method used for the group who used highlighter for marking was to mark out letters with the pens. Characters, places and times were set as keywords and the subjects were requested to mark them.

Also, the marking color to be used for characters was set as orange, for places as purple and for times as green.

After finishing the silent reading time, a memory test for characters (8 sections), places (5 sections), and time (4 sections) which appeared in the sentences was carried out. Then differences between the group who used highlighter pens and the group who did not use highlighter pens were verified. Figure 2 shows the sentences without marking. Figure 3 shows the marking actually given by the subjects.

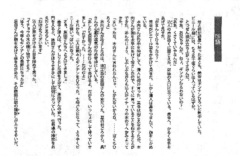 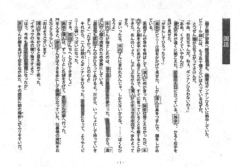

Fig. 2. Sentences in the Japanese language without marking

Fig. 3. Sentences in the Japanese language marked by a subject

2.4   Investigation of Memory Amount

Figure 4 shows results of the test which was conducted for each group after the silent reading. The test was in narrative form where the subjects wrote characters, places and times (sections to know time) that they memorized. The number of appearances of keywords in the sentences was 8, 5 and 4 respectively.

2.5   Experimental Method

Experiment II Marking Experiment of Arithmetic.

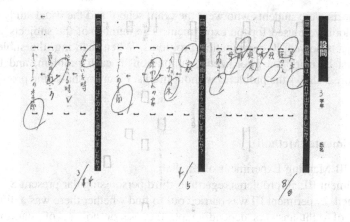

Fig. 4. Memory amount test

Experiment II was carried out to find whether there was difference in the number of right answers in arithmetic computation problems (four fundamental rules of arithmetic mixed problems) depending on the use or no use of marking with high-lighter pen.

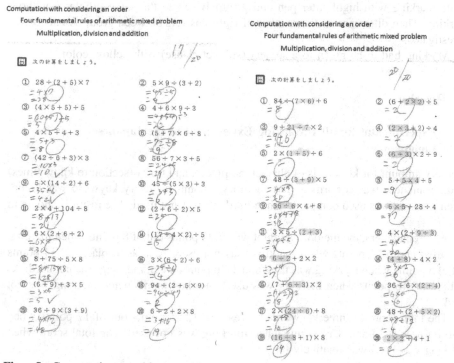

Fig. 5. Computation problems without marking

Fig. 6. Computation problems with marking

The subjects were students who went the cram school and the usual study rooms of the cram school were used for the experiment. The number of the subjects was 45.

The subjects solved 20-computation problems. When marking, the subjects were requested first to mark the prioritized computation in each problem, and then start solving. Figure 5 shows the problems without marks. Figure 6 shows the problems with marks.

2.6   Experimental Method

Experiment III Marking Experiment of English.

In experiment III, 50 problems regarding third person singular present S of English were presented. Experiment III was carried out to find whether there was a difference in the number of right answers depending on the use or no use of marking with a highlighter pen. In this experiment, subjects (subject clauses) were marked to accurately recognize whether third person singular present S was necessary or not. The subjects were separated in groups as follow and the test was conducted twice.

Group A: 1st time (without marking) + second time (with marking) 28 subjects.

Group B: 1st time (without marking) + second time (without marking) 26 subjects.

First, grammatical explanations for third person singular present S were given to each group before conducting the test. Then, each group solved problems without marking with highlighter pen. Next without break, group A solved the same problems while marking with highlighter pen and group B solved the same problems without marking. Then difference of the number of right answers between group A and B was investigated.

Marking had to be given to a subject (subject clause) with yellow color.

3   Results

3.1   Experimental Result I Marking Experiment of the Japanese Language

Memory amount for keywords of characters, places, and times (section to know times) in the sentences was confirmed. The memory amount for every keyword was higher when marking was used compared when marking was not used. The result is shown in Fig. 7.

As to characters, the memory amount was 7.25 points out of 8 points when marking was used and 6.14 points when marking was not used. Also as to places, 2.54 points out of 5 points when marking was used and 1.36 points when marking was not used. As to times, 2.46 points when marking was used and 0.64 points when marking was not used.

The total score of three keywords scores was 12.25 points out of 17 points when marking was used and 8.14 points when marking was not used. The total score when marking was used was relatively high.

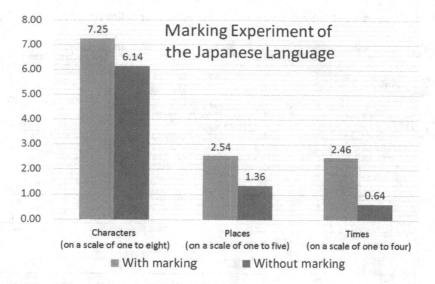

Fig. 7. Results of the memory amount of each keyword in marking experiment of the Japanese language.

It was confirmed that there was difference in the memory amount but the difference was not so remarkable when one keyword memory was measured but there was a large difference when several keywords memories were measured (Figs. 8, 9 and Table 4).

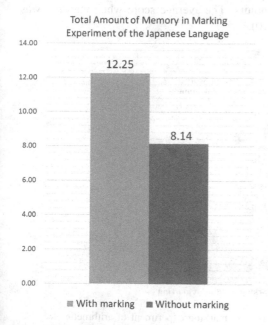

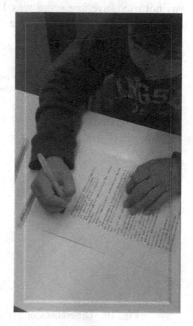

Fig. 8. Total amount of memory in marking experiment of the Japanese language

Fig. 9. Subject at the time of marking experiment

Table 4. Comparison of Subjects scores and average scores depending on the use of marking

with marking						without marking					
Grade	Name	Characters (on a scale of one to eight)	Pieces (on a scale of one to five)	Times (on a scale of one to four)	Total	Grade	Name	Characters (on a scale of one to eight)	Pieces (on a scale of one to five)	Times (on a scale of one to four)	Total
The third grade at a junior high school	K.D	8	0	1	9	The third grade at a junior high school	I.H	7	2	1	10
The third grade at a junior high school	N.A	7	4	2	13	The third grade at a junior high school	K.Y	7	4	1	12
The third grade at a junior high school	T.M	7	2	2	11	The third grade at a junior high school	M.S	7	0	2	9
The second grade at a junior high school	Y.A	7	0	2	9	The third grade at a junior high school	S.M	8	1	1	10
The third grade at a junior high school	Y.M	6	3	1	10	The third grade at a junior high school	T.D	7	2	2	11
The third grade at a junior high school	H.A	8	5	4	17	The sixth grade at a elementary school	T.A	6	0	1	7
The third grade at a junior high school	S.T	8	4	3	15	The sixth grade at a elementary school	I.R	5	3	1	9
The third grade at a junior high school	T.M	6	2	0	8	The sixth grade at a elementary school	K.R	6	2	2	10
The third grade at a junior high school	A.T	6	3	1	10	The sixth grade at a elementary school	K.U	6	1	1	8
The second grade at a junior high school	K.A	6	2	2	10	The sixth grade at a elementary school	B.M	4	0	0	4
The fifth grade at a elementary school	T.H	8	4	4	16	The sixth grade at a elementary school	S.K	6	3	1	10
The sixth grade at a elementary school	K.E	6	2	4	12	The sixth grade at a elementary school	S.R	8	2	0	10
The second grade at a junior high school	Y.T	8	1	2	11	The sixth grade at a elementary school	Y.A	5	1	0	6
The second grade at a junior high school	K.Y	8	4	4	16	The second grade at a junior high school	M.Y	5	0	0	5
The second grade at a junior high school	T.E	8	4	1	13	The second grade at a junior high school	K.A	6	2	0	8
The second grade at a junior high school	M.D	7	2	4	13	The second grade at a junior high school	M.M	5	0	0	5
The second grade at a junior high school	S.M	8	0	4	12	The second grade at a junior high school	N.R	1	0	0	1
The sixth grade at a elementary school	O.Y	8	3	3	14	The second grade at a junior high school	K.A	7	1	0	8
The second grade at a junior high school	T.T	6	1	0	7	The second grade at a junior high school	K.R	7	0	0	7
The first grade at a junior high school	O.T	8	1	4	13	The second grade at a junior high school	S.N	8	1	0	9
The first grade at a junior high school	N.S	8	3	3	14	The third grade at a high school	N.K	8	2	1	11
The first grade at a junior high school	K.J	8	3	3	14	The third grade at a high school	N.M	6	3	0	9
The first grade at a junior high school	K.F	6	4	3	13						
The first grade at a junior high school	Y.H	8	4	0	12						
The first grade at a junior high school	F.K	8	2	4	14						
The first grade at a junior high school	I.H	7	3	4	14						
The first grade at a junior high school	O.M	7	2	3	12						
The first grade at a junior high school	M.Y	7	3	1	11						
Total		203	71	69	343	Total		135	30	14	179
Average		7.25	2.54	2.46	12.25	Average		6.14	1.36	0.64	8.14

3.2 Experimental Results II Marking Experiment of Arithmetic

Differences in the number of right answers were confirmed depending on the use of marking. When marking was used, average score was 18.76 points and when marking was not used, average score was 17.53 points. The average score when marking was used clearly showed higher value (Fig. 10).

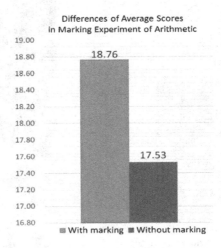

Fig. 10. Differences of average scores in marking experiment of arithmetic

3.3 Experiment Results III

Marking Experiment of English.

In third person singular present S judgment test, differences of the number of right answers in the second test depending on the use of marking were confirmed.

In the case of Group A (1st time without marking, second time with marking), average score increased remarkably from 27.82 to 43.

In group B (1st time without marking, second time without marking), average score decreased from 38.19 points to 37.46 points. Therefore, it is considered that marking tends to increase attentional capacity by enhanced recognition of important points. In group B, the average score was decreased. This can be because of the decreased attentional capacity due to increased level of fatigue (Fig. 11).

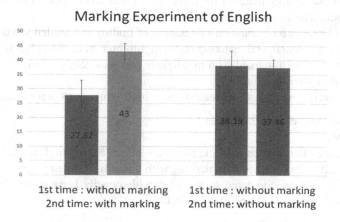

Fig. 11. Results of marking experiment of english

4 Impression Evaluation

Impression evaluation in five stages using SD method was carried out to find what kind of impression would be given to the subjects by marking with a highlighter pen. Evaluation Items is shown in Table 5. Also the subjects were requested to select a suitable writing material for marking important points or sections from choices of pencils, mechanical pencils and highlighter pens. Also, a test which showed two rows consisting of same several letters on paper was presented to the subjects. The letters in rows seemed to be arranged in a random manner but included the same word. The letters which formed the word was marked with highlighter pen in one row and marked with pencil (underline) in the other row. The subjects were requested to describe their impression of easiness to find the word in each row. Their impression was confirmed. The question is shown in Fig. 12.

According to the evaluation by SD method, 82 % (41 out of 50) answered very impressive/impressive to a certain degree for a question as to an impression and 76 % (38 out of 50) answered very effective and effective to a certain degree for a question as to learning effects.

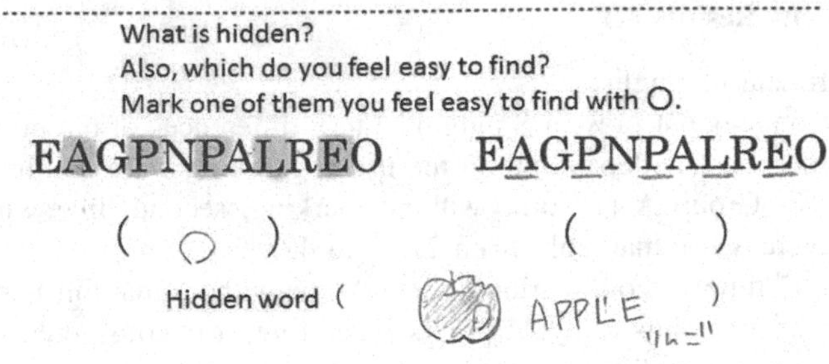

Fig. 12. Question with marking and question with underline

As to suitable writing material for marking, 45 subjects out of 50 (90 %) selected highlighter pen. The result is shown in Table 6.

As to the impression evaluation of easiness of finding the hidden word depending on marking with pencil and marking with highlighter pen, 50 subjects out of 50 answered that the word marked with highlighter pen was easy to find.

The result is shown in Table 7.

In free description, they wrote reasons why highlighter pens were good as follow:

1. Easy to see and easy to understand,
2. Firstly see,
3. As letters are often written in black, marked sections are highlighted and easy to see and so on. It was suggested that marking with a highlighter pen promoted feeling of easy understanding compared to marking with pencils because highlighter pens accentuated and emphasized marked sections.

Table 5. Evaluation items

Feel bright	Feel dark
Joyful	Not joyful
Can concentrate	Can not concentrate
Impressive	Unimpressive
Easy to use	Difficult to use
Effective on leaning	Ineffective on leaning

Table 6. Suitable writing material for marking

Pencil	Mechanical pencil	Highlighter pen
1	4	45

Table 7. Comparison of Impression between highlighter pen marking and underline marking

Marking with highlighter pen	Marking with underline
50	0

5   Conclusion

In this study, it was verified that marking keywords or important points in questions with highlighter pen could have learning effects and contribute to necessary memory ability, attentional capacity and cognitive capacity of learners (elementary school students, junior high school students, and high school students) by experiments using the story test in the Japanese language, arithmetic computation problems and third person singular present S judgment problems in English.

The results show clear differences by marking with highlighter pen, that is, increased memorized keywords of the story in the Japanese language, the higher number of right answers in arithmetic computation and the increased number of right answer in the English test.

Therefore, it appears that marking with highlighter pen can improve academic performance of learners. This can meet one of the major objectives of the learners and marking with a highlighter pen can be expected to enable enhanced leaning effects in fields of memory ability, attentional capacity, cognitive capacity or computational ability.

References

1. Suzuki, R., Kimura, M., Horie, Y., (Nihon University), Ouchi, K., (Japan Color Research Institute): Marking effects with fluorescence color. Ergonomics vol. **38**
2. Mori, T.: Effects of silent reading and vocal reading upon memory for prose. Jpn J. Educ. Psychol. **28**, 57–61 (1980)
3. Tajika, H., Ihida, J.: Children's understanding and memory for arithmetic word problems. Jpn. J. Educ. Psychol. **37**, 126–134 (1989)

Process Analysis of *Kyo Karakami* Manufacturing

Seiji Senda[1]([✉]), Erika Suzuki[2], Tetsuo Kikuchi[2], Mitsunori Suda[3],
and Yuka Takai[4]

[1] Karacho Co., Ltd., Kyoto, Japan
moet0527@me.com
[2] Toyugiken Co., Ltd., Kanagawa, Japan
{erika-suzuki,tetuo-kikuchi}@toyugiken.co.jp
[3] Kyoto Institute of Technology, Kyoto, Japan
mitsunorisuda04@gmail.com
[4] Osaka Sangyo University, Osaka, Japan
takai@ise.osaka-sandai.ac.jp

Abstract. This study is to clarify technique of expert in *Kyo Karakami* manufacturing by using process analysis and the eye motion analysis. *Kyo Karakami* manufacturing consists of *"Some"* process and *"Kata-oshi"* process. *"Some"* process and *"Kata-oshi"* process divided by 4 and 5 phases, respectively. From interview to expert, *"Some"* process divided by 3 steps. In *"Some"* process, expert worked almost same time at each steps. In *"Kata-oshi"* process, expert gave time "phase a" which provide total working time shortening.

Keywords: *Kyo karakami* · Traditional hand crafts · Process analysis · Eye motion analysis

1 Introduction

Karakami is a decorative paper made by coating washi paper with various colors and printing it with a pattern using mica [1–3]. *Karakami* originated in China and spread to Japan during the Nara period. At the time, *Kara-kami* was prized by highborn nobles and was used primarily as writing paper. However, Chinese-made *Kara-kami* was in itself a precious commodity and difficult to obtain. Japanese-made imitations of *Karakami* appeared during the Nara period; these were mainly used by sutra copying offices and for similar documents. The type of *Karakami* used in the Kyoto area for *fusuma* panels and related items is referred to as *Kyo Karakami*. In those days, most *Karakami* was made in Kyoto, and the *Kara-kami* produced there was called *"Kyo Karakami."* Popular during the Heian period, *Kyo Karakami* was used in *shoji* doors. While it fell out of favor temporarily during the Sengoku period, it flourished again between the Muromachi and Edo periods, when it was used for fusuma panels and wallpaper. It is thought that there were 13 producers of *Karakami* in Kyoto in 1839. After the Meiji period, demand for *Karakami* fell, as mechanization advanced and

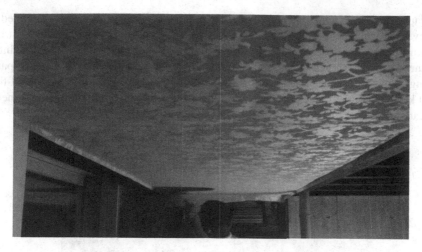

Fig. 1. An example of *Kyo Karakami* for ceiling

lifestyles changed. In addition, many *Karakami* producers lost their tools in major fires or wartime destruction. For this reason, only one *Karakami* producer, *Karacho*, is still able to create *Kyo Karakami* using traditional techniques. *Karacho* creates the *Karakami* used in such historical structures as the Katsura Imperial Villa and Nijo Castle. The *Karkami* used in these buildings is of a particular design that is required for restorations. Protecting the techniques *Karacho* cultivated over many years and ensuring that they are passed on to the next generation is vital for keeping Japanese culture alive. In the past, *Karakami* artisans began their training after graduating from junior high or high school. In recent years, the school entrance patterns of young Japanese people have changed, with a higher rate of students going on to college. As a result, some artisans now begin training after graduating from college. For this reason, artisans tend to be over 30 years old by the time they complete their training and are ready to practice. We believe that this training period is a bit too long for modern young people and we hope it can be shortened.

Some study about support for traditional handicrafts technique has been reported [4–6]. However, research of *Karakami* has never reported before. Therefore, purpose of this study is to clarify technique of expert in *Kyo Kara-kami* manufacturing. The process analysis and the eye motion analysis were conducted.

2 *Kyo Kara-Kami* Manufacturing

2.1 Process

Kyo Karakami manufacturing consists of two processes. One is "*Some*" process which Japanese paper is colored by paint. Two is "*Kara-oshi*" process which after "*Some*" process Japanese paper is printed by block. In "*Kata-oshi*" process, craft worker rubs on Japanese paper with the flat of themselves hand. Normally, we are inclined to believe that using baren provides good print at "*Kata-oshi*" process. Whereas strong rubbing is not good for printing. If strong rubbing done, pattern will be not print to Japanese paper as shown in Fig. 2. But transfer caused by deficiency of water in paint. Strong rubbing deprives water from paint, so paint viscosity becomes high, and then paint keeps sticking at block. For such reasons that *Kyo Karakami* manufacturing needs delicate hand works.

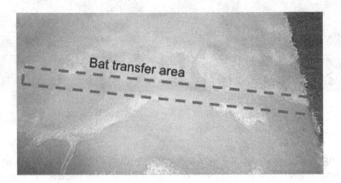

Fig. 2. Bat transfer example of *Kyo Karakami* by too mach pressure

2.2 Material

Kyo Karakami is using Japanese paper; especially *Echizen* Japanese paper is suitable. In "Some" process, paint solved by past and water is used. In "*Kata-oshi*" process, paint solved by *Kira* (mica), past and water is used. Mixing *Kira* has the effect of emphasizing printed pattern in angle of watching.

2.3 Tools

In "*Some*" process, the brush is used as shown in Fig. 3. The brush size is changed depending on Japanese paper size.

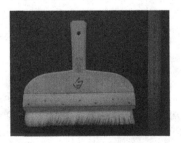

Fig. 3. Brush for "*Some*" process

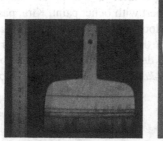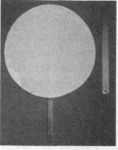

Fig. 4. Brush and *Hurui* for "*Kata-oshi*" process

In "*Kata-oshi*" process, the block is used for printing pattern. *Karacho* has more than 600 design blocks [3]. Almost block fixed place of use. Dedicated tool called "*Furui*" is used for putting paint on the block. The *Furui* made by the bamboo loop and the gauze. At first, mixed paint is colored by the brush to the *Furui*, and then paint on the *Furui* is colored to the block. Figure 4 shows the brush and the *Furui* for "*Kata-oshi*" process.

3   Method

3.1   Experimental Outline

In this study, crafts worker performed "*Some*" and "*Kata-oshi*" process. During these processes, we recorded video and measured eye motion.

3.2   Participants

Participants were two *Kyo Karakami* artisans. 26 years career artisan (man) is called expert. 2 years career artisan (woman) is called non-expert. Two participants were artisan of *Karacho*. *Karacho* was established in the 17th century and is the only *Kyo Karakami* factory today. *Karacho* has only two artisans today. So, just two artisans can become participants of this study.

3.3   Experimental Environment

The experiment was conducted on December 18, 2014 at *Karacho* factory. The participants performed "*Some*" and "*Kata-oshi*" processes same of daily work.

3.4   Materials and Tools

For "*Some*" process, *Echzen* Japanese paper and white color paint were used. The white paint mixed by expert with white paint, past and water. The participants use same white paint.

For "*Kata-oshi*" process, Japanese paper after "*Some*" process and ocher color paint were used. The ocher paint mixed by expert with ocher paint, Kira, past and water. The participants use same white paint. The block pattern was selected "*Takara-zukushi*" as shown in Fig. 5. *Takara-zukishi* pattern draws various treasures for example "fish", "gavel", "sacred gem" in checker board design [3]. *Takara-zukushi* pattern is difficult printing compared to the other *Kyo Kara-kami* blocks by reason of a lot of convex area.

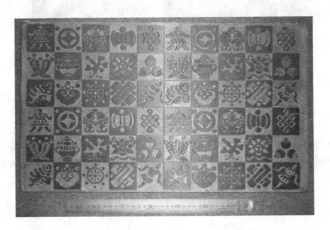

Fig. 5. Block of "*Takara-dukushi*"

3.5   Measurements

The participants' motions while working were recorded by a digital camcorder. All work hours were measured from the recorded video.

The participants' eye motions were measured by eye tracking instruments (Talk Eye II: Takei Scientific Instruments Co., Ltd.). The sampling rate was 60 Hz.

4   Results

4.1   Process Analysis

Total working time in "*Some*" process of expert and non-expert were 40.4 s and 34.6 s, respectively. "*Some*" process was divided by 4 phases as follows. Figure 6 shows schematich images and photos of 4 phases.

Phase A: The Japanese paper is brushed horizontal direction, at the same time the brush is moved from far side to near side.

Phase B: The Japanese paper is brushed horizontal direction, at the same time the brush is moved from near side to far side.

Phase C: The Japanese paper is brushed vertical direction, at the same time the brush is moved from right side to left side.

Phase D: The Japanese paper is brushed vertical direction, at the same time the brush is moved from left side to right side.

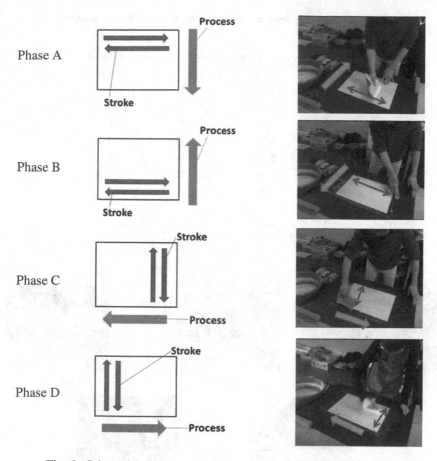

Fig. 6. Schematich images and photos of 4 phases in "*Some*" process.

Table 1 lists working sequence and working time. Expert has done 10 sequences. On the other hand, non-expert finished 7 sequences. Expert have not done phase D. Non-expert have not done phase C.

Total working time in "*Kata-oshi*" process of expert and non-expert were 61.7 s and 73.8 s, respectively. "*Kata-oshi*" process was divided by 5 phases as follows. Figure 7 shows photos of 5 phases.

Phase a: The paint is put into the brush.
Phase b: To paint by the brush to the *Furui*.
Phase c: To color by the *Furui* to the block.
Phase d: The Japanese paper is put on the block.
Phase e: The Japanese paper is rubbed by hands and *Karkami* pattern print to the
        Japanese paper.

Table 1. Working sequence and working time of "*Some*" process

Sequence no.	Expert		Non-expert	
	Phase no.	Phase time (sec.)	Phase no.	Phase time (sec.)
1	A	4.90	A	3.69
2	B	4.43	B	3.47
3	C	3.51	D	4.59
4	A	2.74	B	3.71
5	C	4.72	D	4.86
6	A	5.10	A	6.44
7	C	3.91	D	7.79
8	A	3.09	–	–
9	B	4.01	–	–
10	A	3.97	–	–

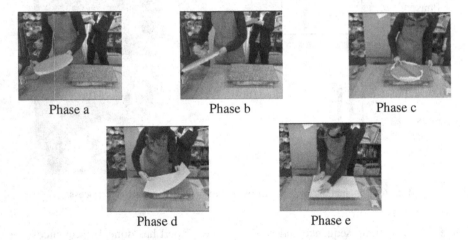

Phase a   Phase b   Phase c

Phase d   Phase e

Fig. 7. Photos of 5 phases in "*Kata-oshi*" process

Table 2 lists working sequence and working time. Expert has done 11 sequences. On the other hand, non-expert finished 9 sequences. Non-expert have done once phase a, b, d. Expert have done repeat phase b, d.

4.2   Eye Motion Analysis

Figure 8 shows line of sight at phase A and C in "*Some*" process. In phase A and B with to brush horizontal direction, line of sight of expert and non-expert was focused on where the brush would move to next. In phase C and D with to brush vertical direction, line of sight of expert was always in center of Japanese paper. On the other hand, line of sight of non-expert was focused on where the brush would move to next.

Table 2. Working sequence and working time of "*Kata-oshi*" process

Sequence no.	Expert		Non-expert	
	Phase no.	Phase time (sec.)	Phase no.	Phase time (sec.)
1	a	2.54	a	5.41
2	b	1.70	b	6.24
3	c	10.0	c	16.7
4	a	8.20	d	11.7
5	b	1.84	e	14.7
6	d	9.09	c	4.90
7	e	12.5	e	3.72
8	c	5.47	c	5.48
9	e	1.47	e	4.89
10	c	4.81	–	–
11	e	4.05	–	–

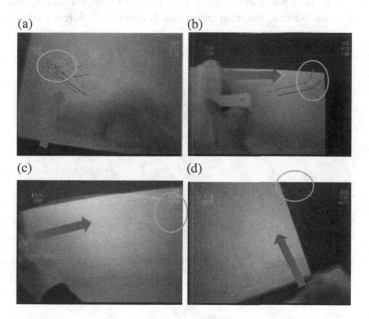

Fig. 8. Line of sight in "*Some*" process at (a) expert; phase A, (b) expert; phase C, (c) non-expert; phase A, (d) non-expert; phase C.

Figure 9 shows line of sight at phase e in "*Kata-oshi*" process. Line of sight of expert and non-expert was focused on where the hands would move to next.

(a)   (b)

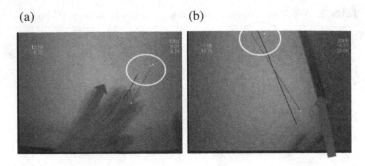

Fig. 9. Line of sight in "*Kata-oshi*" process at (a) expert; phase e, (b) non-expert; phase e

4.3   Printed *Kyo Karakami*

Kyo Karakami made by each participant was shown in Fig. 10. But transfer was observed in end part of *Kyo Karakami* printed by non-expert. Sometime *Kyo Karakami* is made by big Japanese paper as shown in Fig. 1. In this case, one *Karakami* pattern is printed many times. So that, but transfer on end is due to a deficiency of continuity of pattern.

(a)   (b)   (c)

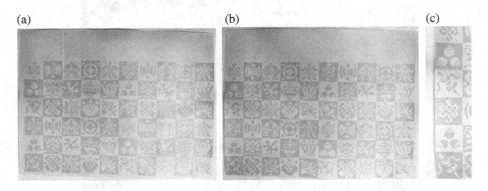

Fig. 10. Kyo *Karakami* made by (a) expert, (b) non-expert, (c) magnified non-expert

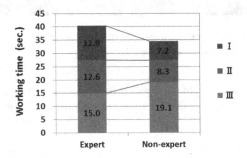

Fig. 11. Working time in step (1)-(3)

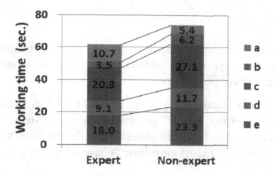

Fig. 12. Working time in phase a-e

5 Discussions

We interviewed expert as *"Some"* process. Expert said the most important point of *"Some"* process is to put paint into the brush with pushing out bristles in paint. In addition, he said "Some" process can divide 3 steps; (1) To spread paint, (2) To fit seamlessly into paper, (3) To take out brush lines. If artisan brush not enough paint, step (1) could not be done good condition. Expert divides sequence of two participants. Expert sequences divide into step (1)-(3) as sequence 1-3, 4-6, 7-10, respectively. Non-expert sequences divide into step (1)-(3) as sequence 1-2, 3-4, 5-7, respectively. Figure 11 shows working time in step (1)-(3). Each step working time of expert was almost same. Working time at step (1) and (2) of non-expert was shorter than that of expert. Working time at step (3) of non-expert was longer than that of expert. Non-expert could not put paint into brush; therefore working time of step (1) and (2) was shorter. Moreover, non-expert could not judge finishing job so fast, therefore working time of step (3) was longer.

In phase C and D, line of site of expert was always in center of Japanese paper. Expert said I checked paper condition by peripheral vision in order to lighten his workload. We found out expert's head didn't move and non-expert's head moved every time in phase C and D.

We interviewed expert as *"Kata-oshi"* process. Expert said the most important point of *"Kata-oshi"* process is same as *"Some"* process, to put paint into the brush with pushing out bristles in paint. If artisan brush enough paint, to brush the *Furui* will be enough, and phase c does not need long time. Working time in each phase of *"Kata-oshi"* process is shown in Fig. 12. Working time in phase a of expert was around two times longer than that of non-expert despite total working time of expert was shorter than that of non-expert. We guessed this tendency occurred by expert' mind. Careful work at phase a will provide total working time shortening.

6 Conclusions

This study is to clarify technique of expert in *Kyo Kara-kami* manufacturing by using process analysis and the eye motion analysis. The most important findings of this research can be summarized as follows:

(1) *"Some"* process and *"Kata-oshi"* process divided by 4 and 5 phases, respectively.
(2) From interview to expert, *"Some"* process divided by 3 steps.
(3) In *"Some"* process, expert worked almost same time at each steps.
(4) In *"Kata-oshi"* process, expert gave time "phase a" which provide total working time shortening.

References

1. Senda, K.: Kyo Karakami by Karacho. Sen'i Gakkaishi **51**(5), P218–P219 (1995)
2. Senda, K.: Kyo Karakami by Karacho. Gakugei Shuppan-sha Co., Ltd, Kyoto (1994)
3. Senda, K.: The Design of Kyo-Karakami. Shokosha, Karacho, Kyoto (2011)
4. Sano, S., Ueda, T., Terada, T., Izumi, Y., Nishijima, S.: Fundamental study of evaluation method of nailing by the 3D motion analysis for improving the skill. J. Life Support Eng. **20** (1), 3–8 (2008)
5. Umemura, H., Ishikawa, J., Endo, H., Abe, K., Matsuda, J.: Analysis of expert skills on burner works in glass processing. Jpn. J. Ergon. **47**(4), 139–148 (2011)
6. Onodera, T., Kuriyama, H., Takamura, N., Aoki, S., Irie, T., Marumo, M.: Research on skill transfer support system experienced technician. In: Proceedings of 29th Fuzzy System Symposium, WF2-3, pp. 947–950 (2013)

Exploring How People Collaborate with a Stranger:
Analyses of Verbal and Nonverbal Behaviors in Abstract Art Reproduction

Haruka Shoda[1,2](✉), Tomoki Yao[1], Noriko Suzuki[3], and Mamiko Sakata[1]

[1] Department of Culture and Information Science, Doshisha University,
Tataramiyakodani 1–3, Kyotanabe 610-0394, Japan
hshoda@mail.doshisha.ac.jp
[2] Japan Society for the Promotion of Science, Kojimachi 5-3-1,
Chiyoda 102-0083, Japan
[3] Faculty of Business Administration, Tezukayama University, Tezukayama 7-1-1,
Nara 631-8501, Japan

Abstract. We explored human-to-human communication when two people collaboratively attempt to reproduce an abstract painting. We examined the effects of friendship (i.e., stranger versus friend) and the task's three phases (i.e., first, second, versus third) on verbal and nonverbal behaviors. In our experiment, pairs of strangers ($n = 24$, 12 pairs) and friends ($n = 24$, 12 pairs) reproduced three abstract paintings. We measured the duration of their conversations, gestures, and painting behaviors, and the behaviors were labeled based on Traum (1994). The results showed that the amount and the functions of painting differed as a function of friendship. Since friends seemed more likely to focus on the efficient completion of the task, painting functions as a means of communicating images to partners. On the other hand, since strangers attempt to minimize conflicts with their partners, they start painting after discussing what to paint next.

Keywords: Collaboration · Friendship · Time-series change · Nonverbal behaviors · Abstract art reproduction

1 Introduction

Human-to-human communication is constructed by sharing information by voice, gestures, facial expressions, and so forth (e.g., Mehrabian, 1971). Mutual communication between two agents occurs in every scene of daily life. Especially in the context of human care, the importance of how caregivers or counselors communicate with their clients is increasing due to aging worldwide societies (United Nations, 2012). In such a context, caregivers or counselors often repeatedly do multiple tasks with clients who might express abstract information that is not easily understood through verbal or gestural messages. Even though we use verbal (i.e., contents of utterances), vocal (i.e., intonation), and gestural information

© Springer International Publishing Switzerland 2015
V.G. Duffy (Ed.): DHM 2015, Part I, LNCS 9184, pp. 379–388, 2015.
DOI: 10.1007/978-3-319-21073-5_38

(i.e., body movement) to share ideas with others, such abstract information as images and impressions can be communicated more effectively by drawing on a canvas (Åkerman et al., 2010). In other words, drawing or painting provides additional information to support vocal and gestural information. In the present study, we show that painting with a partner is one useful way for sharing abstract ideas between two agents.

Caregivers or counselors may experience another problem at their first meeting with clients: the difficulty of performing collaborative tasks with a stranger. Even if the first collaboration with the stranger did not go well, conflicts can generally be eliminated by repeatedly doing the task (e.g., Fujiwara et al., 2010). By comparing communication transitions in strangers and acquaintances (or friends) by repeating tasks, we propose appropriate strategies for communicating with new clients at first meetings.

In the present study, we conducted a basic study to obtain clinical implications in caregiver-and-client communication, particularly in sharing abstract impressions or images. Through collaborative reproduction tasks, we explored how two university students communicated impressions and/or images about an abstract painting to each other. We examined the effects of friendship (friends versus strangers) and the task's repetition (i.e., phases: first, second, third) on the participants' verbal (i.e., conversation), gestural, and painting behaviors. By analyzing the contents of conversation and painting, we identified the functional differences in communication between strangers and friends.

2 Method

2.1 Participants

A total of 48 graduate and undergraduate students from ages 18 to 23 ($M = 20.52, SD = 1.29$) participated in the experiment and were assigned to a stranger ($n = 24$; 12 pairs) or friend pair ($n = 24$; 12 pairs). Pairs of strangers obviously did not know each other before the experiment; each of the friend pairs had had close relationships for at least one year. For each group, we set six same-sex and six different-sex pairs.

2.2 Stimuli

As experimental stimuli to be presented to the participants, we chose three abstract paintings based on our preliminary experiment in which non-art majors reproduced art and evaluated the task's difficulty. We used three paintings by Cubist painter Georges Braque (1882–1963): *Nude Reclining on the Pedestal* (1931), *Still Life with Guitar* (1935), and *The Window Shade* (1954). In Cubist art, objects are depicted fragmentarily, and images and impressions are very subjective (Dohi, 1984).

2.3   Procedure

In the experiment, each participant concentrated for one minute on an abstract painting and had three minutes to reproduce it from memory on A4-sized Kent paper using pastel crayons. Participants memorized the paintings by themselves but reproduced the work completely in collaboration with their partner. The task was repeated three times in which the presentation order of the paintings was counter-balanced. We video-taped the upper torso of all participants and their paintings by three digital video cameras (HDR-XR550V, Sony).

2.4   Parameters

From the 9-min recordings per participant, we extracted verbal and nonverbal behaviors using annotation software called ELAN (EUDICO Linguistic Annotator; Lausberg and Sloetjes, 2009). We measured the duration of each conversation, gesture, and painting based on the following criteria:

Conversation (in Sec). We measured the duration of both participants' utterances, which were sandwiched between more than 500-ms silent intervals. Such fillers as ums, laughter, and mumblings to themselves were removed.

Gestures (in Sec). We extracted both participants' representational gestures that spatially expressed target objects (e.g., McNeill, 1987). We included finger movements on paper as gestures through which they attempted to express an object's shape and/or size.

Painting (in Sec). We measured the painting durations, which were sandwiched between more than 500-ms non-painting behaviors. They were defined as the duration that pastel crayons touched and moved on the paper; static (non-moving) states were excluded even if the crayon touched the paper.

2.5   Functions of Conversation and Painting

We classified each of the three parameters into one of the following tags (Table 1) according to Traum's grounding theory (1994). That work focused on discourse, but we also applied tags to the painting, in line with Takeoka, Shimojima, and Katagiri (2003).

The second author conducted these classifications, and two volunteers independently reclassified them, confirming the high reliability of these measurements (Cohen's κs = .625 and .629). Furthermore, we categorized the functions of repair, req repair, req ack, cancel A, and cancel B in the conversations into adjustment functions, because they are used in conversation when the pair participants adjusted or summarized their own ideas.

Table 1. List of tags attached to each participant's conversation and painting behaviors.

Tag	Definition
Init	Initial presentation of information
Cont	Continuation of previous act by same person
Ack	Acknowledgment of partner's presenting actions and/or information, such as okay, yes, and all right
Repair	Correction of information presented with init
Req repair	Request for a correction to partner
Req ack	Request for an acknowledgment by partner
Cancel A	Rejection of information from partner
Cancel B	Rejection of one's own suggestion
Ack–init	Acknowledgment occurring with Initiation
Other	Others

3   Results

3.1   Duration of Conversations, Gestures, and Painting

Figure 1 shows the mean duration of each parameter, computed for pairs of strangers and friends in each phase. The time length before painting and the painting duration with conversation were also computed. Friends appear to paint more (Fig. 1C) and talk more while painting (Fig. 1E) than strangers. The conversation (Fig. 1A) and gesture (Fig. 1B) amounts appear to decrease, but painting appears to increase as a function of the task's phase.

To confirm the above results, we conducted a 2 (friendship as a between-subject factor) × 3 (phase as a within-subject factor) mixed analysis of variance for each parameter. For each conversation and gesture (Fig. 1A, B), the main effect of the phase was significant, but those of friendship and two-way interaction were not significant, conversation: $F(1, 46) = 0.90, p = .35, \eta_p^2 = .02$ (friendship), $F(2, 92) = 8.50, p < .001, \eta_p^2 = .16$ (phase), $F(2, 92) = 0.49, p = .62, \eta_p^2 = .01$ (friendship × phase); gestures: $F(1, 46) = 1.12, p = .30, \eta_p^2 = .02$ (friendship), $F(2, 92) = 12.47, p < .001, \eta_p^2 = .21$ (phase), $F(2, 92) = 1.06, p = .35, \eta_p^2 = .02$ (friendship × phase). Post-hoc t-tests with Bonferroni's correction showed that participants took more time in the first phase than in the second (conversation: $p = .004$; gesture: $p = .002$) and third phases (conversation: $p = .004$; gesture: $p < .001$). The differences between the second and third phases were not significant (conversation: $p = 1.00$; gesture: $p = .30$).

For painting (Fig. 1C), the main effects of friendship and phase were significant but the two-way interaction was not, $F(1, 46) = 8.96, p = .004, \eta_p^2 = .16$ (friendship), $F(2, 92) = 15.03, p < .001, \eta_p^2 = .25$ (phase), $F(2, 92) = 0.32, p = .73, \eta_p^2 = .007$ (friendship × phase). As shown in Fig. 1C, friends spent more time painting than strangers. Post-hoc t-tests with Bonferroni's correction showed

□ Strangers   ■ Friends

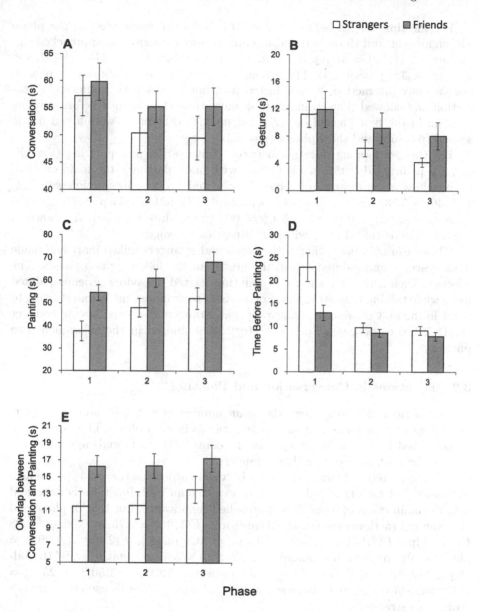

Fig. 1. Mean duration computed for each pair of strangers and friends in each phase for conversation (A), gestures (B), painting (C), time length before painting (D), and overlap between conversation and painting (E). Error bars indicate standard errors.

that participants spent less time painting in the first phase than in the second ($p = .006$) and third phases ($p < .001$). No significant difference was found between the second and third phases ($p = .14$).

For the time length before painting (Fig. 1D), the main effect of the phase was significant and those of friendship and two-way interaction approached significance, $F(1, 22) = 3.91, p = .06, \eta_p^2 = .15$ (friendship), $F(2, 44) = 10.31, p < .001, \eta_p^2 = .32$ (phase), $F(2, 44) = 2.38, p = .10, \eta_p^2 = .10$ (friendship × phase). For two-way interaction, we conducted post-hoc t-tests with Bonferroni's correction and showed that strangers took more time than friends before starting to paint in the first phase ($p = .06$), but no such differences were found in the second ($p = .56$) and third phases ($p = .52$).

For the overlapping duration between conversation and painting (Fig. 1E, i.e., the painting duration while talking with one's partner), the main effect of friendship was significant, but those of phase and two-way interaction were not, $F(1, 46) = 5.53, p = .02, \eta_p^2 = .11$ (friendship), $F(2, 92) = 1.33, p = .27, \eta_p^2 = .03$ (phase), $F(2, 92) = 0.16, p = .85, \eta_p^2 = .003$ (friendship × phase). As shown in Fig. 1E, friends talked more while painting than strangers.

These results indicate that both friends and strangers talked more and made more gestures and painted less in the first than the following two phases. The effects of friendship were shown for painting-related behaviors. Friends painted more while talking than strangers. Friends only took more time before starting to paint in the first phase only, indicating that strangers discussed how to conduct the task before painting. Such a strategy went unused in the subsequent two phases.

3.2   Functions in Conversation and Painting

Conversation. Figure 2 shows the mean number of init, ack, and the adjustment functions for pairs of strangers and friends in each phase. The values were standardized by the mean duration of the conversations. Friends appear to use each of these functions more than strangers.

We conducted a 2 (friendship as a between-subject factor) × 3 (phase as a within-subject factor) mixed analysis of variance for each function. For init and ack, the main effect of friendship approached significance, but that of phase and two-way interaction were not significant, init: $F(1, 46) = 3.75, p = .06, \eta_p^2 = .08$ (friendship), $F(2, 92) = 1.13, p = .33, \eta_p^2 = .02$ (phase), $F(2, 92) = 1.09, p = .34, \eta_p^2 = .02$ (friendship × phase); ack: $F(1, 46) = 3.58, p = .06, \eta_p^2 = .07$ (friendship), $F(2, 92) = 0.47, p = .63, \eta_p^2 = .01$ (phase), $F(2, 92) = 1.50, p = .23, \eta_p^2 = .03$ (friendship × phase). As shown in Figs. 2A and B, friends used init and ack more than strangers.

As for the adjustments, we found that the main effects of friendship and phase and the two-way interaction were all significant, $F(1, 46) = 44.85, p < .001, \eta_p^2 = .49$ (friendship), $F(2, 92) = 4.94, p = .009, \eta_p^2 = .10$ (phase), $F(2, 92) = 4.44, p = .01, \eta_p^2 = .09$ (friendship × phase). Post-hoc t-tests using Bonferroni's correction showed for each phase that friends used adjustment more than strangers ($ps < .001$). These results indicate that friends engaged in more interactions than strangers for presenting new information (i.e., init), acknowledging their partner's ideas (i.e., ack), and adjusting ideas with their partner.

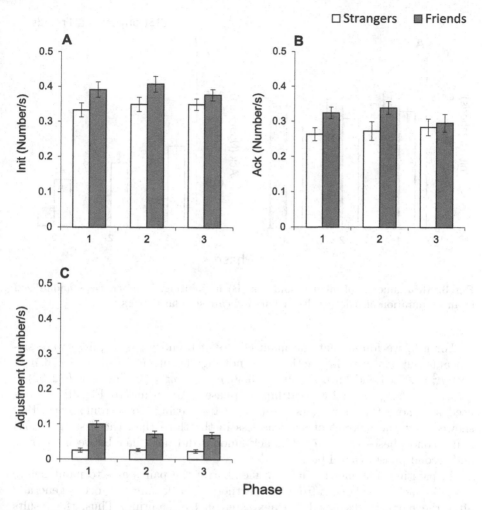

Fig. 2. Mean number of init (A), ack (B), and adjustment (C) in conversations. Number was standardized by mean duration of conversations. Error bars indicate standard errors.

Painting. Figure 3 shows the mean number of the init and ack functions for strangers and friends in each phase. The values were also standardized by the mean duration of painting. Interestingly, strangers appeared to use ack more but init less than friends.

To confirm this, we conducted a 2 (friendship as a between-subject factor) × 3 (phase as a within-subject factor) mixed analysis of variance for each function. For init, the main effect of friendship approached significance, but that of phase and two-way interaction were not significant, $F(1, 46) = 3.16, p = .08, \eta_p^2 = .06$ (friendship), $F(2, 92) = 0.36, p = .70, \eta_p^2 = .008$ (phase), $F(2, 92) = 0.02, p = .98, \eta_p^2 < .001$ (friendship × phase). As shown in Fig. 3A, friends used init more than strangers.

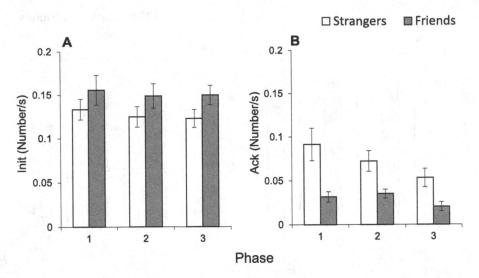

Fig. 3. Mean amount of init (A) and ack (B) in painting. Number was standardized by mean duration of painting. Error bars indicate standard errors.

For ack, we found that the main effects of friendship and phase were significant, but two-way interaction was not significant, $F(1, 46) = 16.56, p < .001, \eta_p^2 = .27$ (friendship), $F(2, 92) = 3.40, p = .04, \eta_p^2 = .07$ (phase), $F(2, 92) = 1.13, p = .33, \eta_p^2 = .02$ (friendship × phase). According to Fig. 3B, friends used ack more than strangers. Post-hoc t-tests using Bonferroni's correction showed that the amount of ack was less in the third than the first ($p = .04$) and second phases ($p = .07$). The ack amount did not differ between the first and second phases ($p = 1.00$).

In painting, init means that one member of the pair starts to paint before obtaining acknowledgment from the partner; but ack functions occur generally after the partners discussed the next step in the painting. Thus, the results indicate that friends tended to start painting without discussing what to paint next, but strangers tended to reproduce the painting after such discussion.

4   Discussion

In the present study, we found communication differences between friends and strangers in terms of the duration they spent on painting, the overlapping duration of their conversation and painting, and the time they spent before painting. These results indicate that painting-relevant behaviors differed as a function of friendship.

Friends spent more time painting and talked more while painting. Our analyses of communicative functions show that friends used more inits in painting, suggesting that for them, painting presents information in a similar way as conversation and gestures do. The behavior of friends reflects their prior shared experiences (Chelune et al., 1984). Even if something goes wrong with the task, they might have a strategy to solve the problem, or for most cases they actually share a relationship that permits mistakes by partners. Friends might use fewer cognitive resources to adjust their relationships with their partner, enabling them to focus on the efficient completion of tasks by directly expressing their ideas on paper.

On the other hand, strangers spent more time before starting to paint in the first phase and tended to paint after obtaining their partner's acknowledgment (shown in the ack function in painting), indicating that strangers are unlikely to use painting as a communication medium like friends. For strangers, painting is the output of verbal and/or gestural communication. According to Simons and Peterson (2000), relationship or emotional conflicts are perceptions of interpersonal incompatibility and typically include tension, annoyance, and animosity among group members. Such a relationship conflict is likely to occur when they lack adequate information about other members (Fujiwara et al., 2012). In our collaborative reproduction task, all of the pair members might have different impressions even if they were exposed to the same painting, due to the abstract nature of Cubist art. Even so, conflict among people sharing close relationships is easily solved (Fujiwara et al., 2012). However, strangers might experience such conflicts with their partners because they lack information about each other. To avoid conflicts, they are likely to verbally defend their own impressions in advance and acknowledge the entreaties of their partner by painting.

In conclusion, strangers and friends show different strategies in sharing the abstract information contained in Cubist paintings. Strangers tend to choose a style that emphasizes verbal question and painting answers (i.e., insisting that they remember verbally and start painting based on it) to avoid relationship conflicts. In contrast, friends tend to talk and paint together to efficiently complete tasks. These results suggest several implications for clinical applications. Turn-taking by talking and painting might be useful when a caregiver shares information at first meeting with clients. Future work will investigate whether this can be applied to real contexts.

Acknowledgments. The contents of this study are based on the second author's master thesis. We thank Yuejun Zheng, who supervised and generously supported the second author's master thesis. We also thank 48 students at Doshisha University for their participation in our experiment, Koshi Nishimoto and Yu Ohshima for checking the validity of our measurements, and Haru Nitta and Kana Shirai for their valuable inputs for this study.

References

Åkerman, P., Puikkonen, A., Virolainen, A., Huuskonen, P., Häkkilä, J.: Sketching with strangers: in the wild study of Ad-hoc social communication by drawing. In: Proceedings of the 2010 ACM Conference on Ubiquitous Computing, pp. 193–202 (2010)

Chelune, G.J., Robison, J.T., Kommor, M.J.: A cognitive interaction model of intimate relationships. In: Derlega, V.J. (ed.) Communication, Intimacy, and Close Relationships, pp. 11–40. Academic Press, Orlando (1984)

Dohi, Y.: The Birth of Abstract Art. Hakusuisha, Tokyo (1984). (in Japanese)

Fujiwara, K., Daibo, I., Maeda, N., Yokoyama, H., Maeda, T., Kishino, F., Kitamura, Y., Hayashi, Y.: Transitional features of multiple conversations: the influence of dyadic conversation on following triadic conversation. IEICE Technical report (HIP), 110, 79–84 (2010). (in Japanese)

Fujiwara, K., Daibo, I., Matsuyama, S.: The communication behavior and interpersonal perception in task oriented small group (2): communication behavior and interpersonal relationships. IEICE Technical report (HCS) 111, 79–84 (2012). (in Japanese)

Lausberg, H., Sloetjes, H.: Coding gestural behavior with the NEUROGES-ELAN system. Behav. Res. Meth. Instr. 41, 841–849 (2009)

McNeill, D.: Psycholinguistics: A New Approach. Harper and Row, New York (1987)

Mehrabian, A.: Silent Messages. Wadsworth, Belmont (1971)

Simons, T.L., Peterson, R.S.: Task conflict and relationship conflict in top management teams: the pivotal role of intragroup trust. J. Appl. Psychol. 85, 102–111 (2000)

Takeoka, A., Shimojima, A., Katagiri, Y.: Turn-taking in graphical communication: an exploratory study. In: Proceedings of the Fourth SIGdial Workshop on Discourse and Dialogue, pp. 34–38 (2003)

Traum, D.R.: A Computational Theory of Grounding in Natural Language Conversation. Unpublished Ph.D. Dissertation, Department of Computer Science, University of Rochester (1994)

United Nations: 2009 Energy Statistics Yearbook. Department for Economic and Social Information and Policy Analysis,Statistics Division, United Nations, New York (2012)

Process Analysis of Expert and Non-expert Engineers in Quartz Glass Joint Process

Masamichi Suda[1(✉)], Toru Takahashi[2], Akio Hattori[2], Yuqiu Yang[3],
Akihiko Goto[4], and Hiroyuki Hamada[5]

[1] Kyoto Institute of Technology, Kyoto, Japan
Masamichi_suda@daico.co.jp
[2] Techno Eye Corporation, Kyoto, Japan
{takahashi,yoshi_suda}@daico.co.jp
[3] College of Textiles, Donghua University, Shanghai, China
amy_yuqiu_yang@dhu.edu.cn
[4] Department of Information Systems Engineering,
Faculty of Design Technology, Osaka Sangyo University, Osaka, Japan
gotoh@ise.osaka-sandai.ac.jp
[5] Advanced Fibro-Science, Kyoto Institute of Technology, Kyoto, Japan
hhamada@kit.ac.jp

Abstract. Quartz glass is a special glass material known as "King of Glass". The silicon purity of the quartz glass is very high, therefore it is excellent in heat resistance, chemical resistance and optical transparency as compared to other glasses, such as borosilicate glass. In this study, the differences in the working process between engineers with different years of experience during the "joint-process" of quartz glass material were analyzed. "Joint-process" is one of "fire-process" and is of heating and jointing glass cylinders during rotating using a dedicated glass lathe machine. It is found that these differences in the process of heating joint of glass cylinder have effects on the accuracy of finial production and the manufacturing efficiency.

Keywords: Ergonomics and sustainability · Quartz glass · Process analysis · Fire process · Mechanical property evaluation

1 Introduction

Quartz glass is a special glass material known as "King of Glass". The silicon purity of the quartz glass is very high, therefore it is excellent in heat resistance, chemical resistance and optical transparency as compared to other glasses, such as borosilicate glass.

At present, it is used in the production field of leading-edge. Now researches are carried out to develop it as key components of special manufacturing equipment, scientific instruments and analysis equipment that require high-precision, high purity, the high light transmittance. However, due to its high heat resistance, it is difficult to be processed into various shapes. As a result, manufactured quarts glass products, generally, might be different even in one batch. To respond to such products for precision instruments, it is preferable to select the heat molding process by flame called "fire-process" in many cases. "fire-process" is the process of forming a softening point of

© Springer International Publishing Switzerland 2015
V.G. Duffy (Ed.): DHM 2015, Part I, LNCS 9184, pp. 389–398, 2015.
DOI: 10.1007/978-3-319-21073-5_39

heated quartz glass material by a mixed combustion flame of hydrogen and oxygen. Therefore, a technique for forming a glass material softened by heating is required, and now it is done by human hand processing of engineers. While skilled human technique of long time experience is required in order to produce high precision and an efficient products. Therefore digitizing and analysis of the work of expert engineers with high level of hand skill is needed to increase the processing technology of the engineers less skilled and take advantage in the manufacture of high-precision products. In this study, the differences in the working process between engineers with different years of experience during the "fire-process" of quartz glass material were analyzed. Fire-process is of heating joint glass cylinders during rotating using a dedicated glass lathe machine. The working behaviors of three operators were recorded by videos during "fire-process". And the thickness of jointed part of final products was measured by ultrasonic equipment to evaluate the quality of the jointed situation. And a test piece of processing area was measured mechanical properties. It is found that these differences in the process of heating joint of glass cylinder have effects on the accuracy of finial production and the manufacturing efficiency.

As we all know, quartz glass has been applied in many fields such as optical equipment, medical appliance, and space industry due to its excellent performance in heat resistance, chemical resistance and optical transparency. Therefore, high working accuracy was required when people want to get a special shape. However, Because of the high heat resistance, it's difficult for quartz glass to be shaped. To meet the requirement of manufacturing quarts glass products, the process of heat molding by flame called "fire-process" was selected. "fire-process" is forming a softening point of heated quartz glass material by a mixed combustion flame of hydrogen and oxygen. Operators do all the processes by controlling the rotating disk of glass lathe which can change the position of object and the temperature of flame. The technique for forming a glass material softened by heating was done by hand processing engineers. Finally, the quality of products may be different because of different efficiency of engineer. Accumulating the experience of manufacture is a long time work which can't be quantified. With the problem of aging of skilled operators is becoming more and more serious, youth who can inherit the crafts will decrease. In order to pass down the excellent technique of skilled engineer in a shot time, digitalization of the work behavior and technique is highly required. Therefore, in this study, the "fire-processing" of glass material with high processing difficult of quartz glass, the comparison in the working process of the technology among different experience operators has been discussed. Meanwhile, the effect of processing technology on thickness of quartz tube was analyzed.

2   Material and Experimental Method

The "fire-process" is the generic term of processes such as bending, stretching, expanding glass which was previously heated by fire. When manufacturing the product, glass tube was fixed on dedicated rotating disks, then the glass tube was heated and the disk were rotated simultaneously. This method is often used today.

In this study, the heating jointing process had been carried out as experimental method. Recently, the inevitable trend of manufacturing the products into large-scale, complex, high-precision and keeping the product accuracy stability make it important to adjust the handcraft and machine operation to achieve high-quality products. Meanwhile, only to change a machine makes no contribution to improve the operability and accuracy, thus the processes of operators with different experience in identical condition of experiment were mainly discussed.

Two quartz glass tubes had been prepared to be connected by glass lathe with the combination heating flame including hydrogen and oxygen. The sizes of quartz tube were as follow: outside diameter is 33 mm, inside diameter is 30 mm, and length is 378 mm. The machine used to conduct all processes was called "GLASS LATHE". Ultrasonic thickness tester type is CTS-30 A with 0.01 mm measurement precision. Because of the distribution of thickness of tube was uneven. Before the experiment was carried out, the measurement of thickness of glass tube was conducted around center of tube at every 10 mm interval. Because thickness of every unprocessed tube has little difference, the measurement mentioned previously can assist to record the tiny changes of thickness of the tube before and after the processing. Measurement points was shown in Fig. 1.

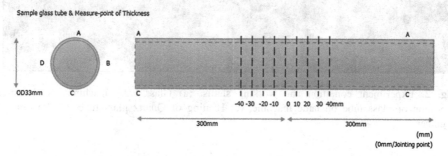

Fig. 1. Measure-point of Thickness in glass tube sample

Figure 2(a–d) show experiment condition and working status where Fig. 2(a) shows the working status of glass lathe machine for quartz glass fire-process. In the glass lathe machine, Left-Chuck was stationary and Right-chuck was controlled by Right-Chuck Handle. The two chucks were rotating simultaneously. When jointing two tubes, the right-chuck move from right to left is to make two separated tubes more closely. Figure 2(b) show installed condition of glass tube on lathe machine. As it is shown in Fig. 2(c), the burner was settled between two chucks and faced two tubes which can move horizontally to heating the arbitrary part of tube. The flame with 2000°C which can soften the quartz glass was generated by the combination of hydrogen and oxygen. Additionally, the position of operator was shown in Fig. 2(d).

From the very beginning of the experiment, quartz glass tube was divided into two parts from the centre of length direction, and then the two parts of tubes were fixed on right-chuck and left-chuck respectively and jointed into one tube by heating flame.

Operator completed three tubes each time, when conductor gave the command of beginning, they started to working in process usual. For avoiding the bad effect on operators, others were not permitted to watch their actions when they entered the working condition.

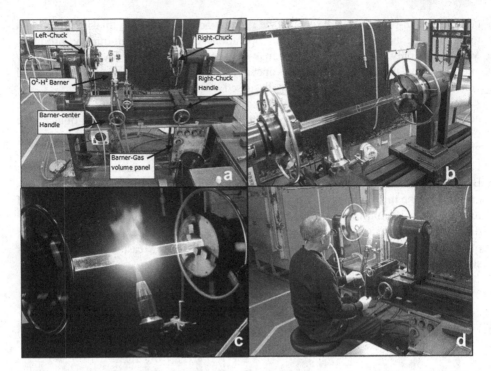

Fig. 2. Experiment condition and working status: (a) Glass lathe machine; (b) Installed condition of glass tube on lathe machine; (c) Heating of Quartz glass tube; (d) Position of engineer.

3 digital cameras were applied to record the operator's action from start to end, which helped researchers could carry out the analysis their actions.

3   Operators' Information

In this study, three different experience operators were invited as subjects where expert-advance has 54 years of experience, expert has 20 years of experience, non-expert has 5 years of experience (Table 1).

Table 1. Subjects information

Type	Years of process experience
Expert-Advance(Exp-A)	54 years
Expert(Exp-B)	20 years
Non-Expert	5 years

Three operators was selected from engineers who works on fire process every day and their experiment of operate was continuous for many years.

4 Results

First of all, the processes which was recorded from video with which corresponding time is used to make the chart graph to analyze the action of operators. Chart graphs show three operator's processing schedules.

The processes of jointing were 'Non-processing' 'Fin-heating Right' 'Fin-heating Left' 'Carbon tool process' 'Heating of joint area' 'Jointing' 'Pre-heating Right' 'Pre-heating Left' respectively as they were shown in Fig. 3(a–c).

There were different proportions of Time-cost of each process in the graph in three charts which may reveal the efficiency of operations. For example, the ratio of 'the No-operation time' to 'the Total Time' among three engineers is Exp-A (0 %) < Non-Exp(8.7 %) < Exp-B(15.9 %).

Figure 4 show the total time of three operators, and it's obvious that the shorter time they used, the higher proficiency they had. Total used time of expert-A was 4 min and 15 s averagely, however, Non-Exp was 6 min 15 s averagely, and they had a difference value of 2 min and 12 s. The difficulties was known from the operators that if it takes too much times, the shape of tube would collapse which could make the process fail.

Also, the proportions of theses processes based on total processing time of three operators were shown in Fig. 5. The huge disparity between Exp-A and Exp-B can be seen from the 'Pre-heating Right' and 'Pre-heating Left' which shows that it took Exp-A 47 s, Exp-B 1 min 4 s, but Non-Exp only 5 s averagely for Pre-heating respectively. Meanwhile, it can be seen that for Exp-A there is almost no 'Non-processing' time, while that of Exp-B and Non-Exp were 29″ and 1′1″ respectively. And it can be known from video that the Non-Exp were observing by eyes and confirming next processing step.

The thicknesses changes of glass tubes of each operators were measured after processing and the results shown in Fig. 6. The trend that there was no huge disparity in the amount of change from start to end around joint part of Exp-A's processes. However, the changes of Non-Exp were that joint part became thicker while vicinity of the point where there is 10 mm from center sharply thinned, which was also can be seen from Exp-B case but not so obviously.

With respect to total length of each subject were also measured at the start to end of process. The results were shown in Fig. 7. It's obvious that the total length of Exp-B tube shortened −0.49 mm, that of Non-Exp tube shortened +0.04 while that of Exp-A tube shortened −2.2 mm.

The average bending strength of 4-point bending test results shown in Fig. 8.

Typical data of the material manufacturer is $65 \sim 95$ N/mm^2. The average value of this 3, Exp-B was 58.37 N/mm^2, Non-Exp was 47.33 N/mm^2. For these, the average value of the Exp-A was 70.21 N/mm^2.

5 Analysis

It can be inferred from the whole process as the chart graph shows, in order to make a easy condition for processing, experienced operator would spend some time in Pre-heating the joint part and the area around there. Although heating the glass for a

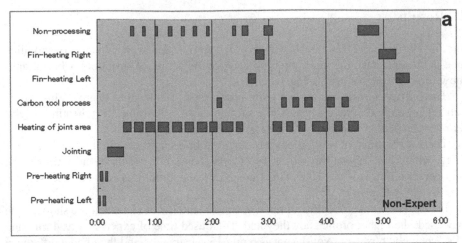

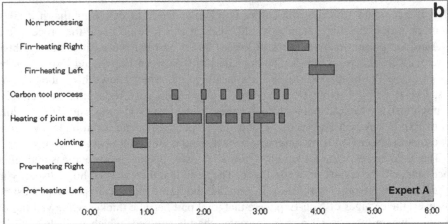

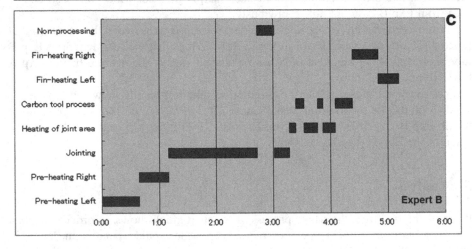

Fig. 3. Process time chart: (a) Non-expert; (b) Expert A; (c) Expert-B

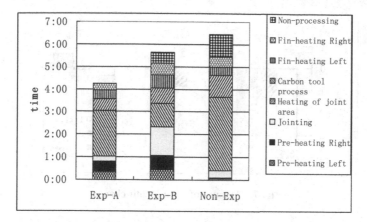

Fig. 4. Average of process time

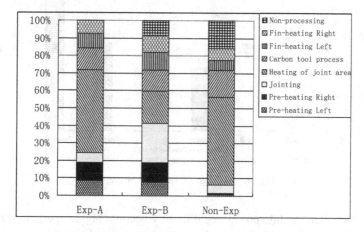

Fig. 5. Percentage of process time

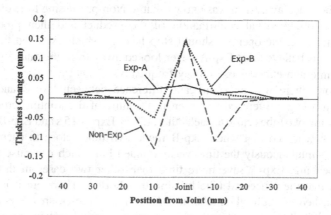

Fig. 6. Thickness changes of quartz glass tube after process among Non-Exp, Exp-A, Exp-B

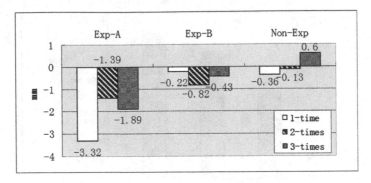

Fig. 7. Amount of total length change

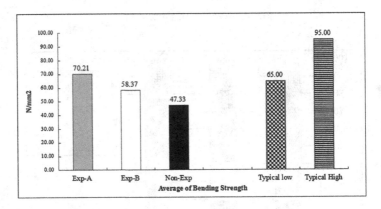

Fig. 8. Average of bending strength

long time can soften it while processing difficulty become high, experienced operators like Exp-A, Exp-B could still control the shape of quartz tube perfectly.

Now sight was focused on that the Non-processing time of Exp-A was extremely short. From the video analysis it was known that in Non-processing time of Exp-B and Non-Exp were doing visual confirmation of the product and then proceeding the process. In that case, the operator should stop heating which extended the total processing time. It is believed that Exp-A never looked away from the quartz glass during processing while non-expert looked away frequently.

Furthermore, there was no significant difference between Exp-B and Exp-A in procedure, but a large difference was seen in the time of the jointing process. In the process of putting two tubes close to each other, it took Exp-A 15 s and Exp-B 1 min 16 s.

It can be considered that when Exp-B made two tubes close to each other with heating tubes simultaneously the time was extended but which can raise risk failing. Relatively speaking, Exp-A save more time than other two cases in this procedure which shows that the processed tube became the shortest. Therefore it is considered that Exp-A pushed the right glass tube in order to make a thick area. Pre-arrangement can be adopted for forming uniformly thick portion with subsequent processes.

In this way, Exp-A has the highest operant level that he has ability of integrating lots of processes as a whole which including control the processing condition and pushing the glass tube to make the thick area etc. It can decrease the time costs. However, Non-Exp didn't have the experience like Exp-A which increased the processing time.

Practician a operation is the highest level, he can offer several ongoing operation of the process (processed at the same time grasp the processing state, and then the joint of the quartz tube at the same time to push yes joints thickening) integration done at the same time, to shorten the processing time successfully.

Comparing the processing of Exp-A and Exp-B, the change of the glass tube thickness after processed in Exp-A was less than Exp-B. Although it is generally recognized that carbon tool process make effects on glass tube thickness control, there is no obvious evidence can prove that the carbon tool process is not changed by consciously operating of engineer. To consider the factor of controlling the thickness of tube is the series procedure of 'Pre-heating-Jointing-Heating around' with combining Exp-A's Pre-arrangement and jointing methods. With respect to the timing and discharge amount of air processed by operators themselves with blowing air into the glass tube from their mouth, the experiments haven't been conducted yet. It is necessary to analyze the air discharge aspect in the future.

And In this study we could test the bending strength of this sample pieces. As a result of the fact destructive testing, four-point bending strength of the Exp-A was very close to the Typical-data provided by the material manufacturer. Therefore, even in comparison to the original material and the sample Exp-A was Joint, it can be said that a quality very close in strength. As shown Exp-A thickness measurement results after Processing, it is believed that this result was born because it was more uniform about wall thickness compared to the other two engineers.

6 Conclusion

In this study, the analysis of "fire-process" was carried out to find the difference between Non-Expert and Expert-B.

The result shows that there was a clear difference in the product quality based on skill maturity. Especially, the proficient operators can operate several processes simultaneously and use short-term eye view confirmation to judge the situation of glass tube and then process immediately which can improve the efficiency and high quality. However, Non-Exp did those processes step by step without synthesize them well which increase the total processing time.

7 Further Experiment

In this study, the data were obtained by carrying out three operators as subjects and let them processing three quartz glass tubes respectively to analyze the results. But it was only a pilot and continuing to investigate the correlation experiments is necessary.

The data of operator's air discharge, timing and measurement of change amount in the product shape in processing have not been conducted yet. Considering further experimental method and carry out new analysis for improve the quality of processing quartz glass products is highly required.

References

1. Cibiel, G.: "Ultra stable oscillators dedicated for space applications: oscillator and quartz material behaviors vs. radiation". In: 2006 IEEE, International Frequency Control Symposium and Exposition. IEEE (2006)
2. Rongkai, H.: "Research on the forming technique and surface treatment process of quartz glass bulbs for arc tubes". In: 2011 Second International Conference on Mechanic Automation and Control Engineering (MACE). IEEE (2011)
3. Cobbold, G.W.N., Underdown, A.E.: Some practical applications of quartz resonators. Inst. Electr. Eng. Proc. Wirel. Sect. Inst. 3(9), 151–162 (1928)
4. Kaplan, W., Elderstig, H., Veider, C.: A novel fabrication method of capillary tubes on quartz for chemical analysis applications. In: Proceedings, IEEE Workshop on. Micro Electro Mechanical Systems, 1994, MEMS 1994. IEEE (1994)
5. Booth, C.F.: The application and use of quartz crystals in telecommunications. J. Inst. Electr. Eng. Part III: Commun. Eng. 88(2), 97–128 (1941)

Comparison of Eye Movement During the Polishing Process of Metallographic Sample Between Expert and Nonexpert

Takuya Sugimoto[1(✉)], Yuka Takai[2], Hiroyuki Nishimoto[3],
and Akihiko Goto[2]

[1] Kyoto Institute of Technology, Kyoto, Japan
t-sugi@koyo-kinzoku.com
[2] Osaka Sangyo University, Osaka, Japan
takai@ise.osaka-sandai.ac.jp,
hiroyuki.nishimoto@outlook.com
[3] Takeda Pharmaceutical Company Limited, Tokyo, Japan
gotoh@ise.osaka-sandai.ac.jp

Abstract. The carburizing process requires metallurgical inspection by means of polished metallurgical mounts. Metallographic preparation for a metallurgical mount is an important process for the quality assurance of the carburizing process. The purpose of this study is to clarify the expert's characteristics of polishing process based on the eye movement analysis. Two inspectors with 20 (hereinafter referred to as "expert") and 0.5 years (hereinafter referred to as "nonexpert") of experience in metallographic preparation were interviewed and their eye movement analyzed. As a result, the expert made pressure adjustments and cleaning the surface and supplying alumina as needed while performing the polish.

Keywords: Polish · Metallographic preparation · Eye movement analysis

1 Introduction

The most common heat treatment process for hardening ferrous alloys is known as carburizing. Usually one or more test specimens for quality assurance accompany the carburizing process. The quality assurance of the carburizing process requires metallographic analysis of case depth, core hardness, intergranular oxidation, network carbide, and retained austenite with an optical microscope at × 100–1000 magnification by means of metallographic mounted samples. An accurate metallographic analysis is very important for heat treater to develop their process or improve their product reliability [1–3].

To achieve an accurate analysis, the true microstructure of the carburized part must be preserved during the metallographic sample preparation. Unfortunately, case-hardened part such as carburized part has several hardness variations in a single part that would normally require difficult grinding/polishing operations, especially with complicated shape part such as gear part. As a result, harmful scratches or the rounding or the specimen has occurred on the polished surface. If the sample has such problem, it leads wasting of time and money because re-grinding and polishing operations are

© Springer International Publishing Switzerland 2015
V.G. Duffy (Ed.): DHM 2015, Part I, LNCS 9184, pp. 399–410, 2015.
DOI: 10.1007/978-3-319-21073-5_40

required. Metallographic preparation consists of sectioning, mounting, grinding and polishing, and etching. Herein, we focus on the grinding and polishing process.

Grinding and polishing of a mounted sample removes sectioning damage and creates a polished surface for evaluation. This process is usually performed manually (handheld) or by automated method with many sizes of an abrasive.

In fact, the surface finishes of metallurgical samples of carburized gears differ between expert and nonexpert preparations even though grinding and polishing are performed by semi-automated machine. In other words, it is difficult for a nonexpert to continuously supply stable conditions (i.e., minimum scratch and limited edge rounding) for a metallographic sample. In particular, a case-hardened gear part such as a carburized gear is difficult to grind and polish because the grinding and polishing rate varies depending on the hardness of the mount, which consists of metal and mount materials although mirror finishes and edge retention are required for near-surface inspections. Many techniques for grinding and polishing are contained in standards or technical documents [4–8]. Metallographic preparation for thermal sprayed sample has been studied [9]. However, no research has focused on the difference between the grinding and polishing of metallographic sample by experts and nonexperts. This research compares and contrasts the eye movements of an expert and non-expert as they each perform grinding for metallographic sample, then clarifies the characteristics of the work of the experts.

2 Measurement Method

The subjects were a researcher with 20 years of experience (the expert) and another one with 2.5 years of experience (the non-expert). A 9310 (AMS6265) gear (pitch diameter: 24.5 mm), cut into a quarter of a gear consisting of four teeth, was used as a sample. The subjects were given samples that had already undergone heat embedding, the final step before grinding and polishing, which were to be performed by the expert and non-expert using a semi-automatic grinding machine (by Refinetec, STO-228 K). The grinding sheet used was P120, P400 SiC grinding sheet. The polishing was done by P1200's SiC grinding sheet and 5 µ, 0.3 µm of alumina. Eye movements were measured with Talk Eye II by Takei Scientific Instruments Co., Ltd. at a sampling rate of 30 Hz. The final roughness measurement was performed with an ultra-precision measurement system (Talysurf PGI by Taylor Hobson). After the grinding work was completed, the subjects were interviewed as needed, and researchers studied what eye movements of the expert corresponded to a surface finish that had minimal inconsistencies.

3 Results

3.1 The Position of Subject's Hand and Line of Vision

Figure 1 shows the position of the subject's hand and line of vision during the SiC grinding.

P120. The expert's line of vision was on the rotation speed adjustment control of the grinding board for 9.1 s, 10.2 s after he began the grinding work. During that time, his hands stayed on the control, and after 19.5 s, his eyes were focused on the pressure control handle until 29.4 s. Until the grinding work was done at 81.7 s, the expert's eyes went back and forth 8 times between the pressure control handle and the rotation speed adjustment control. The expert's hands stayed on the pressure control handle for 19.1 s from 17.3 s, gradually increasing the pressure, and never returning to the pressure control handle.

On the other hand, after staying on the pressure control handle for 1.8 s from 1.1 s, the non-expert's eyes never returned to the pressure control handle until the end of the grinding work, his eyes instead going between the grinding board and elsewhere. The non-expert's hands were on the pressure control handle from 1.0 s for 1.8 s, but they never went back there.

P400. The expert's eyes were on the pressure control handle 1.2 s after he began grinding and went back and forth 11 times between the pressure control handle and the grinding board or the clock until he completed the grinding work. His hands stayed on the pressure control handle for 25.0 s from 6.9 s, applying pressure gradually.

The non-expert, on the other hand, had his hands on the pressure control handle from 2.2 s for 1.8 s, but never to return until after the grinding was complete at 40.8 s. His eyes went back and forth between the grinding board and the clock. His hands were on the pressure control handle from 2.3 s for 1.8 s, but after that, they never returned to the pressure control handle.

P1200. The expert's eyes stayed on the pressure control handle for 1.8 s, 2.2 s after the grinding rotation board began operating. Until the end of the grinding work, his gaze traveled from the pressure control hand to the grinding board or the clock four times. The expert's hands were on the pressure control handle for 19 s from 4.9 s onward, gradually increasing the pressure.

On the other hand, the non-expert's gaze stayed for 2 s on the pressure control handle 1.1 s after the grinding rotation board began operating. From then on, his gaze never went back to the pressure control handle until after the grinding work was complete, but went back and forth between the grinding rotation board and elsewhere. The non-expert's hands were on the pressure control handle for 1.8 s from 2.0 s, and after setting the pressure until the grinding work was done, they never went back to any grinding work.

Figure 2 shows the position of the subject's hand and line of vision during the Alumina polishing.

5 μm. The expert's gaze stayed on the rotation speed adjustment control for 4 s, 0 s after the grinding rotation board began operating. His hands were on the rotation speed adjustment control for 4 s from 0 s, adjusting the rotation speed. From 7.1 s, the expert's gaze went back and forth five times between the pressure control handle and the grinding rotation board for 17.9 s. The expert's hands were on the pressure control handle for 6.8 s from 11 s, gradually applying pressure. From 23.8 s until 90.1 s, his gaze traveled back and forth between the alumina bolt and the rotation board eight times. During this time, his hands were on the alumina bolt and water supply nozzle, reaching for the alumina twice and water once for rinsing purposes.

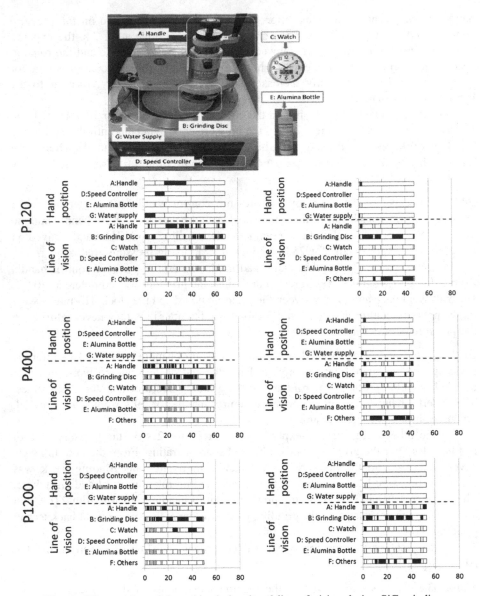

Fig. 1. The position of the subject's hand and line of vision during SiC grinding

The non-expert's eyes stayed on the pressure control handle from 0 s for 1.8 s, but never went back there until the end of the grinding work. His eyes went back and forth four times between the grinding board and the alumina bolt from 3.0 s, reaching for the alumina three times, the water once.

0.3 μm. The expert's eyes stayed on the grinding board from 0 s for 9.9 s, his hands on the water supply nozzle from 0 s to 9.8 s, cleaning the grinding board. His gaze went

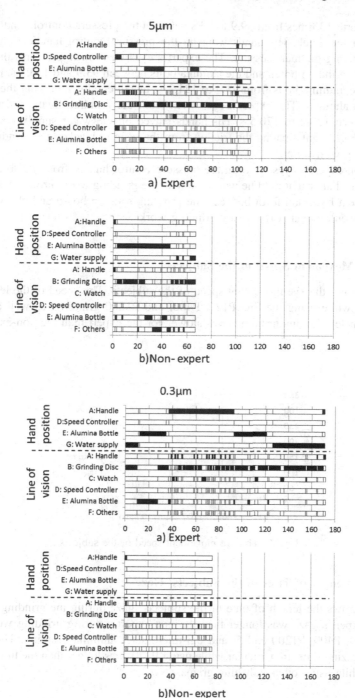

Fig. 2. The position of subjct's hand and line of vision during Alumina polishing

back and forth 13 times from 39.9 to 93 s between the pressure control handle and the grinding or the clock. His hands were on the pressure control handle from 37.2 to 92.8 s, applying gradual pressure. The expert's eyes went back and forth three times between the grinding board and the alumina bolts between 93.9 and 123.3 s. His hands were on the alumina bolts from 93.9 to 121.2 s, incrementally supplying the grinding board with alumina. The expert's eyes went from the grinding board and the clock twice between 123.2 to 170.5 s. His hands stayed on the water supply nozzle from 126.4 to 169.1 s, anticipating the friction from the resin to blacken the grinding board and cleaning with water.

The non-expert's eyes were on the pressure control handle from 1.2 to 2.1 s, but never returned after that until he was done with the grinding work. From 3.8 s onward, his gaze went back and forth between the grinding rotation board and elsewhere, but his hands would never perform any grinding work.

3.2   Eye Movement Speed of the Subjects

Figure 3 shows the eye movement speed of the subjects. The speed of the left eyeball movement while using the SiC P120, P400, and P1200 grinding, as well as 5- and 0.3-micrometer alumina grinding, was slower for the expert than the non-expert.

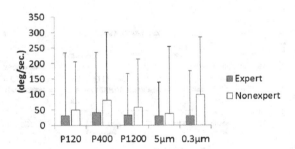

Fig. 3. The eye movement speed of the subjects

3.3   The Length of Time of the Subjects' Gaze

Figure 4 shows the length of time of the subjects' gaze during the grinding work.

The expert's gaze was longer than the non-expert's during grinding work, using SiC's p120, P400, P1200 and 5- and 0.3-micrometer alumina grinding. The expert's length of gazing time, in particular while using P120, was longer than the time he spent looking while using other polishing grains.

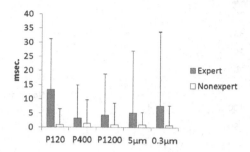

Fig. 4. The length of time of the subjects' gaze

3.4 Characteristic Movements of the Subjects' Eyeballs During Grinding Work

Figure 5 shows characteristic movements of the subjects' eyeballs during grinding work. While adjusting the grinding pressure, the expert fixed his gaze on the grinding handle itself and let it follow the rotation of the handle. Furthermore, while increasing the pressure by rotating the handle, the expert let his gaze go back and forth between the grinding board and the handle. The non-expert, by comparison, moved his gaze to where he was about to set the handle, and unlike the expert, didn't allow his gaze to follow the movement of the handle. Also, the non-expert's gaze while adjusting the pressure didn't go back and forth between the grinding board and the handle.

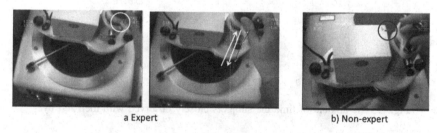

a Expert   b) Non-expert

Fig. 5. Characteristic movements of the subjects' eyeballs during adjusting pressure

3.5 The Speed of the Subjects' Left Eyeball Movement

Figure 6 shows the speed of the subjects' left eyeball movement while observing the polished surface. After grinding work with all the SiCs was complete, the expert was slower than the non-expert. Especially after grinding with P400 and P1200, the expert was more than four times slower than the non-expert.

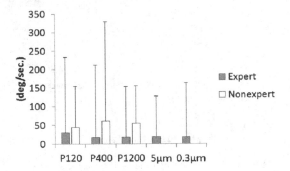

Fig. 6. The speed of the subjects' left eyeball movement while observing the polished surface

3.6 The Amount of Time the Subjects Closely Observed with their Left Eye While Inspecting the Polished Surface

Figure 7 shows the amount of time the subjects closely observed with their left eye while observing the polished surface. The expert's length of time with SiC grinding with P120, P400 and P1200 was longer than that of the non-expert.

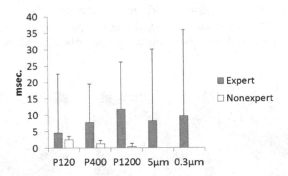

Fig. 7. The amount of time the subjects closely observed with their left eye

3.7 The Characteristics of the Eyeball Movements While Inspecting the Polished Surface

Figure 8 shows the characteristics of the eyeball movements of the subjects while inspecting the polished surface. When inspecting the polished surface, the expert maintained greater distance from the object than the non-expert and kept his gaze steady. Furthermore, the expert tilted the sample to change the angle of the lighting as he inspected. When asked about this, the expert responded that he was looking at the overall balance of the scratches at different angles, rather than confirming each scratch. The non-expert, on the other hand, kept the object closer, his gaze moving about as he inspected. When asked about this, the non-expert responded that he was checking to see the scratches from the previous sandpaper, but wasn't looking for the overall balance.

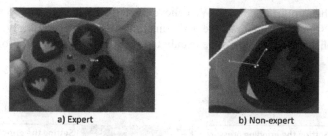

a) Expert   b) Non-expert

Fig. 8. The characteristics of the eyeball movements of the subjects while inspecting the polished surface.

3.8 The Roughness (RMAX) of the Final Average Finish

Figure 9 shows the roughness (RMAX) of the final average finish of the subjects' works – four places on the tooth surface, three places on the dedendum. The average roughness of the expert's work was 1.12 micrometers, whereas that of the non-expert was 2.34 micrometers. The results of t-test show that the expert's finish was significantly less rough ($p < 0.05$).

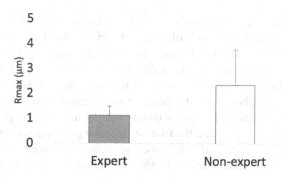

Fig. 9. The roughness (RMAX) of the final average finish of the subjects' works

4 Discussion

Figure 10 shows the flow chart showing the characteristic of subject's grinding work. What was characteristic about the expert's grinding and polishing work was that immediately after he began operating the grinding machine, his hand was on the handle, gradually increasing pressure. Furthermore, during that time, the expert's gaze went back and forth between the handle and the grinding board as he checked on the rotation of the holder, which affixes the sample in place, and the water flow during wet grinding. When asked about this, the expert explained that he was making sure the holder was rotating smoothly, while also listening to the sound the grinding machine was making and gradually increasing the pressure, trying not to cause deep scratches in the unpolished surface. The sound generated during grinding work, other than the grinding noise, is that of the bearing or the motor. We believe the expert was listening to the vibrating and grinding sounds of the machine and adjusting his work accordingly. As a result, cutting by polishing grains was done evenly to create a finish with little roughness and inconsistency.

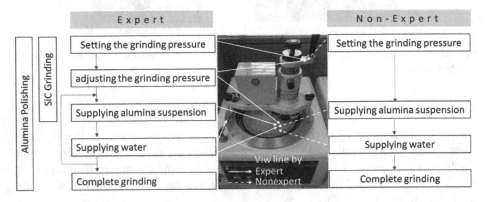

Fig. 10. Flow chart showing the characteristic of subject's grinding work

On the other hand, the non-expert's gaze at the handle was for setting purposes only, and he chose a higher pressure setting than the expert did. He didn't look for any feeling of resistance from the handle, nor listen to the sound generated from the grinding, nor observe the rotation of the holder to see if it would pick up speed then slow down. While the non-expert was aware of the fact that a higher pressure setting would cause deeper scratches or tilt the grinding surface and leave large scratches on the finish, he lacked the ability to make adjustments. As a result, the polishing grains left deep grooves on the surface, and the friction from the grinding generated resistance that caused the rotation speed of the holder to seesaw between acceleration and deceleration. As the holder continued its fast/slow rotation, the resin with its low level of hardness, and the pearlite in the metal areas were deeply scratched, but not the hard martensite layer on the surface of the metal, which made for a rougher and inconsistent finish compared with the expert's.

Furthermore, what was interesting about the expert's gaze while working with 5 and .3 micrometers of alumina is that after he adjusted the pressure, his eyes were mainly on the polishing rotation board. We think that the expert was observing whether the alumina suspension would blacken as a result of the black epoxy getting shaved by the alumina because the test fragment was being impacted. Concluding that an increase in the blackness of the alumina suspension was evidence of effective alumina polishing, after the black color in the suspension liquid increased, the expert added water to clean the top of the polishing board. Seeing the black color of the epoxy mixing with the alumina suspension due to friction, the expert thought that the surface would get big scratches. That is why, after the suspension liquid darkened considerably, he added water and after that, additional alumina suspension. The non-expert, on the other hand, was watching the polishing board and elsewhere, but without checking in on whether the epoxy, which was eroding due to friction, would mix right into the alumina suspension.

Also, what was notable about the expert's gaze while observing the polished surface was that his eyes barely moved and that he inspected the surface as he tilted it. Because of this, we believe, the amount of time the expert spent looking at the specimen was longer than that of the non-expert. By tilting the surface of the specimen to change the angle of the light's reflection and reveal the scratches, the expert was looking for evenness in the overall unpolished surface. The expert's concern was dealing with the scratches that materialized during the cutting of the specimen, erasing scratches that were created two steps before the final polishing process and to confirm that the scratches from the just-completed abrasion showed up in a well-balanced way on the surface. The non-expert was only concerned about the scratches that occurred during cutting the specimen and whether there were scratches left over from two steps back. The non-expert was poring over the entire surface, moving his eyes to check every single scratch. As a result, the speed of the non-expert's eyeball movement was faster than that of the expert, and he spent a shorter amount of time looking.

5 Conclusion

In this research, we observed the way an expert and non-expert performed polishing work on a metal testing specimen and compared their eye movements and their actual polishing motions. And the results show: (1) while performing the polish, the expert made pressure adjustments in considering with the rotation rate of specimen holder, the sound of polishing machine, and the flow of water. On the other hand, the non-expert lacked the ability to make pressure adjustments and left it at the same setting; (2) during alumina polishing, the expert cleaned the surface and supplied alumina as needed, anticipating that the eroded epoxy would mix into the suspension liquid.; (3) the expert's method of studying the unpolished surface involved not moving his gaze, tilting the specimen to observe the surface under changing light. Furthermore, the expert was checking to see, in addition to the amount of scratches present, whether the scratches were scattered across the surface evenly.

References

1. Netsushorigijutsunyuumon, vol. 3. The japan society of heat treatment (2001)
2. Sugioka, N., Kitada, M., Nishijima, M.: Metallurgical microstructure of the spear blade manufactured from the end of muromachi period to the edo period. Jpn. Inst. Met. Mater. 75 (5), 185–191 (2013)
3. Tanaka, M., Kitada, M., Nishijima, M.: Microstructure and nonmetallic inclusion in Japanese percussion lock gun fabricated in the late edo period. Jpn. Inst. Met. Mater. 74(12), 779–787 (2010)
4. Soshikishashinnotsukurikat, vol. 1, Zairyo gijutsu kyoiku kenkyukai (2008)
5. Metallography and Microstructure, vol. 9. ASM Handbook (2004)

6. Hayes, B.S., Gammon, L.M.: Optical Microscopy of Fiber-Reinforced Composites. ASM International, Materials Park (2010). First printing
7. Standard Guide for Preparation of Metallographic Specimen, ASTM E3-01. ASTM International (2007)
8. Samuel, L.E.: Metallographic Polishing by Mechanical Methods. ASM International, Materials Park (2003)
9. Smith, M.F.: A comparison of techniques for the metallographic preparation of thermal sprayed samples. J. Therm. Spray Tech. **2**, 287–294 (1993)

Omotenashi in the Japanese Bridal Market

Shigeyuki Takami[1(✉)], Aya Takai[1], Takuya Sugimoto[2], Masamichi Suda[2],
and Hiroyuki Hamada[2]

[1] Takami Bridal Co., Ltd., Kyoto, Japan
{shigeyuki,a-takei}@takami-bridal.com
[2] Kyoto Institute of Technology, Kyoto, Japan
t-sugi@koyo-kinzoku.com, masamichi_suda@daico.co.jp,
hhamada@kit.ac.jp

Abstract. *Omotenashi* is the Japanese approach to exceptional hospitality. In particular, the *Takami Style of Omotenashi* strives for the continuous improvement of customer satisfaction in the bridal market. While the price of weddings and bridal services are equivalent to purchasing luxury cars or other high end items, bridal clients are willing to pay large amounts of money for services that are not tangible items. Questionnaires were provided to brides and grooms with the purpose of discovering ways to increase customer satisfaction for bridal services.

Keywords: *Omotenashi* · Customer satisfaction · Bridal market · Bridal industry · *Takami style*

1 Introduction

1.1 About the Bridal Industry

The Bridal Industry is significantly unique when compared to other industries. Most industries have a repeat client base that will continuously return for items they need or services they receive. For instance, restaurants, hotels, and retail stores depend on return customers. These types of businesses have clients who could possibly return any given number of times. On the contrary, although a client experiences exceptional services during a wedding ceremony, the chances of those clients returning for the same services are close to none, because in most cases, a wedding is a once in a lifetime event.

The monetary cost of a single wedding is comparable to purchasing high luxury items such as cars and jewelry. However, the difference with weddings in comparison to these other purchases is that upon completion of the ceremony clients are not left with a tangible product. It would be difficult to find many other industries other than the Bridal Industry, where clients willingly spend such large sums of money. Time is thus well spent researching what aspects constitute good customer service, especially given that there is very little existing data (or even dissertations) outlining Bridal Industry research.

V.G. Duffy (Ed.): DHM 2015, Part I, LNCS 9184, pp. 411–418, 2015.
DOI: 10.1007/978-3-319-21073-5_41

2   Methods

There are multiple ways to approach researching customer satisfaction. Customer satisfaction is defined as, "the state of mind that customers have about a company and its products or services when their expectations have been met or exceeded (http://www.qualtrics.com/)." According to this definition, customer service involves a client's opinions, and thus questionnaires are the method of choice for collecting information.

It is important to note that *Omotenashi* is a key component in improving customer satisfaction. However, in order to meet clients' increasing demands for exceptional service, one must keep up with new ways to be innovative and new styles of *Omotenashi* should be implemented. A higher quality of customer service, which is the *Takami Style of Omotenashi* aims to "make people and society happy," The *Takami Style of Omotenashi* is an ideology that involves gathering as many 'thank yous' from clients, and reciprocating that feeling of gratitude with exemplary approaches of tradition, to perpetuate an ever evolving bridal culture. An enduring theme of the Takami Style is *authenticity* whereas no "real" monetary price or brand value can be ascribed to authenticity. Especially when it comes to customer service, authenticity is a quality constantly pursued, and achieved through trials of care, patience, courage, passion, and effort throughout time (http://www.chosakai.or.jp/).

Based on the *Takami Style*, a questionnaire needs to be created and administered with the intent to correct any negative experiences customers may have, and to ensure the highest quality of *Omotenashi* is expressed.

3   The Definition of *Omotenashi*

Wedding trends in the Japanese Bridal Market are often polarizing, and feature contrasting themes and traditions. Unlike many other nations, residents of Japan are generally not religious, thus wedding styles largely reflect current trends. Wedding trends include a Western vs traditional Japanese wedding, or non-traditional themes that include fairy tale weddings.

For the last few decades, the Western style wedding (a Christian-based wedding in a formal chapel with the bride wearing a white wedding gowns and a tuxedo for the groom) with a reception to follow in a banquet room in a luxurious hotel, an upscale restaurant, or special wedding facility have been popular arrangements.

Another mainstream wedding style is a traditional Japanese or Shinto style wedding. The attire for a Shinto-style wedding are a wedding kimono or *shiromuku* for a bride, and a *haori* and *hakama* for a groom, which is a fresh look that is interesting and profoundly representative of traditional culture.

In either Western style or Japanese style, people see that an important quality of service is hospitality. On one hand it is generally agreed upon that hospitality in the Japanese wedding service has improved over time, however on the other hand, the understanding and value of *Omotenashi* in Japanese culture has also changed.

Omotenashi is usually translated merely as hospitality in English. However, the definition of *Omotenashi* in Takami Bridal has a more significant meaning, and exemplifies the ultimate level of hospitality, which not only offers clients satisfaction but also touches the clients' hearts.

Marriage is a momentous occasion in an individual's life, and for most intended to be a once in a lifetime event. With this point in mind, if we are unable to understand our clients' perspectives and their individual stories leading up to marriage, and fail to provide the *Takami Style of Omotenashi*, we would have missed our mark. Every other wedding company offers wedding coordination services. However, we can offer something greater as part of the experience of our *Omotenashi*, which people will never forget in their lifetime.

We continue to receive commendations and 'thank yous' from many satisfied customers throughout the years, as a result of Takami Bridal's commitment to *Omotenashi*. As a result some clients return decades later when their children are planning their weddings, stating they wanted their children to experience the same excellent Takami Style service that they had received at their wedding many years ago.

Given this example, *Omotenashi* could also then be attached to a memory passed on from generation to generation through stories. In the Japanese culture, the traditional values of honor, duty and the fulfillment of one's wishes are deeply instilled within each member of the Takami Bridal organization, and aide of providing our international customers with exceptional customer service. Those values are the core or heart of the company, and are commonly understood as the "company philosophy." Every member of Takami Bridal is inspired to follow through with services that create unforgettable memories to last the lifetime of every customer. One of Takami Bridal's unique approaches to customer service includes owning and operating fine dining restaurants in addition to offering wedding services. Each of our wedding facilities all throughout Japan, and including Hawaii, operate wedding banquets, as well as a fine dining restaurant open to the public all at the same site. By doing so, we are able to offer clients a complete quality experience, as well as executing Omotenashi by providing an opportunity for clients to return to the place where they were married. Many clients also return to celebrate other significant events and special occasions at the restaurant, including wedding anniversaries, marriage proposals, and birthdays. We invite our customers to return to our restaurant where the breathtaking view of the ocean serves as a sentimental memory of the day they celebrated their marriage vows, as well as a reminder of how important it is to appreciate one another.

To understand *Omotenashi* based on data and figures, starting this year Takami Bridal began to administer a new survey to clients called the NSP survey. Through this questionnaire our goal is to understand the quality level of customer service that we provide, as well as our clients' reactions to those services across different wedding facilities. As a whole it is important to understand how our *Omotenashi* motivates customers to bring other customers to our company in the future.

4   Analysis of Questionnaire

The questionnaire is marked by 6 scores: 3 is the highest, 0 is average and -3 is the lowest score. The questions are organized in the following categories:

1. Before the wedding day, evaluate the person in charge in application and meeting
    1.1. Attitude of the person in charge at wedding and banquet
    1.2. Attitude of the person in charge at the dress and tuxedo rental shop
    1.3. Attitude of the person in charge as photographer
2. At the day of wedding
    2.1. Facilities
        2.1.1. Wedding hall or chapel – Atmosphere, location, and appearance
        2.1.2. Access to the wedding hall or chapel
        2.1.3. Banquet hall – Atmosphere, location, and interior
    2.2. Wedding
        2.2.1. Contents of Wedding
        2.2.2. Correspondence of minister
        2.2.3. Choir
3. At the banquet
    3.1. Contents of the banquet
    3.2. Progression
    3.3. Performance (candle light service, cake cut ceremony, etc.)
4. Net Promoter Score (NPS)

5   Results of the Questionnaire

The results of the questionnaire are shown in Tables 1 and 2. Table 1 shows the weddings in Tokyo and Table 2 shows the weddings in Fukuoka.

There are 2 different locations that compare the number of weddings. Tokyo has a larger population than Fukuoka. Both Tables 1 and 2 show that most of clients are satisfied. The factors that are marked with a 3 in each category are necessary for maintaining the highest standard of *Omotenashi* in the Takami Style. Figures 1 and 2 indicate the satisfaction and dissatisfaction of the customers. According to Fig. 1, the average score of 2.2.2 given to the correspondence of minister is the lowest score in the Tokyo region. As reflected in Fig. 2, 1.2 is the lowest score applied to the attitude of the person in charge at the dress and tuxedo rental shop in Fukuoka. However, Fukuoka also scored a high average of 2.2.2.

Each province is represented in different colors. The data provided is based on an average of collected data between the dates of October 2014 to January 2015, and is subject to change entirely within an average of five or so years.

Table 1. The results of the questionnaire in Tokyo (Resource from Takami bridal)

			Application and Meeting before wedding			At the day of wedding									NPS
						1) Facilities			2) Wedding			3) Banquet			
Tokyo			Attitude of the person in charge at wedding and banquet	Attitude of the person in charge at rental dress and tuxedo shop	Attitude of the person in charge at photographer	Wedding hall or chapel of atmosphere, location and appearance	Access to the wedding hall or chapel	banquet hall of atmosphere, location and interior	Contents of wedding	Corresponds nos of minister	choir	Contents of banquet	Progression	Performance (Candle light service, cut in cake etc)	
Year	Wedding Date Month	Day	1–1)	1–2)	1–3)	2–1)-1	2–1)-2	2–1)-3	2–2)-1	2–2)-2	2–2)-3	2–3)-1	2–3)-2	2–3)-3	
2014	9	7	1	1	2	3	1	3	3	2	2	3	3		8
2014	9	13	3	0	0	3	3	3	3	3	3	3	3		7
2014	9	13	-2			3	1		2	2	2				7
2014	9	15	3	3	3	3	3	3	3	2	3	3	3	3	10
2014	9	14	0	3	0	3	3	3	3	2	3	3	3	2	8
2014	10	4	2	2	1	3	2	3	2	1	0	2	1		9
2014	10	4	1	3	1	3	3	3	3	1	2	3			9
2014	10	11	2	-2	0	2	1	2	1	-1	1	1	2	0	7
2014	10	12	2	0	1	1	2	1	3	2	1	3	2		6
2014	10	13	3	3	3	3	3		3	3	3				10
2014	10	18	2	3	3	3	3	3	-1	-3	3	3	3	3	9
2014	10	25	2	2	2	3	2	2	2	1	1	2	2		8
2014	11	8	3	3	3	3	3	3	3	3	3	3	3	3	10
2014	11	15	3	3	3	3	1	3	3	3	3	3	3	3	9
2014	11	22	3	3	3	3	2	3	3	3	0	3	3		10
2014	11	23	1	2	0	2	2	0	1	-1	0	1	0		4
2014	11	29	3	3	3	3	2		3	3	3				9
2014	11	30	3	3	3	2	2	2	2	2	2	3	3	3	9
2014	12	6	1	3	3	3	2	3	3	3	3	3	3	3	9
2014	12	6	2	1	2	3	2	2	1	0	2	3	2		9
2014	12	13	3	3	3	3	3	3	3	3	3	3	3	3	10
2014	12	13	3	3	3	3	3		3	3	3				10
2014	12	28	3	2	2	3	3	1	3	2	3	3	3	2	10
2014	12	28	1	1	3	2	3	2	3	3	3	3	3	2	9
2015	1	3	0	3	0	3	3		3	3	3				10
2015	1	10	0	3	0	3	3	3	2	0	1	3	3	3	9
2015	1	17	2	2	2	3	3	3	2	2	2	2	2	2	9
2015	1	17	3	3	2	3	3	3	0	2		2	3		9
2015	1	18	3	3	3	3	3	3	3	3	3	3	3		10
2015	1	24	3	3	3	3	3	3	3	3	3	3	3	3	10
AVG			2.185	2.407	2.478	2.8	2.433	2.625	2.448	1.964	2.462	2.68	2.696	2.692	8.766667

Table 2. The results of the questionnaire in Fukuoka (Resource from Takami bridal)

Fukuoka			Application and Meeting before wedding			挙式当日に関して									NPS
						1) Facilities			2) Wedding			3) Banquet			
			Attitude of the person in charge at wedding and banquet	Attitude of the person in charge at rental dress and tuxedo shop	Attitude of the person in charge at photographer	Wedding hall or chapel of atmosphere, location and appearance	Access to the wedding hall or chapel	banquet hall of atmosphere, location and interior	Contents of wedding	Correspondence of minister	choir	Contents of banquet	Progression	Performance (Candle light service, out in cake etc)	
Year	Wedding date Month	Day	1-1)	1-2)	1-3)	2-1)-1	2-1)-2	2-1)-3	2-2)-1	2-2)-2	2-2)-3	2-3)-1	2-3)-2	2-3)-3	
2014	9	13	3	3	2	2	3	3	3	3	3	3	3	2	9
2014	10	11	3	3	3	3	3	3	3	3	3	3	3		10
2014	10	14	3	3	3	3	3	3	3	3	2	3	3	3	10
2014	10	18	2	2	2	3	3	3	2	2	2	2	2		8
2014	11	2	3	-3		3	1	-1	3	3	3	3	3		5
2014	11	16	3	2	3	2	0	2	3	3	3	1	2		8
2014	9	14	1	-1	1	2	2	2	2	2	2	0	2		10
2014	11	23	3	3	3	3	3	3	3	3	3	3	3		10
2015	1	11	0	3	3	3	1	3				3	3		8
2015	1	24	3	3	2	1	3	2	2	3	3	3	3	3	9
AVG			2.667	1.8	2.444	2.5	2.444	2.3	2.667	2.778	2.667	2.667	2.7	2.667	8.7

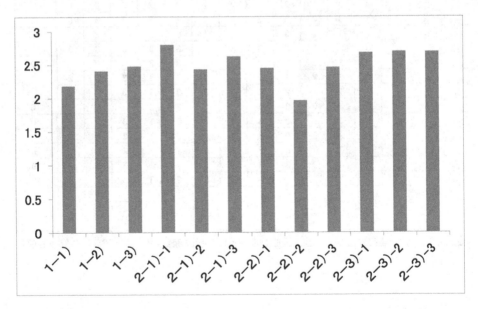

Fig. 1. The strong and weak points of service in Tokyo (Resource from Takami Bridal)

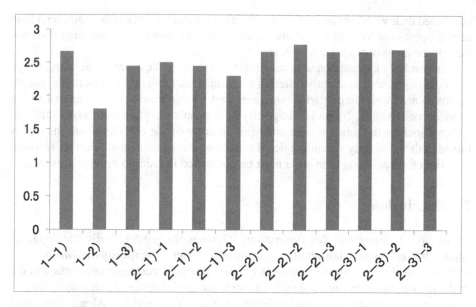

Fig. 2. The strong and weak points of service in Fukuoka (Resource from Takami Bridal)

6 Areas of Consideration

As a result of the questionnaire, there are many areas that scored the highest mark of 3, however these areas can be prioritized within categories. In other words, it needs to evaluate and improve the line of questioning or even consider the timing of which the questionnaire is given to the client. For instance, it is generally known that wedding clients are generally satisfied until the actual wedding day, so depending on when the client was given the questionnaire, the results will be determined based on what the client was feeling at that time.

Here is another example illustrating the importance of timing: By chance a bride may run into another bride at the chapel or wedding hall while filling out the questionnaire, by which her feedback may become influenced by her disappointment. A wedding is one of the greatest highlight events in her life, so the bride must be the main character at the stage. She does not wish to share the stage with another bride.

A third example in which a client's feelings could be reflected in observations of customer service, is considering the various points of interaction with the client. A client may feel completely satisfied throughout the various stages of their wedding planning, up until a certain point when they come across a negative experience. Thus by administering smaller questionnaires at different points of interaction with the client, it makes it possible to investigate when or where the customers feel the most satisfied or dissatisfied. It is necessary for customers to feel satisfied at every stage throughout the wedding service.

Client demographics also need to be considered when analyzing the data collected from the questionnaires. Figures 1 and 2 reflect information based on clients that conducted their weddings in the Tokyo and Fukuoka areas respectively. However, client demographics for Takami Bridal are various, and the information provided does not include the areas of Nagoya, Kyoto, etc.

The results of the questionnaire may differ as a result of the distances between Tokyo and Fukuoka as well as slightly differing traditional backgrounds. For example, people in Tokyo are more familiar with foreigners and foreign customs as compared to the residents of Fukuoka. Tokyo is a large city with people traveling from many different regions, such as the rural areas in other prefectures outside of Tokyo, and the city is mixed with the slightly varying regional traditions throughout Japan. Further research on a short term and long term scale must be conducted in order to provide accuracy.

7 Conclusion

As discussed throughout this dissertation, *Omotenashi* is specifically the Japanese approach to exceptional hospitality and customer service. Specifically the *Takami Style of Omotenashi* strives for the continuous improvement of customer satisfaction in the bridal market, thus it became urgent for the organization to discover methods of discovering ways to increase customer satisfaction for bridal services. Along with other commemorative events such as anniversaries and the birth of a child, a wedding ceremony is symbolically and sentimentally one of the most significant events in many peoples' lives. Keeping this fact into consideration, along with the acknowledgment of the monetary expense that goes into a wedding, it is imperative for Takami Bridal that clients take away with them a fond memory of their wedding ceremonies.

Takami Bridal's commitment to create a new standard for excellence in customer service, or *Omotenashi,* is a daunting task considering the questionnaires used for research aim to quantify the behaviors of customers, and comprehend the varying levels of customer satisfaction inclusive of all possible differences. The *Takami Style of Omotenashi* must then be suitable and satisfying for all clients regardless of varying demographics or regional differences.

References

1. TAKAMI BRIDAL, Club Fame, 第 2 回高見重光 TAKAMI 代表取締役. http://kyotocf.com/contents/kyotomonsengen/takami_shigemitsu/
2. Qualtrics, About Customer Satisfaction Surveys. http://www.qualtrics.com/research-suite/survey-types/customer-satisfaction-surveys/
3. 一般財団法人　経済産業調査会, 『ほんまもん』の伝承, 2011. http://www.chosakai.or.jp/essay/201111/index.html

A Study on Characteristic of Calligraphy Characters Part 1 Analytical Method with Computer Technology

Zelong Wang[1(✉)], Issei Harima[1], and Zenichiro Maekawa[2]

[1] Advanced Fibro-Science, Kyoto Institute of Technology, Kyoto, Japan
simon.zelongwang@gmail.com
[2] Future-Applied Conventional Technology Center,
Kyoto Institute of Technology, Kyoto, Japan
fwkh1975@mb.infoweb.ne.jp

Abstract. The letter develops as the means that a human being takes the communication and becomes the important element characterizing the racial culture. A variety of letters exist in the world, but it becomes two big flows of a phonogram and the ideograph at the present. The kanji is a representative of the ideographs.

Keywords: Calligraphy character · Characteristic · Analytical method

1 Introduction

The letter develops as the means that a human being takes the communication and becomes the important element characterizing the racial culture. A variety of letters exist in the world, but it becomes two big flows of a phonogram and the ideograph at the present. The kanji is a representative of the ideographs. Kanji was born in China and has the history of 4,000 years. Japan is known as a specific race in the world using the kanji of the ideograph and the hiragana letter of the phonogram at the same time. The Japanese improved a kanji and devised a hiragana letter originally.

The culture to catch the form of the letter as an art object other than a function to perform communication exists in the world. The history of the calligraphy to express a kanji and a hiragana letter with a writing brush style is very old.

An impression to receive from a writing brush style, namely the sensitivity evaluation is subjective and is hard to quantify it.

In late years, with development of the sensitivity engineering including the handwriting study by the sensitivity evaluation, the study for the quantification is advancing [1–3]. However, the study that pursued the characteristic of the shape of the writing brush style in detail from a quantitative point of view is not found.

Therefore, in this study, we suggest technique to evaluate the characteristic of the shape of the writing brush style quantitatively.

This study is classified into three parts. Part1 treats the analytical method with computer technology. Part2 treats one character of calligraphy Letter "kanji" and "hiragana". Part3 treats the writing paper with calligraphy letter works.

V.G. Duffy (Ed.): DHM 2015, Part I, LNCS 9184, pp. 419–428, 2015.
DOI: 10.1007/978-3-319-21073-5_42

2 The Establishing of Brush Letter Evaluated System

2.1 The Synopsis of Brush Letter Evaluated System

The new brush letter evaluated system was proposed and designed to quantitative the calligraphy product, which was written on paper.

As always, the quality of calligraphy product was evaluated and judged by experienced masters according to their experience and intuition, which is a very subjective relied on the evaluators' status and reputation. The new brush letter evaluated system was used to establish an evaluation index of synthesis quantify method by numerical method.

The calligraphy is a visual art related to writing. It is the design and execution of lettering with a broad tip instrument or brush form to signs in an "expressive, harmonious, and skillful manner", which was created and developed on Asia, especially in China and Japan. The Japanese character was originated from China, adopted and used Chinese characters. However, during this long period, Japanese have formulated some native characteristic forms. Therefore, current brush letter evaluated system was focused on the Chinese "Kanji" and Japanese "Hiragana", which was designed to obtain a quantified analysis of this evolution. The three types of Chinese "Kanji" of "Kaisho", "Gyosho", "Sousho" and Japanese "Hiragana" were paid attention to compare according to the order of calligraphy development. The characteristic of "sumi" length distribution and the stability index were calculated and used to analysis the length of the line and balance index in order to establish a quantitative evaluated benchmark.

2.2 The Proposed of Brush Letter Evaluated System

Writing brush works is expressed with characters by writing brush on paper. Character by writing brush is style written by writing brush. When the writing brush is lowered and strongly pushed to the writing paper, width of the line of character grows big. When the tip of the writing brush completely leaves the writing paper, line disappears. Digitizing construction of written paper is done as preprocessing of proposed system. Next, the length of the line and balance index of writing brush characters were carried out by using numeric written paper.

The program's analysis process of brush letter evaluated system was shown as following:

1. Written paper is regarded as two dimensional plane and is divided into many square elements. The image of written paper was produced by scan machine, all the image data was changed into the same designed size.
2. The data of RGB color image was changed to gray image data. The density of "sumi" was digitized in numerical value from 1 to 255 and is substituted for each element as the property value of the element.
3. In order to examine the distribution of section length of "sumi" line (black ink) at any incline angle, new software program is proposed.

4. The outline is taken out from "sumi" line by linking the element between "sumi" part and blank part. And the data of gray image was changed into write and black colors by binaryzation method ("Sumi" area is 0, the blank is 255).
5. Writing brush character was inclined angle θ (θ = 0, 15, 30...150, 165). Section length at any angle θ was by using new program as shown in Fig. 1.
6. New software program was proposed in order to obtain the breadth distribution of "sumi" line in writing brush character. The breadth distribution was summarized by two methods. The "Method-1" was applied to analysis the single character in part-2, which was calculated based on interval "sumi". And the "Method-2" was used to analysis the whole writing paper of "Hiragana" in part-3, which was calculated based on continued "sumi" on one line as shown in Table 1.
7. The degree of stability S of writing brush character also was an important element for new soft ware program, which was calculated according to Eq. 1.
8. Additionally, full situation of "sumi" is examined by "sumi" area in block cell.
9. Finally, Writing brush character is evaluated from viewpoint of 5 items, that is, ①Stability index, ②Sumi area, ③Vertical/horizontal ratio, ④Diagonal to right/Horizontal ratio, ⑤Diagonal to left/Horizontal ratio (Table 1).

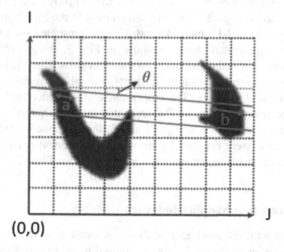

Fig. 1. The scanning and calculation method of brush letter evaluated system

Table 1. The example of calculated method for "Method-1" and "Method-2"

	Method-1	Method-2
Breadth-1	a = 1	a + b = 3
Breadth-2	b = 2	–

Equation

1. $J_G \geq \frac{m}{2}$:

$$S_I = \frac{V}{nm}\left\{\left(1 - \frac{I_G}{n}\right) + \alpha\left(1 - \frac{I_G}{m}\right)\right\}$$

2. $J_G < \frac{m}{2}$:

$$S_I = \frac{V}{nm}\left\{\left(1 - \frac{I_G}{n}\right) + \alpha\left(\frac{I_G}{m}\right)\right\} \tag{1}$$

S_I :   Stability Index
(I_G, J_G) :   Coordinate of center of figure
V :   "sumi" area of character

3 The Verification of Brush Letter Evaluated System

3.1 The Verification of the Breadth Distribution of "Sumi"

The four different types of images separated into two basic types, quadrate and empty circle, had been calculated by new program in order to prove the program's validity, which were illustrated in Figs. 2, 3, 4 and 5. According to the Fig. 2, the results of solid quadrate shape by "Method-1" and "Method-2" were presented the same distribution. In case of separate quadrated shape as show in Fig. 3, the breadth of "sumi" by "Method-1" was concentrated distribution on the short parts. But, the breadth of "sumi" by "Method-2" was concentrated on longer parts, and all distribution was similar with the "Method-2" of solid quadrate. The empty circle shape calculated results based on two methods were shown in Fig. 4. The separated empty circle of two methods also was shown in Fig. 5. As shown in Figs. 4 and 5, the continued empty circle and the separated empty circle were presented a similar distribution. It is can confirm that the program was correct based on four graphic verification for Figs. 2, 3, and 4.

3.2 The Verification of Stability Index (S)

Nine "sumi" types with the same area at different location were applied to verify the stability index program as shown in Fig. 6. According to Fig. 6, the "sumi" for nine types were consist of three layers, the "sumi" areas were located at three location of left, right, and middle side among each layer. The total size of graphic verification was 10*10, and the background was white color with the value of 255. And each "sumi" area made up by four pixels with black color with the value of 0, which were marked with yellow color as shown in Fig. 6. The verification result of stability index (S) was shown in Fig. 7. The upper layer was shown smaller stability value than middle and lower layers. And the lower layer was presented largest stability value. Therefore, the result of program was met the original design. The stability index was considered as a degree that the calligraphy was not easy to move under gravity force.

Method-1

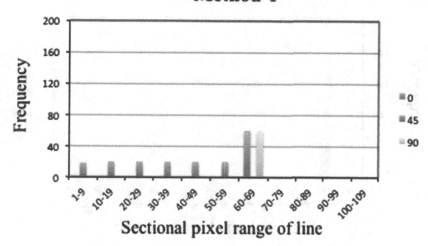

Method-2

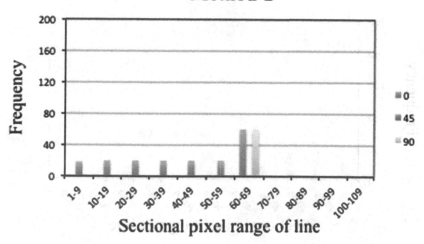

Fig. 2. The graphic verification of solid quadrate shape

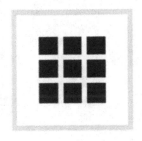

Method-1

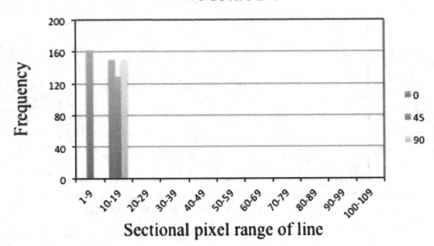

Method-2

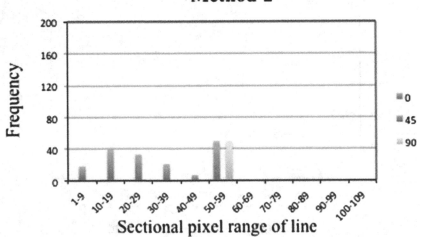

Fig. 3. The graphic verification of separate quadrated shape

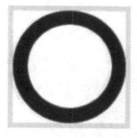

Method-1

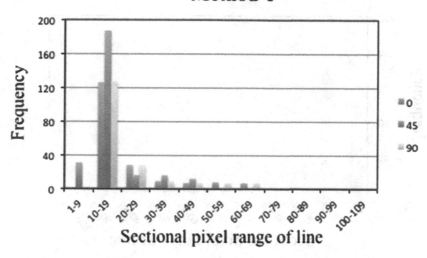

Method-2

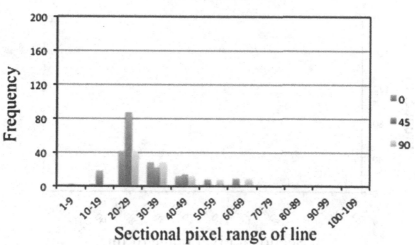

Fig. 4. The graphic verification of empty circle shape

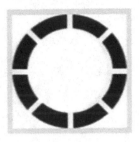

Method-1

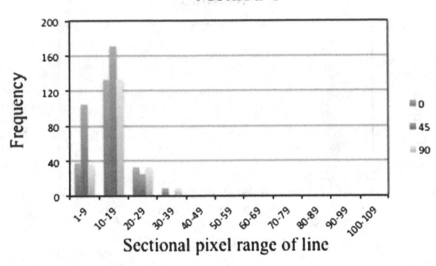

Method-2

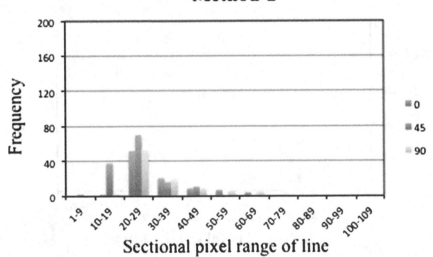

Fig. 5. The graphic verification of separated empty circle shape

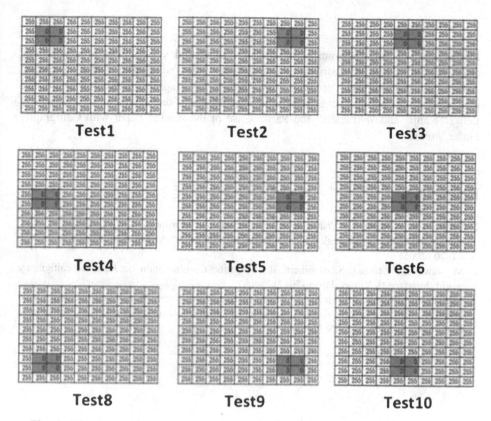

Fig. 6. Nine "sumi" types with the same area at different location (Color figure online)

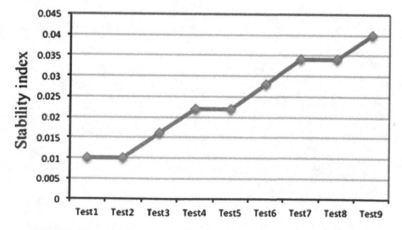

Fig. 7. The stability index result of nice types' graphic verification

4 Conclusion

In this research, the program of brush letter evaluated system was proposed. The characteristic of breadth distribution and stability index were calculated by program. Afterwards, the proposed program was verified by graphic verification tests. The program will be applied to characterize the Part-2 Case of one Character of Calligraphy Letter "Kanji" and "Hiragana" and Part-3 Case of the writing paper with Calligraphy Letter works.

References

1. Park, O.-S., Nonaka, T., Nishiwaki, T., Maekawa, Z., Morimoto, K., Kurokawa, T.: Subjective and objective evaluation for the beauty of HIRAGANA. Jpn. Soc. Kansei Eng. **5**(2), 63–70 (2005)
2. Maekawa, Z., Yamada, S., Hagihara, R.: Scientific Consideration on Japanese calligraphy world, Interface21 Kyoto, Japan (2012)
3. Maekawa, Z., Wang, Z., Yamada, S.: Motion analysis of weaving 'Kana-Ami' technique with different years of experience. In: Proceedings of Japan International SAMPE Symposium & Exhibition, SAMPE JAPAN (2013)

A Study on Characteristic of Calligraphy Characters Part 2 Case of One Character of Calligraphy Letter "Kanji" and "Hiragana"

Zelong Wang[1(✉)], Mengyuan Liao[1], Kayo Yokota[1],
Riichi Hagihara[2], and Zenichiro Maekawa[3]

[1] Advanced Fibro-Science, Kyoto Institute of Technology, Kyoto, Japan
simon.zelongwang@gmail.com
[2] Hagihara sanngyo goshi Co., Tokyo, Japan
rihyaku@gmail.com
[3] Future-Applied Conventional Technology Center,
Kyoto Institute of Technology, Kyoto, Japan
fwkh1975@mb.infoweb.ne.jp

Abstract. During long history of Kanji in china, "Kaisho" (Regular script), "Gyosho" (Semi-cursive script), "Sousho" (Cursive script) were born from 3rd century to 5th century. The Japanese improved a kanji and devised a Hiragana originally. "Kaisho" letter is form not to transform. "Gyosho" letter is the form transformed a little than it. "Sousho" letter is the form transformed more. Hiragana letter has thin, long and smooth form. 4 kinds of calligraphy letters are analyzed by using proposed system and characteristic of calligraphy letters were thrown into relief from three viewpoints. The technique to evaluate the characteristic of the shape of the writing brush style quantitatively is proposed in this study. This study is classified into three parts. Part-2 treats one character of calligraphy Letter "Kanji" and "Hiragana". 188 characters are analyzed by using the proposed technique in part-1.

Keywords: Kanji · Hiragana · Iroha poem · One calligraphy character

1 Introduction

1.1 Characteristic of One Character 3 Kinds of "Kanji" and "Hiragana"

During long history of Kanji in china, "Kaisho", "Gyosh", "Sousho" were born from 3rd century to 5th century. The Japanese improved a kanji and devised a Hiragana (平仮名) originally. "Kaisho" letter is form not to transform. "Gyosho" letter is the form transformed a little than it. "Sousho" letter is the form transformed more. Hiragana letter has thin, long and smooth form.

The culture to catch the form of the letter as an art object other than a function to perform communication exists in the world. The history of the calligraphy to express a kanji and a hiragana letter with a writing brush style is very old.

As shown in Fig. 1, when the writing brush is lowered and strongly pushed to the writing paper, width of the line of character grows big. When the tip of the writing brush completely leaves the writing paper, line disappears.

V.G. Duffy (Ed.): DHM 2015, Part I, LNCS 9184, pp. 429–436, 2015.
DOI: 10.1007/978-3-319-21073-5_43

An impression to receive from a writing brush style, namely the sensitivity evaluation is subjective and is hard to quantify it. 4 kinds of calligraphy letters are analyzed by using proposed system shown in Part-1.

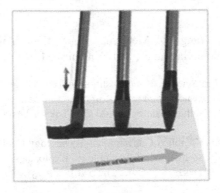

Fig. 1. Relationship between movement and width of line by writing brush

1.2   Iroha Poem

The "Hiragana" letter consists of 48 characters. Iroha poem is very famous Japanese poem written during 11th century, This poem has the characteristic made without repeating 47 hiragana letters. This poem is the song which sang of Buddhism-like mutability. The author of this song is missing. This poem has been used as handbook for Japanese to do writing practice hiragana since 11 century. Iroha poem translated into English was quoted from the site of Watanabesato, as shown as follows.

As colors smell but fall. Who are eternal in our world? Today, I went through deep mountain of existing form, and saw a shallow dream without being drunken.

1.3   Influence of Illusion on the Character by Writing Brush Comparison Between 3 Kinds of Kanjis and Hiragana

In order to compare hiragana with 3 kinds of kanjis, each one character of calligraphy letter of iroha poem is taken up in this study. 188 characters are analyzed, as shown in Table 1. Three kinds of kanjis, that are, "Kaisho", "Gyosho" and "Sousho", which derived each Hiragana are illustrated in 47 ways of cases at this table. The calligraphy letter adopted in this study is selected from the Dictionary for three types of calligraphy letter[1]. As shown in Table 1, it is clearly to find an evolved trend from square and upright feeling to randomize and flow feeling step by step for the same character of calligraphy letter among "Kaisho", "Gyosho", "Sousho" and "Hiragana".

---

[1] Takada, C.: Dictionary for five types of calligraphy letters, Houshokai (1998).

2   Result and Discussion

As proposed in Part-1 with "Method-1", influence of illusion on the character by writing brush could be considered by analytical method with computer technology. Therefore, averaged ink element ratio among 188 characters to horizontal part in diagonal left, vertical and diagonal right parts summary results were illustrated in Fig. 2. In general, all Kanjis and Hiragana showed most ink element distribution in diagonal left direction, following by diagonal right part and vertical part. As well know, diagonal left part and diagonal right part is a pair of symmetrical evaluation indicators, which could support character's structure symmetry judgment. According to plotting in Fig. 2, comparative smaller difference between diagonal left and right parts were clarified in "Kaisho" and Hiragana character type, however "Gyosho" and "Sousho" showed bigger gap. In other words, "Gyosho" and "Sousho" types of

Table 1. Relationship between movement and width of line by writing brush I. Kaisho II. Gyosho III. Sousho IV. Hirakana.

(Continued)

Table 1. (Continued)

#	I	II	III	IV		#	I	II	III	IV
25	和	和	和	わ		37	左	左	左	さ
26	加	加	加	か		38	幾	幾	幾	き
27	与	与	与	よ		39	由	由	由	ゆ
28	太	太	太	た		40	女	女	女	め
29	禮	禮	禮	れ		41	美	美	美	み
30	曾	曾	曾	そ		42	之	之	之	し
31	門	門	門	つ		43	惠	惠	惠	ゑ
32	祢	祢	祢	ね		44	比	比	比	ひ
33	奈	奈	奈	な		45	毛	毛	毛	も
34	良	良	良	ら		46	世	世	世	せ
35	武	武	武	む		47	寸	寸	寸	す
36	宇	宇	宇	う						

character displayed unbalanced impression in left and right direction. Referring to the evolution of character change, it is obvious to find a decreasing ink element trend from "Kaisho" to final "Hiragana", which verified visual impression difference of heavy/thick and light/thin quantitatively.

In Fig. 3, calculated average value of character's total ink elements ("sumi" area) and stability among 188 characters were plotted in group of "Kaisho", "Gyosho", "Sousho" and "Hiragana" for comparison, especially all the value was standardizing by dividing Hiragana value. Among three kinds of Kanjis, both Sumi area and stability parameters showed similar decreasing trend from "Kaisho" to "Sousho". Comparing with Hiragana, "Sousho" still displayed less "sumi" area and stability. In a word, "Kaisho" occupied the largest "sumi" area and best stability among all as a basic character origin. Furthermore, evolved Hiragana still kept a larger "sumi" area and stability than "Gyosho" and "Sousho", thus accepted and adopted by Japanese people finally.

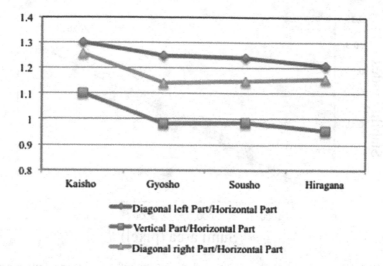

Fig. 2. Average result of Diagonal left part/Horizontal part, Vertical part/Horizontal part, Diagonal right part/Horizontal part, based on four types of 47 characters.

In previous discussion, similar data plotting of "sumi" area and stability overlapped phenomena was found in Fig. 3. In order to clarify the relationship between character's "sumi" area and stability, sets of stability index and "sumi" area data array were arranged in Fig. 4 following with a trend line drawing. It is worthwhile to find a positive correlation between stability and "sumi" area parameter with a linear regression ratio of $R^2 = 0.97$. That is to say, no matter what the type of character showed character's "sumi" area made the great influence on character's visual stability.

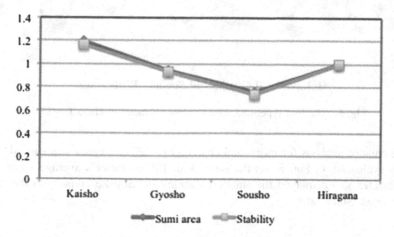

Fig. 3. The average "sumi" area and the stability index in the case based on four types of 47 characters.

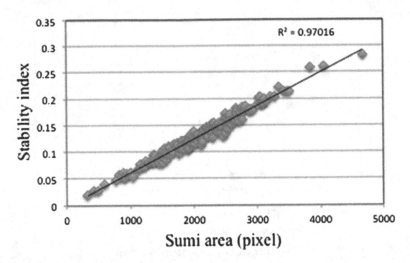

Fig. 4. The relationship between stability index and "sumi" area among four types of 47 characters.

For better understanding of various types of character's structure feature, the first character of iroha poem "い" (Fig. 5) was explained in Figs. 6 and 7 deeply. As showed in Fig. 5, "い" character displayed the largest ratio of diagonal left, diagonal right and vertical parts to Horizontal part in "Sousho" type.

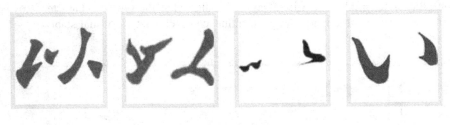

Ⅰ.Kaisho   Ⅱ.Gyosho   Ⅲ.Sousho   Ⅳ.Hirakana

Fig. 5. The four types character the first character of character "い"

The balance analysis for individual character in different types was carried out by stability evaluation in Fig. 6. As the same with 188 character's average value trend, "い" character also displayed the smallest stability in "Sousho" type with the similar data value as "sumi" area.

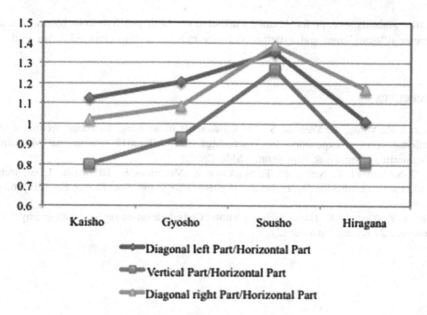

Fig. 6. Average result of Diagonal left part/Horizontal part, Vertical part/Horizontal part, Diagonal right part/Horizontal part, based on four types of characters "い".

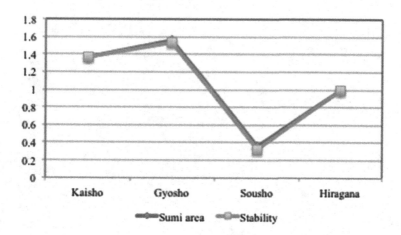

Fig. 7. Sumi's area and the stability index in the case based on four types of characters "い"

3 Conclusions

In this paper, hiragana letter consists of 48 characters and their corresponding Kanji characters of "Kaisho", "Gyosho", "Sousho" and "Hiragana" were analyzed and compared quantitatively by various parts length ratio, character's "sumi" area and structure stability. Finally, Hiragana's evolution process and feature were demonstrated, which clarified that Hiragana could keep comparative larger "sumi" area and structure stability except for Kasho. Furthermore, high positive correlation between character's "sumi" area and structure stability index was also clarified in the end.

References

Maekawa, Z., Wang, Z., Yamada, S.: Motion analysis of weaving 'kana-ami' technique with different years of experience. In: Proceedings of ASME 2012 International Mechanical Engineering Congress & Exposition, ASME (2012)

Park, O.-S., Nonaka, T., Nishiwaki, T., Maekawa, Z., Morimoto, K., Kurokawa, T.: Subjective and objective evaluation for the beauty of HIRAGANA. Jpn. Soc. Kansei Eng. 5(2), 63–70 (2005)

Maekawa, Z., Yamada, S., Hagihara, R.: Scientific Consideration on Japanese calligraphy world, Interface 21 Kyoto, Japan (2012)

A Study on Characteristic of Calligraphy Characters Part 3 Case of the Writing Paper with Calligraphy Letter Works

Zelong Wang[1(✉)], Riichi Hagihara[2], and Zenichiro Maekawa[3]

[1] Kyoto Institute of Technology Advanced Fibro-Science, Kyoto, Japan
simon.zelongwang@gmail.com
[2] Hagihara Sanngyo Goshi Co, Osaka, Japan
rihyaku@gmail.com
[3] Kyoto Institute of Technology Future-Applied Conventional Technology Center, Kyoto, Japan
fwkh1975@mb.infoweb.ne.jp

Abstract. The technique to evaluate the characteristic of the shape of the writing brush style quantitatively is proposed in this study. This study is classified into three parts. Part3 treats the writing paper with calligraphy letter works. 8 kinds of calligraphy letter works from songbook "Hyaku ninn isshu" are used in the part3 of this study.

Keywords: Calligraphy character works · Stability index · Songbook of hyaku ninn isshu

1 Introduction

1.1 Characteristic of Calligraphy Letter Works

In Japan, the history of the calligraphy to express a kanji and a hiragana letter with a writing brush style is very old. "Kaisho" is form not to transform. "Gyosho" is the form transformed a little than it. "Sousho" is the form transformed more.

The Japanese improved a kanji to assume China the origin and devised a hiragana letter originally. The hiragana letter has thin, long and smooth form. In addition, the hiragana has coupling form to lead to the next character. The "Hiragana" letter lets Japanese heart feel at ease and beauty.

Writing brush works is expressed with Characters by writing brush on paper. The hiragana works has a characteristic bigger than the kanji works. The kanji characters form a line orderly in the kanji work. On the other hand, the hiragana characters form a line irregularly in the hiragana works.

The characteristic of hiragana is shown as follows,

① Character is continued
② Characters form a line irregularly
③ "Sumi" is light and dark
④ Blank is the important element of the work.

© Springer International Publishing Switzerland 2015
V.G. Duffy (Ed.): DHM 2015, Part I, LNCS 9184, pp. 437–444, 2015.
DOI: 10.1007/978-3-319-21073-5_44

1.2   The Songbook: Hyaku Ninn Isshu

8 kinds of calligraphy letter works used in this study is chosen among "Hyaku ninn isshu"."Hyaku ninn isshu" is the songbook which "Teika Hujihara" (1162~1241) chose the song of 100 poets from the 7_{th} century to the 13_{th} century by one poem each and gathered. 8 calligraphy letter works are shown from Figs. 1, 2, 3 and 4. The songs translated into English were quoted from the site of fusau.com, as shown as follows:

1-h Many years ago in the ancient capital of Nara,
Cherry blossoms thrived in eight-layered petals.
Today in the Palace with its nine royal portals,
Cherish them we do in this noble spring gala.

2-h At Shinobu, Michinoku clothes are dyed so randomly,
Only God knows what patterns come out and how.
Who, then, put me off my usual balance of emotion?
It's you I hold so dear, I'm dying to be dyed in your colors.

3-h Here I live, dear old friends, near deer's abodes southeast of Kyoto.
Name's Ujiyama I hear people call worthy hiding place of world-weary men.

4-h What a cruel fate it is for me to see you still.
Now that you're out of reach, I wish you were out of sight.
I'd hate to hate your face, I'd hate to face my fate.

5-h Of course you know Ibukiyama?
Famed source of moxa herbs:
Curing bodies by burning aching spots.
Of course you don't know my heart
Burning in stealth thinking about you.

6-h White as frost first down on the wintry ground
Mocking my bewildered eyes unable to say which is which,
Chrysanth, are you inviting me, "Pick me up, if you can"?

7-h Wind-induced snow of flowers timelessly white in spring
Might be pleasant to see, but well, whiter still is my hair
Reduced in volume with the passage of time,
No spring ever visits me again.

8-h Premature name as one in love
Stood out in the way of love to be won.
What fun is there in having it known
To anyone else than you I've held so secretly dear?

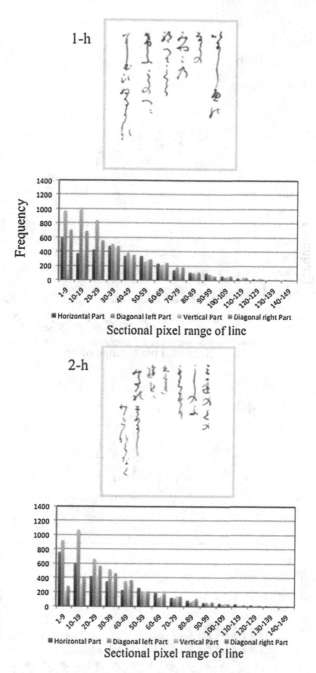

Fig. 1. The hiragana works of h-1 and h-2

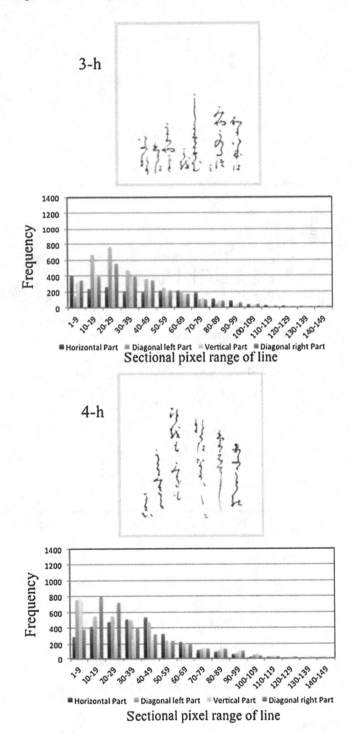

Fig. 2. The hiragana works of h-3 and h-4

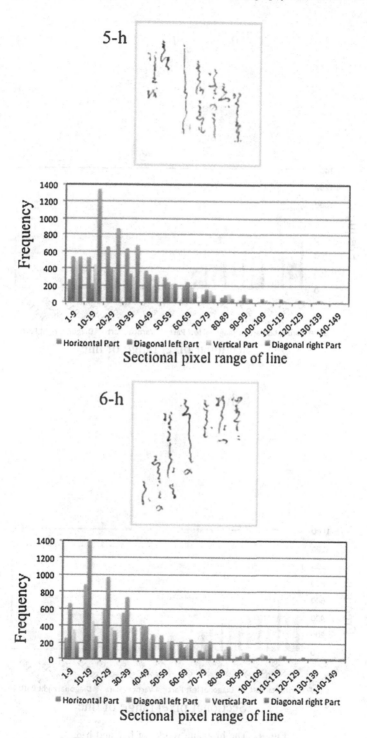

Fig. 3. The hiragana works of h-5 and h-6

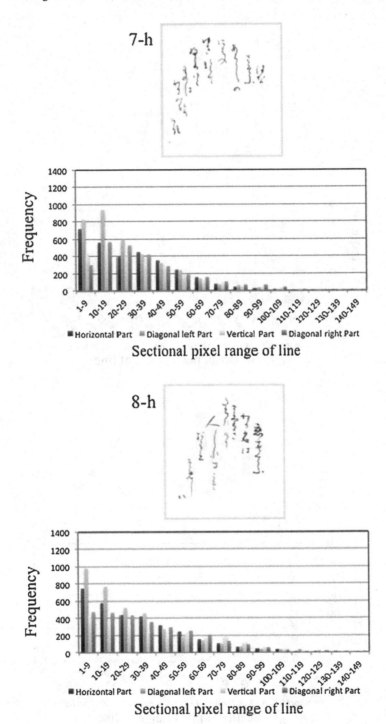

Fig. 4. The hiragana works of h-7 and h-8

2 The Proposed Evaluation Method

The blank part on paper is important in the hiragana works. Therefore, this proposed evaluation method is applied to the whole including blank. The hiragana works are classified in 8 kinds, as shown from Figs. 1, 2, 3 and 4. The characters are written in the slanted line part.

New software program is proposed with "Method-2" in order to obtain the degree of overall instability is of hiragana works. Full situation of "sumi" is examined by "sumi" ratio in block cell among horizontal part, diagonal left part, vertical part and diagonal right part.

(1) Written paper is regarded as two dimensional plane and is divided into many square elements.
(2) The density of "sumi" is digitized in numerical value from 1 to 256 and is substituted for each element as the property value of the element.
(3) The center of figure is obtained.
(4) The degree of instability is of hiragana work is calculated. The degree of instability is shown as follows.
(5) Calligraphy works is evaluated by using Is.

3 Result and Discussion

As showed from Figs. 1, 2, 3 and 4, 8 kinds of Hiragana works distributions histogram of horizontal part, diagonal left part, vertical part and diagonal right part were illustrated respectively. The final stability index of those 8 hiragana works was plotted in Fig. 5. It is worthy to note that 3-h and 4-h have the largest stability index than other works, but 7-h displayed the smallest one. According to the original work writing style and overall feeling, large numbers of hiragana characters wrote in 3-h and 4-h were located in center or downside of work paper, however, characters in 7-h showed a bent moon shape upside. Referred to 5-h and 6 h, it is clearly to find a symmetric group

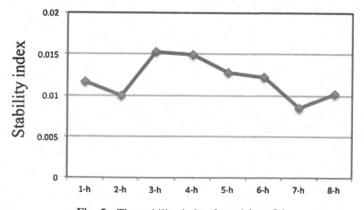

Fig. 5. The stability index from 1-h to 8-h

based on work's writing style, which one is written from right down side to left up side and the other one is written from right up side to left down side. Corresponding stability index of 5-h and 6 h showed the very similar value. As a conclusion, it is demonstrated that the whole hiragana work stability index was affected by hiragana characters arrangement in work paper but not writing flow or shape style, in which more characters located in center or center down side displayed more stable performance.

4 Conclusions

In this paper, hiragana works with 8 kinds of various writing style and characters location arrangement were characterized by horizontal, diagonal left, vertical and diagonal right sumi ratio analysis. Finally, 8 kinds of hiragana works' stability were calculated and compared. It was clarified that work with larger number characters placed in down or center down side displayed more stable performance. In a word, writing style is one important factor for whole work paper beauty evaluation, but how to arrange the characters' location with blank area is more important for whole work's stability, visual comfort and aesthetic feeling.

Reference

1. Oikawa, O.: The technology of scattered writing, Hyaku ninn isshu, Eiwa Co. (1986)

Author Index